a LANGE medical book

Correlative Neuroanatomy

twenty-second edition

Stephen G. Waxman, MD, PhD
Professor and Chairman
Department of Neurology
Yale University School of Medicine
New Haven, Connecticut

Neurologist-in-Chief
Yale-New Haven Hospital
New Haven, Connecticut

Jack deGroot, MD, PhD
Professor Emeritus, Anatomy and Radiology
University of California School of Medicine
San Francisco, California

APPLETON & LANGE
Norwalk, Connecticut

95 96 97 98 / 10 9 8 7 6 5 4 3 2 1

Prentice Hall International (UK) Limited, *London*
Prentice Hall of Australia Pty. Limited, *Sydney*
Prentice Hall Canada, Inc., *Toronto*
Prentice Hall Hispanoamericana, S.A., *Mexico*
Prentice Hall of India Private Limited, *New Delhi*
Prentice Hall of Japan, Inc., *Tokyo*
Simon & Schuster Asia Pte. Ltd., *Singapore*
Editora Prentice Hall do Brasil Ltda., *Rio de Janeiro*
Prentice Hall, *Englewood Cliffs, New Jersey*

ISBN 0-8385-1091-4
ISSN 0892-1237

Acquisitions Editor: John Dolan
Production Editor: Christine Langan
Designer: Elizabeth Schmitz

PRINTED IN THE UNITED STATES OF AMERICA

ISBN 0-8385-1091-4

90000

9 780838 510919

Table of Contents

SECTION III. SPINAL CORD & SPINE

SECTION IV. ANATOMY OF THE BRAIN

SECTION V. FUNCTIONAL SYSTEMS

SECTION VII. DISCUSSION OF CASES

Preface

Neuroscience is in a uniquely exciting phase. The past few decades have been remarkably productive in terms of teaching us about the nervous system, and the pace of progress is quickening. Each month we learn more and more about the nervous system: how it is built, how it functions, and how it develops. Neuroscience is, moreover, becoming increasingly relevant to medicine and is contributing to our understanding of the pathophysiology, diagnosis and treatment of neurological disorders such as Parkinson's disease, multiple sclerosis, stroke, and psychiatric disorders including depression, manic-depressive illness, and schizophrenia. More is on the horizon and it is not far off.

Thus, an understanding of the nervous system and its anatomy is essential to all basic scientists and to clinicians, not just neurologists and psychiatrists. Indeed, clinicians in all specialties need to know about the nervous system because disorders involving the brain, spinal cord, and peripheral nerves are very prevalent, eg, affecting 25% of patients in most general hospitals at some time during their hospital stay.

This book provides a brief but comprehensive overview of neuroanatomy together with a synopsis of its functional implications and discussions of its clinical relevance. It is not meant to supplant the longer, more comprehensive textbooks of neuroscience and neuroanatomy. On the contrary, it was written as a more manageable study aid and overview and as a synopsis for students reviewing neuroanatomy.

In this twenty-second edition of *Correlative Neuroanatomy* most of the chapters have been revised extensively and almost one-half have been nearly totally rewritten. This volume was originally written and has been revised for the student. To this end, we have tried to make the core of neuroanatomy as clear and memorable as possible, both in the text and in the large number of accompanying figures and diagrams. Much of the recent progress in neuroscience has been at the cellular and molecular level, and we have included an introduction to these advances. As a basis for understanding the growth and structure of the nervous system, we have extensively revised the chapters on the cellular elements of nervous tissue and on signaling in the nervous system so that they provide an overview of the classification of neurons and glial cells and of the channels, transmitters, and receptors that are responsible for their specialized properties.

Because many students tend to remember *patients* better than facts, we have introduced, whenever possible, Clinical Illustrations that describe or illustrate important points. Moreover, throughout the text, we have provided clinical correlates and have included a large number of computed tomography scans and magnetic resonance images, both of the normal brain and spinal cord and showing common pathologic entities, such as stroke, intracerebral hemorrhage, and tumors of the brain and spinal cord. We have also written a new chapter entitled, "Introduction to Clinical Thinking," which appears early in the text. This chapter introduces the student to the logical processes involved in sequential clinical thinking about the nervous system ("Where is the lesion? What is the lesion?") and provides a basis for thinking about neuroanatomy in terms of its implications for disorders of the brain, spinal cord, and peripheral nerves.

Over 50 new figures and diagrams have been included in this edition, many in color. These figures were drawn with the student in mind. Much of what we learn in neuroanatomy has a spatial aspect, and these figures were designed to provide clear, explicit, and easy-to-remember diagrams and drawings of important pathways, structures, and mechanisms. Similarly, 21 new tables have been included in this edition. As with the figures, we used color liberally in these tables, in order to make them as clear and easy-to-remember as possible. The figures and tables in this book have been designed so that by understanding them, the student will understand the essentials of neuroanatomy.

Thanks are due to many colleagues and friends who helped with this volume. Susan Spencer, MD, Pierre Fayad, MD, and Thomas N. Byrne, MD provided cases from their clinical experience, and made helpful suggestions with respect to the text. Jeffery D. Kocsis, PhD made important suggestions that improved the figures.

Special acknowledgment is due to Lena Lyons, MA, who labored in a most able and efficient way over the many new figures that illustrate this book. Carolyn Catanuto, as always, provided invaluable and expert assistance in all aspects of production of this volume. John J. Dolan of Appleton & Lange also deserves special thanks—he was involved with this edition from its inception, and his counsel, insight, and encouragement were invaluable.

Thanks are also due to Matthew Waxman and David Waxman for their help. Merle Waxman provided, throughout the production of this book, not only her usual encouragement and support, but also exhortations to remember to keep the *student's* perspective and needs foremost. If Jack DeGroot were here, he undoubtedly would thank Paula deGroot—in many ways, the two functioned as one.

Stephen G. Waxman, MD, PhD
New Haven
October 1994

Dedication

The twenty-second edition of *Correlative Neuroanatomy* is dedicated to Joseph G. Chusid, MD, Professor Emeritus, Department of Neurology, New York Medical College, and Director Emeritus, Department of Neurology, St. Vincent's Hospital and Medical Center, New York City.

Correlative Neuroanatomy was the first book published by Lange Medical Publications in 1938. Dr. Chusid joined Dr. Jack Lange and Dr. Joseph McDonald on the fourth edition, published in 1947. He worked on the book for the next 17 editions, creating a 45-year authorship unprecedented in medical publishing. Dr. Chusid was a pioneer in medical authorship. He helped establish both Lange Medical Publications and *Correlative Neuroanatomy* as a standard in medical student education.

During Dr. Chusid's tenure, the book sold tens of thousands of copies worldwide and was translated into Italian, Japanese, Spanish, Portuguese, Polish, German, Serbo-Croatian, French, and Indonesian.

For several editions, Dr. Chusid revised the book by himself and was able to broaden the scope of the book in relation to the expanding importance of neuroanatomy and neurology. As a leading researcher and teacher, Dr. Chusid sought to make *Correlative Neuroanatomy* both current in its coverage and accessible to students, a trademark that the book continues to embrace today.

The publishers and authors express their gratitude to Joseph G. Chusid for his dedication to *Correlative Neuroanatomy,* to Lange Medical Publications, to medical education, and to the field of neurology. We are honored to dedicate this edition to him.

Jack deGroot

This volume was to be co-authored by deGroot and Waxman. It was a collaboration I had greatly anticipated.

After agreeing to revise the 22nd edition, Jack and I spent many evenings on the phone discussing everything from chapter responsibilities to the detailed text and illustration changes planned for *Correlative Neuroanatomy.* These discussions were followed by a trip to the West Coast, where I was welcomed into Jack's home in San Francisco, spending a day working on the new edition.

As we began our work in Jack's home, which overlooked the Twin Peaks, the first thing that struck me about Jack was the engaging twinkle in his eyes. Very much of a gentleman, and by way of introduction, he shared the story of his own education.

Jack deGroot grew up in Indonesia. During World War II, he was imprisoned in a war camp for one year. He was a medical student at the time, and many of his professors were also prisoners of war. Thus, Jack received "personalized" instruction in neuroanatomy. He never forgot the importance of effective interactions between student and teacher and vice versa. Teaching became Jack's highest priority during his career, evident first in Texas and then at University of California, San Francisco where he played crucial roles in the education of medical and health-related students.

Jack deGroot was a consummate perfectionist. This was demonstrated in his many books, including *Correlative Neuroanatomy,* which he co-authored with Joseph Chusid. He took pride in getting the details right and in making his works clear and understandable to the student. Jack was truly a dedicated, caring teacher. We planned a set of extensive revisions that would reflect his high standards as an educator, author, and neuroanatomist.

Several weeks after my visit to his home, Jack deGroot died unexpectedly of an intracerebral hemorrhage.

Elegant, collegial, scholarly, and always the gentleman, Jack deGroot was indeed a caring teacher and author. I had looked forward to working with him. Although he was not able to fully contribute to this edition of *Correlative Neuroanatomy,* he was a central part of its planning and of the early writing. In many ways, this volume stands as a tribute to him.

Fundamentals of the Nervous System

1

The human central nervous system, smaller and weighing less than most desk-top computers, is the most complex computing device that exists. In addition to receiving and interpreting an immense array of sensory information and controlling a variety of complex motor behaviors, it engages in deductive and inductive logic. The brain can make complex decisions, think creatively, and "feel" emotions. It can *generalize* and possesses an elegant ability to recognize, which cannot be reproduced by even advanced mainframe computers. The human nervous system, for example, can immediately identify a familiar face, no matter at what angle it is presented.

Given the complexity of the nervous system and the richness of its actions, one might ask if its function, whether normal or abnormal, as in various neurologic disorders, can ever be understood. Indeed, neuroscience has begun to provide an understanding, in elegant detail, of the organization and physiology of the nervous system and of the alterations in nervous system function that occur in various diseases. This understanding is firmly based on an appreciation of the *structure* of the nervous system and of the interrelation between structure and function. By understanding correlative neuroanatomy, ie, the structure of the nervous system and its implications for its physiology, the myriad of actions of the nervous system, and the disease processes that interfere with normal function of the nervous system can begin to be understood.

GENERAL PLAN OF THE NERVOUS SYSTEM

Main Divisions

A. **Anatomy:** Anatomically, the human nervous system is a complex of two subdivisions.
1. **Central nervous system (CNS)**–The CNS, comprising the brain and spinal cord, is enclosed in bone and wrapped in protective coverings (meninges) and fluid-filled spaces.
2. **Peripheral nervous system (PNS)**–The PNS is formed by the cranial and spinal nerves (Fig 1–1).

B. **Physiology:** Functionally, the nervous system is divided into two systems.
1. **Somatic nervous system**–This innervates the structures of the body wall (muscles, skin, and mucous membranes).
2. **Autonomic (visceral) nervous system (ANS)**– The ANS contains portions of the central and peripheral systems. It controls the activities of the smooth muscles and glands of the internal organs (viscera) and the blood vessels and returns sensory information to the brain.

Structural Units

The central portion of the nervous system consists of a large, complex **brain** and an elongated **spinal cord** (Fig 1–2 and Table 1–1). The brain is further subdivided into the cerebrum, the brain stem, and the cerebellum. The **cerebrum (forebrain)** consists of the **telencephalon** and the **diencephalon;** the telencephalon includes the cerebral cortex (sometimes called "gray matter"), subcortical white matter, and the so-called basal ganglia, which are gray masses deep within the cerebral hemispheres. The **white matter** carries that name because in a freshly sectioned brain, it glistens on account of its high content of lipid-rich myelin; the white matter consists of myelinated fibers and does not contain neuronal cell bodies or synapses (Fig 1–3). The major subdivisions of the diencephalon are the thalamus and hypothalamus. The **brain stem** consists of the **midbrain (mesencephalon), pons,** and **medulla oblongata.** The **cerebellum** includes the vermis and two lateral lobes. The brain, which is hollow, contains a system of spaces called **ventricles;** the spinal cord has a narrow central canal that is largely obliterated in adulthood. These spaces are filled with cerebrospinal fluid (CSF) (see Figs 1–4, 1–5, and Chapter 11.)

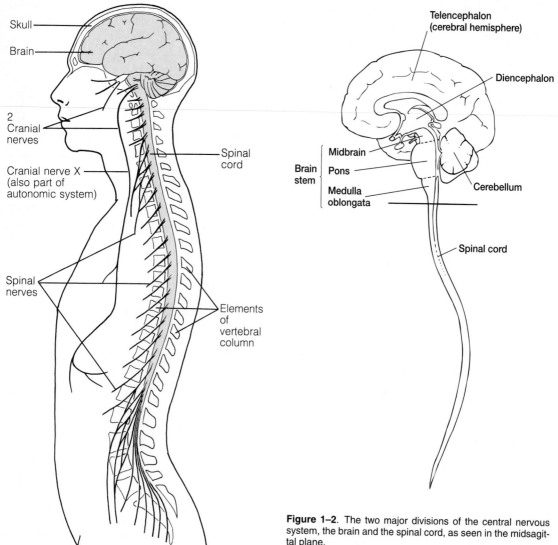

Figure 1–1. The structure of the central nervous system and the peripheral nervous system, showing the relationship between the CNS and its bony coverings.

Figure 1–2. The two major divisions of the central nervous system, the brain and the spinal cord, as seen in the midsagittal plane.

Functional Units

The brain, which accounts for about 2% of the body weight, contains many billions (perhaps even a trillion) of neurons and glial cells (see Chapter 2). The **neurons,** or nerve cells, are specialized cells that receive and send signals to other cells through their extensions (nerve fibers or **axons).** The information is processed and encoded in a sequence of electrical or chemical steps that occur, in most cases, very rapidly (in milliseconds). Many neurons have relatively large cell bodies and long extensions that transmit impulses quickly over a considerable distance. Interneurons, on the other hand, have small cell bodies and short axons and transmit impulses locally. Nerve cells serving a common function, often with a common target, are often grouped together into **nuclei.** These nuclei may originate, relay, modify, or multiply information within the nervous system. Nerve cells with common form, function, and connections that are grouped together outside the central nervous system are called **ganglia.**

Other cellular elements that support and expedite the activity of the neurons are the **glial cells,** of which there are several types. The glial cells outnumber the neurons 10:1.

Connections

Nerve cells convey signals to one another by means of synapses (see Chapters 2 and 3). The chemical transmitters found in most synapses are associated with the

Table 1–1. Major divisions of the central nervous system.

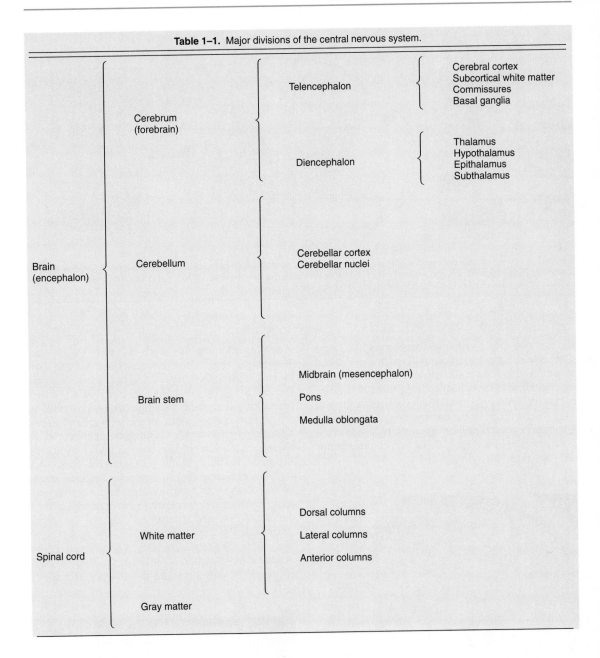

Brain (encephalon)	Cerebrum (forebrain)	Telencephalon	Cerebral cortex Subcortical white matter Commissures Basal ganglia
		Diencephalon	Thalamus Hypothalamus Epithalamus Subthalamus
	Cerebellum		Cerebellar cortex Cerebellar nuclei
	Brain stem		Midbrain (mesencephalon) Pons Medulla oblongata
Spinal cord	White matter		Dorsal columns Lateral columns Anterior columns
	Gray matter		

function of the synapse: excitation or inhibition. A given neuron may receive thousands of synapses, which bring it information from many sources. By integrating the excitatory and inhibitory inputs from these diverse sources and producing its own resultant message, each neuron acts as an information processing device.

The connections, or pathways, between groups of neurons in the central nervous system are in the form of fiber bundles, or tracts **(fasciculi);** these bundles also can be diffusely distributed. Aggregates of tracts, as seen in the spinal cord, are referred to as **columns (funiculi).** Tracts may descend (eg, from the cerebrum

to the brain stem or spinal cord) or ascend (eg, from the spinal cord to the cerebrum). These pathways are vertical connections that in their course may cross **(decussate)** from one side of the central nervous system to the other. Horizontal (lateral) connections are called **commissures.**

Decussation reflects the fact that the nervous system is constructed with bilateral symmetry. This is most apparent in the cerebrum and cerebellum, which are organized into right and left hemispheres, which, at first approximation, are symmetric (as seen later, some higher cortical functions such as language are represented more strongly in one hemisphere than in the

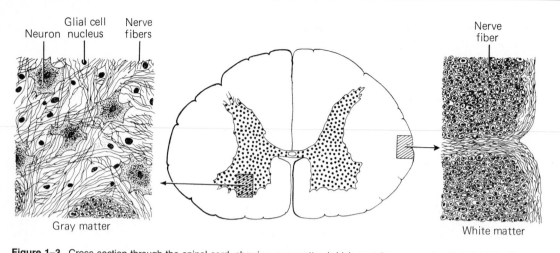

Figure 1–3. Cross section through the spinal cord, showing gray matter (which contains neuronal and glial cell bodies, axons, dendrites, and synapses) and white matter (which contains myelinated axons and associated glial cells). (Reproduced, with permission, from Junqueira LC et al: *Basic Histology,* 7th ed. Appleton & Lange, 1992.)

other, but nevertheless to gross inspection, the hemispheres have a similar structure). Even in more caudal structures such as the brain stem and spinal cord, which are not organized into hemispheres, there is bilateral symmetry, so the right and left sides are mirror images.

A general theme in the construction of the nervous system is **crossed representation:** the right side of the brain receives information about, and controls motor function pertaining to the left side of the world and vice-versa. Thus, visual information about the right side of the world is processed in the visual cortex on the left. Similarly, sensation (eg, touch, joint position sense, etc.) from the body's right side is processed in the somatosensory cortex in the left cerebral hemisphere. In terms of motor control, the motor cortex in the left cerebral hemisphere controls body movements that pertain to the right side of the external world. This includes, of course, control of muscles for the right arm and leg such as the biceps, triceps, hand muscles, and gastrocnemius. There are occasional exceptions to this pattern of "crossed innervation": eg, the *left* sternocleidomastoid muscle is controlled by the *left* cerebral cortex. Notice that, as a result of its unusual biomechanics, contraction of the left sternocleidomastoid rotates the neck to the *right*. Even for the anomalous

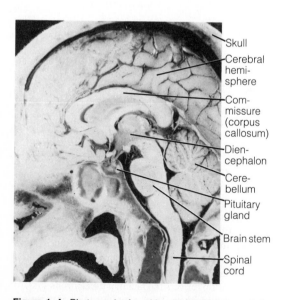

Figure 1–4. Photograph of a midsagittal section through the head and upper neck, showing the major divisions of the central nervous system. (Reproduced, with permission, from de Groot J: *Correlative Neuroanatomy of Computed Tomography and Magnetic Resonance Imagery.* Lea & Febiger, 1984.)

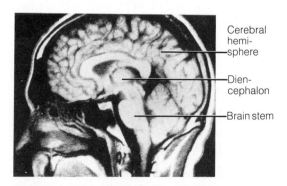

Figure 1–5. Magnetic resonance image (MRI) of a midsagittal section through the head (short time sequence; see Chapter 23). Compare with Figures 1–3 and 11–9.

muscle, then, control of movements relevant to the right side of the world originates in the contralateral left cerebral hemisphere, as predicted by the principle of crossed representation.

The earliest tracts of nerve fibers appear at about the second month of fetal life; major descending motor tracts appear at about the fifth month. **Myelination** (sheathing with myelin) of the spinal cord's nerve fibers begins about the middle of fetal life; some tracts are not completely myelinated for 20 years. The oldest tracts (those common to all animals) myelinate first; the corticospinal tracts myelinate largely during the first and second years after birth.

Although the structural organization of the brain is well established before neural function begins, there is evidence that many of the future connections are set before and shortly after birth. The maturing brain is susceptible to modification if an appropriate stimulus is applied or withheld during a critical period, which can last only a few days or even less (see Chapter 22).

PERIPHERAL NERVOUS SYSTEM

The **peripheral nervous system (PNS)** consists of spinal nerves, cranial nerves, and their associated ganglia (groups of nerve cells outside the central nervous system). The nerves contain nerve fibers that conduct information to (afferent) or from (efferent) the central nervous system. In general, **efferent** fibers are involved in motor functions such as the contraction of muscles or secretion of glands; **afferent** fibers usually convey sensory stimuli from the skin, mucous membranes, and deeper structures.

STRUCTURE, FUNCTION, AND DYSFUNCTION OF THE NERVOUS SYSTEM

Neuroanatomy and the related discipline **neurocytology** describe the structure of the nervous system and its constituent cells. Related aspects of neuroscience, including **neurophysiology** and **neuropharmacology,** focus on the function of the nervous system. **Molecular neuroscience** is providing an understanding, at the molecular level, of the mechanisms responsible for the special properties of neurons and glial cells.

In the clinical domain, a triad of specialties, **neurology, neurosurgery,** and **neuropathology,** focus on the dysfunction of the nervous system and on an understanding of the pathophysiology of neurologic disease together with its diagnosis and treatment. **Neuroradiology,** a modern specialty based on neuroanatomy, uses various refined methods of examination to depict normal or abnormal features of the brain, spinal cord, and nerves and their coverings in order to locate and identify nervous system lesions—which are some-

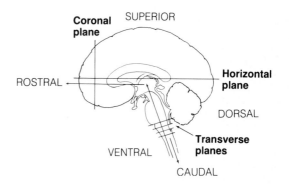

Figure 1–6. Planes (coronal, horizontal, transverse) and directions (rostral, caudal, etc) frequently used in the description of the brain and spinal cord. The plane of the drawing is the midsagittal.

times very small—as an aid to diagnosis. The planes of section and terms used in the study of neuroanatomy and neuroradiology are shown in Figure 1–6.

The advent of new techniques for **functional neuroimaging,** such as positron emission tomography (PET), provides a noninvasive visualization of brain areas that are metabolically active. These techniques are providing new information about the function of various parts of the CNS and about the changes in brain function that occur in various neurologic diseases. This new field will undoubtedly contribute substantially both to neurology and to neuroanatomy.

As outlined throughout this chapter, various aspects of neuroscience are highly interrelated. Central to all aspects of neuroscience, however, is an understanding of the structure of the nervous system. The chapters that follow provide a basis for understanding, in neuroanatomic terms, how the nervous system functions normally as well as how its function is altered in various disorders.

Table 1–2. Terms used in neuroanatomy.

Ventral, anterior	On the front (belly) side
Dorsal, posterior	On the back side
Superior, cranial	On the top (skull) side
Inferior	On the lower side
Caudal	In the lowermost position (at the tail end)
Rostral	On the forward side (at the nose end)
Medial	Close to or toward the middle
Median	In the middle, the midplane (midsagittal)
Lateral	Toward the side (away from the middle)
Ipsilateral	On the same side
Contralateral	On the opposite side
Bilateral	On both sides

REFERENCES

Barr ML, Kierman JA: *The Human Nervous System,* 4th ed. Harper & Row, 1983.

Brodal A: *Neurological Anatomy,* 3rd ed. Oxford Univ Press, 1981.

Carpenter MC, Sutin J: *Human Neuroanatomy,* 8th ed. Williams & Wilkins, 1983.

Geschwind N, Galaburda AM: *Cerebral Lateralization.* Harvard Univ Press, 1986.

Kandel ER, Schwartz JN, Jessell T: *Principles of Neural Science,* 3rd ed. Elsevier, 1991.

Martin JH: *Neuroanatomy.* Elsevier, 1989.

Netter FH: *Nervous System (Atlas and Annotations).* Vol 1: The Ciba Collection of Medical Illustrations. CIBA Pharmaceutical Company, 1983.

Nicholls JG, Martin AR, Wallace BG: *From Neuron to Brain,* 3rd ed. Sinauer, 1992.

Romanes GJ: *Cunningham's Textbook of Anatomy,* 18th ed. Oxford Univ Press, 1986.

Shepherd GM: *Neurobiology,* 2nd ed. Oxford Univ Press, 1988.

Elements of Nervous Tissue

2

Early in the development of the nervous system, a hollow tube of ectodermal neural tissue forms at the embryo's dorsal midline. The cellular elements of the tube appear undifferentiated at first, but they later develop into various types of neurons (nerve cells) and supporting glial cells.

Layers of the Neural Tube

The embryonic neural tube has three layers (Fig 2–1): the **ventricular zone,** later called the **ependyma** around the lumen (central canal) of the tube; the **intermediate zone,** which is formed by the dividing cells of the ventricular zone (including the earliest radial glial cell type) and stretches between the ventricular surface and the outer (pial) layer; and the external **marginal zone,** which is formed later by processes of the nerve cells in the intermediate zone (Fig 2–1B).

The intermediate zone, or mantle layer, increases in cellularity and becomes gray matter. The nerve cell processes in the marginal zone, as well as other cell processes, becomes white matter when myelinated.

Differentiation & Migration

The largest neurons, which are mostly motor neurons, differentiate first. Sensory and small neurons, and most of the glial cells, appear later—up to the time of birth. Newly formed neurons may migrate extensively through regions of previously formed neurons. When glial cells appear, they can act as a framework that guides growing neurons to the correct target areas. Because the axonal process of a neuron may begin growing toward its target during migration, nerve processes in the adult brain are often curved rather than straight. The newer cells of the future cerebral cortex migrate from the deepest to the more superficial layers; the small neurons of the incipient cerebellum migrate first

to the surface and later to deeper layers; the latter process continues for several months after birth.

Once differentiated, neurons do not divide again. Any loss of neurons, whether from normal attrition or pathologic insult, is permanent. This is one reason for the limited degree of functional recovery from neurologic diseases after neurons are destroyed.

NEURONS

Neurons vary in size and complexity. For example, the nuclei of one type of small cerebellar cortical cell (granule cell) are only slightly larger than the nucleoli of an adjacent large Purkinje cell. Motor neurons are usually larger than sensory neurons. Nerve cells with long processes (eg, dorsal root ganglion cells) are larger than those with short processes (Figs 2–2 and 2–3).

Some neurons stretch from the cerebral cortex to the lower spinal cord, a distance of less than 2 feet in infants or 4 feet or more in adults; others have very short processes, reaching, for example, only from cell to cell in the cerebral cortex. These small neurons, with short axons that terminate locally, are called **interneurons.**

Extending from the nerve cell body there are usually a number of branched processes called the **axons** and **dendrites.** The receptive part of the neuron is the **dendrite,** or **dendritic zone** (see section 'Dendrites'); the conducting (propagating or transmitting) part is the axon, which may have one or more collateral branches. The downstream end of the axon is called the **synaptic terminal** or **arborization.** The neuron's cell body is called the **soma** or **perikaryon.** The characteristics of **organelles** within the neuron are summarized in Table 2–1.

Cell Bodies

The cell body is the metabolic and genetic center of a neuron (Fig 2–3). Although its size varies greatly in different neuron types, the cell body makes up only a

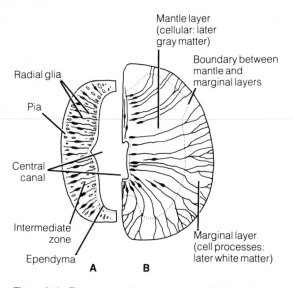

Figure 2–1. Two stages in the development of the neural tube (only half of each cross section is shown). **A:** Early stage with large central canal. **B:** Later stage with smaller central canal.

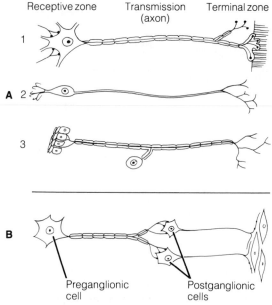

Figure 2–2. Schematic illustration of nerve cell types. **A:** Central nervous system cells: (1) motor neuron projecting to striated muscle, (2) special sensory neuron, and (3) general sensory neuron from skin. **B:** Autonomic cells to smooth muscle. Notice how the position of the cell body with respect to the axon varies.

small part of the neuron's total volume. The cell body contains a **nucleus,** a prominent **nucleolus,** and the **Nissl substance** (endoplasmic reticulum with ribosomes), a protein-synthesizing apparatus. Ribosomes are found in the cell body and proximal dendrites of the neuron; protein synthesis is limited to these regions. Thus, new protein is not made in the axon. Ribosomes are involved in the synthesis of some neurotransmitter substances used away from the cell body, in the synaptic terminal. Synapses from other cells or glial processes tend to cover the surface of a cell body (Fig 2–4).

Dendrites

Most neurons have many dendrites (see Figs 2–2, 2–3, and 2–5). The receptive surface area of the dendrites, the dendritic zone, is usually far larger than that of the cell body. Dendrites receive information via synapses from either the environment (sensory neurons) or other neurons (interneurons and motor neurons). Because most dendrites are long and thin, they act as resistors, isolating electrical events, such as postsynaptic potentials, from each other (see Chapter 3). The branching pattern of the dendrites can be very complex and determines how the neuron integrates synaptic inputs from various sources. Some dendrites give rise to **dendritic spines,** which are small mushroom-shaped projections that act as fine dendritic

branches and receive synaptic inputs. To a large extent, the diversity among neurons depends on the complexity and position of the dendrites and on the position of the cell body.

Axons

A neuron has a single **axon,** which is a cylindrical tube of cytoplasm covered by a membrane, the **axolemma.** A **cytoskeleton** consisting of **neurofilaments** and **microtubules** runs through the axon. The microtubules provide a framework for fast axonal transport (see following section, "B. Axonal Transport"). Specialized molecular motors (**kinesin** molecules) bind to vesicles containing molecules (eg, neurotransmitters) destined for transport, and "walk" via a series of ATP-consuming steps along the microtubules.

The axon is a specialized structure that conducts electrical signals from the initial segment (the proximal part of the axon, near the cell body) to the synaptic terminals. The **initial segment** has distinctive morphologic features; it differs from both cell body and axon. The axolemma of the initial segment contains a high density of sodium channels, which permit the initial segment to act as a **trigger zone.** In this zone, action potentials are generated so they can move along the axon. The initial segment does not contain

Table 2–1. Components of axonal transport.

Component	Rate (mm/day)	Composition
ANTEROGRADE		
Fast	200–400	proteins, lipds, neuro-transmitters
Mitochondria	50–100	mitochondria
Slow (SCb)	2–8	microfilaments, enzymes, clathrin
Slow (SCa)	0.1–1	microtubules, neurofilaments
RETROGRADE		
	200–300	lysosomal breakdown products

Modified, with permission, from Hammerschlag R and Brady ST: Axonal transport. In: *Basic Neurochemistry.* Siegel GJ, Agranoff B, Albers BW, Molinoff PB (editors). Raun, 1989

Nissl substance (see Fig 2–3). In large neurons, the initial segment arises conspicuously from the **axon hillock,** a cone-shaped portion of the cell body. Axons range in length from a few micrometers (in interneurons) to well over a meter (ie, in a lumbar motor neuron that projects from the spinal cord to the muscles of the foot) and in diameter from 0.1 to more than 20 micrometers.

A. Myelin: Many axons are covered by multiple concentric layers of **myelin,** a lipid-rich insulating material produced by Schwann cells in the peripheral nervous system, and by oligodendrocytes (a type of glial cell) in the central nervous system (Figs 2–6 to 2–9). The myelin sheath in peripheral nerves is divided into segments about 1 mm long by small gaps (1μm long) where myelin is absent; these are the **nodes of Ranvier.** The smallest axons are unmyelinated.

B. Axonal Transport: In addition to conducting action potentials, axons transport materials from the cell body to the synaptic terminals **(anterograde transport)** and from the synaptic terminals to the cell body **(retrograde transport).** Because ribosomes are not present in the axon, new protein must be synthesized and moved to the axon. This occurs via several types of axonal transport, which differ in terms of the rate and the material transported (Table 2–1). Anterograde transport may be fast (up to 400 mm/d) or slow (about 1 mm/d). Retrograde transport is similar to rapid anterograde transport. Fast transport involves microtubules extending through the cytoplasm of the neuron.

Both anterograde and retrograde transport are used experimentally to determine how groups of neurons are interconnected. Radioactive or fluorescent substances injected in one area show up anterogradely in another area after a few hours. Horseradish peroxidase is used in retrograde tracing experiments.

An axon can be injured by being cut or severed, crushed, or compressed. Following injury to the axon, the neuronal cell body responds by entering a phase

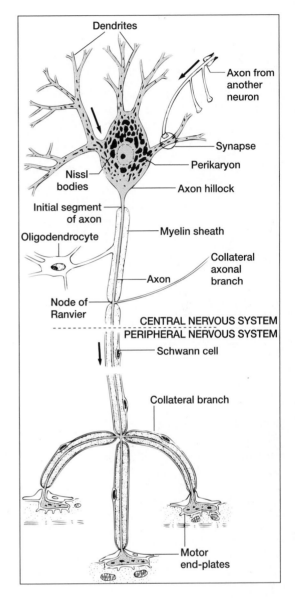

Figure 2–3. Schematic drawing of a Nissl-stained motor neuron. The myelin sheath is produced by oligodendrocytes in the central nervous system and by Schwann cells in the peripheral nervous system. Note the 3 motor end-plates, which transmit the nerve impulse to striated skeletal muscle fibers. Arrows show the direction of the nerve impulse. (Reproduced, with permission, from Junqueira LC, Carneiro J, Kelley RO: *Basic Histology,* 7th ed. Appleton & Lange, 1992.)

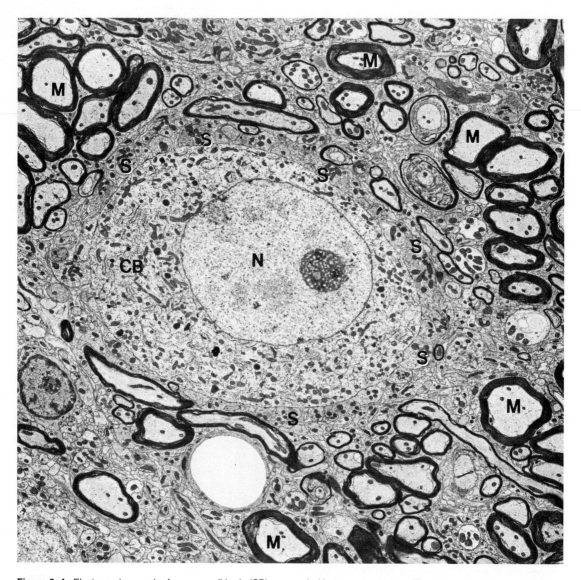

Figure 2–4. Electron micrograph of a nerve cell body (CB) surrounded by nerve processes. The neuronal surface is completely covered by either synaptic endings of other neurons (S) or processes of glial cells (G). Many other processes around this cell are myelinated axons (M). CB, neuronal cell body; N, nucleus. × 5000. (Courtesy of Dr DM McDonald.)

called **chromatolysis.** In general, axons within peripheral nerves can regenerate quickly after they are severed, whereas axons within the CNS do not tend to regenerate. Chromatolysis and axonal regeneration are further discussed in Chapter 22.

Synapses

Communication between neurons usually occurs from the terminal of the transmitting neuron (presynaptic side) to the receptive region of the receiving neuron (postsynaptic side) (Figs 2–5, 2–10, and 2–11). This specialized interneuronal complex is a **synapse,** or **synaptic junction.** As outlined in Table 2–2, some synapses are located between an axon and a dendrite (**axodendritic** synapses, which tend to be excitatory); whereas others are located between an axon and a nerve cell body (**axosomatic** synapses, which tend to be inhibitory). Still other synapses are located between an axon terminal and another **axon;** these **axo-axonic** synapses **modulate** transmitter release by the postsynaptic axon (Fig 2–11). Some large cell bodies may receive several thousand synapses (see Fig 2–4).

Impulse transmission at most synaptic sites involves the release of a chemical transmitter substance (see Chapter 3); at other sites, current passes directly

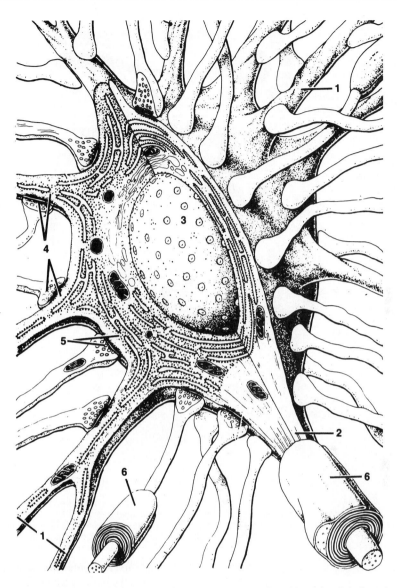

Figure 2–5. Diagrammatic view, in three dimensions, of a prototypic neuron. Dendrites (1) radiate from the neuronal cell body, which contains the nucleus (3). The axon arises from the cell body at the initial segment (2). Axodendritic (4) and axosomatic (5) synapses are present. Myelin sheaths (6) are present around some axons.

from cell to cell through specialized junctions called **electrical synapses,** or **gap junctions.** Electrical synapses are most common in invertebrate nervous systems, although they are found in a small number of sites in the mammalian CNS. Chemical synapses have several distinctive characteristics: synaptic vesicles on the presynaptic side, a synaptic cleft, and a dense thickening on both the receiving cell and the presynaptic side (Fig 2–10). Synaptic vesicles contain neurotransmitters (each vesicle contains a small packet or **quanta** of transmitter). When the synaptic terminal is depolarized (by an action potential in its parent axon),

synaptic vesicles fuse with the presynaptic membrane facing the synaptic cleft, releasing their transmitter (see Chapter 3).

Synapses are very diverse in their shapes and other properties: some are inhibitory and some excitatory; in some, the transmitter is acetylcholine; in others, it is a catecholamine, amino acid, or other substance (see Chapter 3). Some synaptic vesicles are large, some small; some have a dense core while others do not. Flat synaptic vesicles appear to contain an inhibitory mediator; dense-core vesicles contain catecholamines.

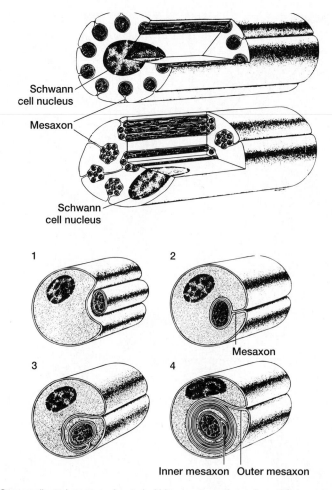

Schwann
cell nucleus

Mesaxon

Schwann
cell nucleus

1   2

Mesaxon

3   4

Inner mesaxon   Outer mesaxon

Figure 2–6. *A:* In the PNS, unmyelinated axons are located within grooves on the surface of Schwann cells. These axons are not, however, insulated by a myelin sheath. ***B:*** Myelinated PNS fibers are surrounded by a myelin sheath that is formed by a spiral wrapping of the axon by a Schwann cell. Panels 1–4 show four consecutive phases of myelin formation in peripheral nerve fibers. (Reproduced, with permission, from Junqueira LC, Carneiro J, Kelley RO: *Basic Histology,* 7th ed. Appleton & Lange, 1992.)

NEURONAL GROUPINGS & CONNECTIONS

Nerve cell bodies are grouped characteristically in many parts of the nervous system. The patterns of grouping are studied by describing the **cytoarchitectonics** (the arrangement of cells in tissue) of the nerve cell bodies. In the cerebral and cerebellar cortices, cell bodies aggregate to form layers called laminas (Fig 2–12). Nerve cell bodies in the spinal cord, brain stem, and cerebrum form compact groups, or **nuclei.** Each nucleus contains **projection neurons** whose axons carry impulses to other parts of the nervous system, and **interneurons** which act as short relays within the nucleus. In the peripheral nervous system, these compact groups of nerve cell bodies are called **ganglia.**

Groups of nerve cells are connected by pathways formed by bundles of axons. In some pathways, the axon bundles are sufficiently defined to be identified as **tracts,** or **fasciculi;** in others, there are no discrete bundles of axons. Aggregates of tracts in the spinal cord are referred to as **columns,** or **funiculi** (see Chapter 5). Within the brain certain tracts are referred to as **lemnisci.** In some regions of the brain, axons are so intermingled that pathways are difficult to identify. These networks are called the **neuropil** (Fig 2–13).

NEUROGLIA

Neuroglial cells outnumber neurons in the brain and spinal cord 10:1. They do not form synapses. These cells appear to play a number of important rules including myelin formation, guidance of developing neurons, maintenance of extracellular K^+ levels, and re-uptake of transmitters after synaptic activity.

Macroglia

The term **macroglia** refers to astrocytes and oligodendrocytes derived from ectoderm. In contrast to neu-

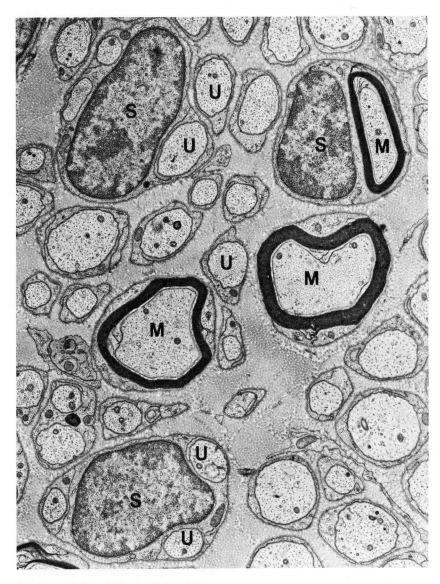

Figure 2–7. Electron micrograph of myelinated (M) and unmyelinated (U) axons of a peripheral nerve. Schwann cells (S) may surround one myelinated or several unmyelinated axons. × 16,000. (Courtesy of Dr DM McDonald.)

rons, these cells may have the capability, under some circumstances, to regenerate.

Astrocytes

There are two types of astrocytes, **protoplasmic** and **fibrillary** (Fig 2–14), but how they differ in function is unclear. Protoplasmic astrocytes are more delicate, contain more protoplasm, and their many processes are branched. They occur in gray matter or as satellite cells in dorsal root ganglia. Fibrillary astrocytes are more fibrous and their processes (containing glial fibrils) are seldom branched. In light microscope preparations, an astrocyte is identified by its irregular oval nucleus

without a distinct cytoplasm. Astrocytic processes radiate in all directions from a small cell body. They surround blood vessels in the nervous system, and they cover the exterior surface of the brain and spinal cord below the pia.

Astrocytes provide structural support to nervous tissue and act during development as "guidewires," which direct neuronal migration. They also play a role in synaptic transmission. Many synapses are closely invested by astrocytic processes, which appear to participate in the re-uptake of neurotransmitters. Astrocytes also contribute to the formation of the blood-brain barrier (see Chapter 11). Although astrocytic processes around capillaries do not form a functional barrier, they

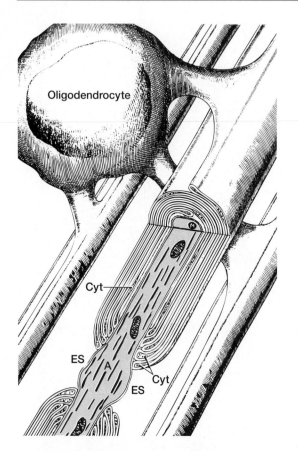

Figure 2–8. Oligodendrocytes form myelin in the CNS. A single oligodendrocyte myelinates an entire family (2–50) of axons. There is little oligodendrocyte cytoplasm (Cyt) in the oligodendrocyte processes that spiral around the axon to form myelin, and the myelin sheaths are connected to their parent oligodendrocyte cell body by only thin tongues of cytoplasm. This may account, at least in part, for the paucity of remyelination after damage to the myelin in the CNS. The myelin is periodically interrupted at nodes of Ranvier where the axon (A) is exposed to the extracellular space (ES). (Redrawn and reproduced, with permission, from Bunge et al: *J Biophys Biochem Cytol* 1961;**10:**67.

can selectively take up materials in order to provide an environment optimal for neuronal function.

Astrocytes act as regulators of electrolyte balance and appear to buffer K^+ (and possibly other ions) in the extracellular space. They form a covering on the entire central nervous system surface and proliferate to aid in repairing damaged neural tissue. These reactive astrocytes are larger and are more easily stained. Chronic repair leads to a **fibrillary gliosis,** sometimes called **glial scarring**.

Oligodendrocytes

These glial cells are identified in light microscope preparations by their round, rather dark nuclei without distinct cytoplasm. They have fewer processes than do astrocytes. Oligodendrocytes predominate in white matter; they form myelin in the CNS and may provide some nutritive support to the neurons that they envelop. A single oligodendrocyte may wrap myelin sheaths around many axons (see Figs 2–8 and 2–9). An oligodendrocyte may myelinate up to 40–50 axons. The fact that a single oligodendrocyte myelinates many axons may account for the paucity of remyelination following loss of myelin in the CNS. In peripheral nerves, by contrast, myelin is formed by **Schwann cells.** Each Schwann cell myelinates a single axon, and remyelination can occur at a brisk pace after injury to the myelin in the peripheral nerves.

Microglia

Microglial cells (rod cells) have an elongated nucleus; they are the **macrophages,** or scavengers, of the central nervous system (Fig 2–14). When an area of the brain or spinal cord is damaged or infected, microglia migrate to the site of injury to remove cellular debris. Some microglia are always present in the brain, but when injury or infection occurs, others enter the brain from blood vessels.

Extracellular Space

There is some fluid-filled space between the various cellular components of the central nervous system. This extracellular compartment probably accounts for, under most circumstances, about 20% of the total volume of the brain and spinal cord. Because transmembrane gradients of ions, such as K^+ and Na^+, are important in electrical signaling in the nervous system (see Chapter 3) the regulation of the levels of these ions in the extracellular compartment (**ionic homeostasis**) is an important function, which is, at least in part, performed by astrocytes. The capillaries within the central nervous system are completely invested by glial or neural processes. Moreover, capillary endothelial cells in the brain (in contrast to capillary endothelial cells in other organs) form **tight junctions,** which are impermeable to diffusion, thus creating a **blood-brain barrier.** This barrier isolates the brain extracellular space from the intravascular compartment.

Clinical Correlation

In **cerebral edema,** there is a definite and often rapid increase in the bulk of the brain. Cerebral edema, which tends to involve the white matter selectively, is either vasogenic (primarily extracellular) or cytotoxic (primarily intracellular). Electron micrographs may reveal massive expansion of the cytoplasm and of glial processes surrounding the capillaries. Therefore, an increase in the volume of the brain in cerebral edema may be caused by increases in the volume of not only the interstitial fluid but also of cells and their processes.

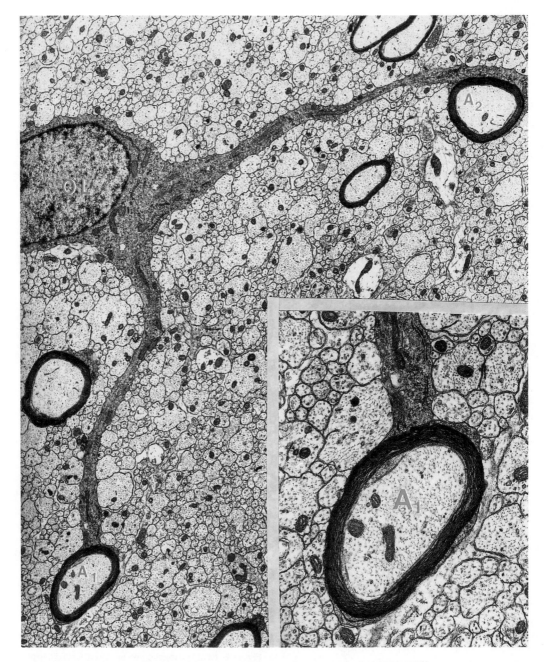

Figure 2–9. Electron micrograph showing oligodendrocyte (OL) in the spinal cord which has myelinated two axons (A_1, A_2). X6600. The *inset* shows axon A_1 and its myelin sheath at higher magnification. The myelin is a spiral of oligodendrocyte membrane which surrounds the axon. Most of the oligodendrocyte cytoplasm is extruded from the myelin. Since the myelin is compact, it has a high electrical resistance and low capacitance so that it can function as an insulator around the axon. × 16,000.

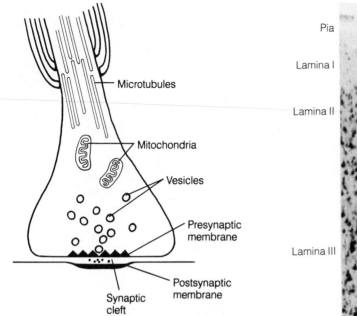

Figure 2–10. Schematic drawing of a synaptic terminal. Vesicles fuse with the presynaptic membrane and release transmitter molecules into the synaptic cleft so that they can bind to receptors in the postsynaptic membrane.

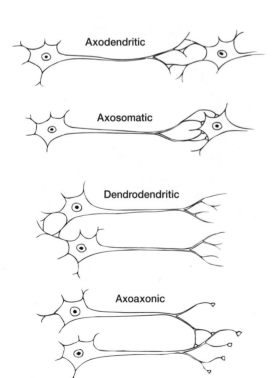

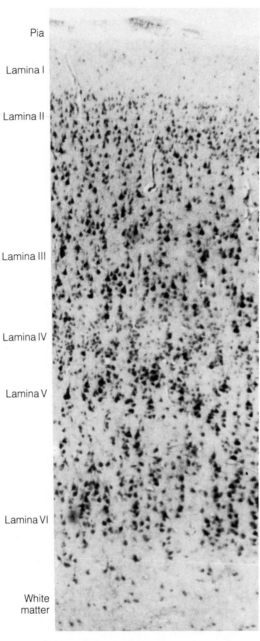

Figure 2–12. Light micrograph of cortical laminas. × 20. Nissl stain.

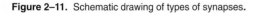

Figure 2–11. Schematic drawing of types of synapses.

Table 2–2. Types of synapses in the CNS.

Type	Pre-synaptic Element	Post-synaptic Element	Function
Axodendritic	Axon terminal	Dendrite	Usually excitatory
Axosomatic	Axon terminal	Cell body	Usually inhibitory
Axoaxonic	Axon terminal	Axon terminal	Presynaptic inhibition (modulates transmitter release in postsynaptic axon)
Dendrodendritic	Dendrite	Dendrite	Local interactions (may be excitatory or inhibitory) in axon-less neurons, eg, in retina

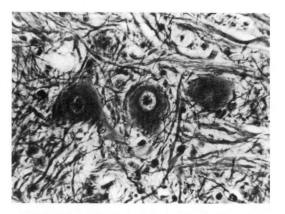

Figure 2–13. Light micrograph of a small group of neurons (nucleus) in a network of fibers (neuropil). × 800. Bielschowsky silver stain.

METABOLIC FEATURES OF THE BRAIN

The adult brain's ability to synthesize certain proteins and lipids is greatly limited, but the dependence on carbohydrate as its main fuel persists. The brain is characterized by a uniquely high overall oxygen consumption, with metabolic activity generally highest in the cortex and cerebellum. The high energy requirement of most portions of the brain is related to the transport of ions, the synthesis of acetylcholine, and the metabolism of glutamic acid. Na^+, K^+-ATPase, which utilizes ATP and thus depends on oxidative metabolism, consumes 25–40% of cerebral energy production. This molecule acts as an ion pump and maintains the gradients of Na^+ and K^+ across neuronal membranes.

Carbohydrate, in the form of glucose, is the principal source of energy for tissue cells of the central nervous system; it serves as a major contributor in building amino acids and fatty acids and is a source of CO_2, which helps regulate pH. Carbohydrate metabolism of nerve tissue is similar to that of muscle. Lactic acid and pyruvic acid appear under anaerobic conditions; they disappear very slowly, and oxygen does not accelerate this process. Very little glycogen storage occurs in neural tissue, and brain extracts react more readily to glucose than glycogen. The respiratory quotient of neural tissue is 1.0, suggesting that ordinarily the tissues of the central nervous system use carbohydrate almost exclusively, burning sugar with oxygen and introducing energy into cells via high-energy phosphate esters. In some circumstances, however, the brain can apparently remain active without either extrinsic or intrinsic carbohydrates.

As might be expected, the adult brain is exquisitely sensitive to lack of oxygen (**anoxia**). Electrical activity is lost within seconds after onset of ischemia, and this is accompanied by loss of consciousness. Within minutes, ionic gradients across neuronal membranes are diminished as the supply of ATP is depleted. Col-

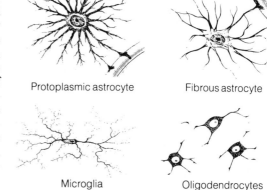

Protoplasmic astrocyte   Fibrous astrocyte

Microglia   Oligodendrocytes

Figure 2–14. Drawings of neuroglial cells specially stained by metallic impregnation. Observe that only the astrocytes exhibit vascular end-feet, which cover the walls of blood capillaries. (Reproduced, with permission, from Junqueira LC, Carneiro J, Kelley RO: *Basic Histology*, 7th ed. Appleton & Lange, 1992.)

lapse of ionic gradients is followed by irreversible nerve cell dysfunction. This can be followed, in turn, by **infarction.** Nerve cell death following anoxia can be delayed by hours to days; this suggests that **secondary cell injury** may lead to neuronal death. It has been hypothesized that this may involve a massive influx of Ca^{2+} into neurons, activating enzymes such as lipases and proteases that destroy the cell.

Low blood glucose levels (hypoglycemia) depress brain metabolism, and patients may become confused or drowsy. These symptoms are often preceded by marked sweating and sometimes hunger. Some patients rapidly develop convulsions and pass into coma. Repeated bouts of hypoglycemia, or a small number of severe episodes, can result in permanent brain damage.

REFERENCES

Abbott NJ: *Glial-Neuronal Interaction.* Ann NY Acad Sci, vol. 633, 1991.

Cajal S: *Histologie du Systeme Nerveux de l'Homme et des Vertebres,* vol. 2. Librairie Maloine, 1911.

Hall ZW (editor): *An Introduction to Molecular Neurobiology.* Sinauer, 1992.

Junqueira LC, Carneiro J, Kelley RO: *Basic Histology,* 7th ed. Appleton & Lange, 1992.

Morrell P (editor): *Myelin,* 2nd ed. Plenum, 1984.

Peters A, Palay SL, Webster H de F: *The Fine Structure of the Nervous System,* 3rd ed. Oxford, 1989.

Siegel G, Agranoff B, Albers RW, Molinoff P: *Basic Neurochemistry,* 4th ed. Raven, 1989.

Waxman SG: *Molecular and Cellular Approaches to the Treatment of Neurological Disease.* Raven, 1993.

Signaling in the Nervous System

3

Neurons are the basic signaling units of the nervous system. Along with muscle cells, neurons are unique in that they are **excitable,** ie, they respond to stimuli by generating electrical impulses. Neurons do this by altering the electrical potential differences that exist between the inner and outer surfaces of their membranes. Electrical responses of neurons (modifications of the electrical potential across their membranes) may be **local,** ie, restricted to the place that received the stimulus, or may be **propagated,** ie, may travel through the neuron and its axon. Neurons communicate with each other via propagated electrical impulses or **action potentials.** This chapter describes the mechanisms underlying electrical excitability in neurons.

MEMBRANE POTENTIAL

The membranes of cells, including nerve cells, are structured so a difference in electrical potential exists between the inside (negative) and the outside (positive). This results in a **resting potential** across the cell membrane, which is normally about −70 mV.

The electrical potential across the neuronal cell membrane is the result of its selective permeability to certain charged ions. Cell membranes are highly permeable to most inorganic ions, but are almost impermeable to proteins and many other organic ions. The difference **(gradient)** in ion composition inside and outside the cell membrane is maintained by *ion pumps* in the membrane, which maintain a nearly constant concentration of inorganic ions within the cell (Fig 3–1 and Table 3–1). The pump that maintains Na^+ and K^+ gradients across the membrane is Na, K-ATPase; this specialized protein molecule extrudes Na^+ from the intracellular compartment, moving it to the extracellular space, and imports K^+ from the extracellular space, carrying it across the membrane into the cell. In carrying out this essential activity, the pump consumes **ATP.**

Two types of passive forces maintain an equilibrium of Na^+ and K^+ across the membrane: A chemical force tends to move Na^+ inward and K^+ outward, from the compartment containing high concentration to the compartment containing low concentration, and an electrical force (the membrane potential) tends to move Na^+ and K^+ inward. When the chemical and electrical forces are equally strong, an **equilibrium potential** exists.

For an idealized membrane that is permeable to only K^+, the **Nernst equation,** which describes the relationship between these forces, is used to calculate the magnitude of the equilibrium potential (ie, the membrane potential at which equilibrium exists). Normally, there is a much higher concentration of K^+ inside the cell ($[K^+]_i$) than outside the cell ($[K^+]_o$) (Table 3–1). The Nernst equation, which would be used to determine membrane potential across a membrane permeable only to K^+ ions, is as follows:

$$E_K = \frac{RT}{nF} \log_{10} \frac{[K^+]_o}{[K^+]_i}$$

where

E = equilibrium potential (no net flow across the membrane)
K = potassium
T = temperature
R = gas constant
F = Faraday constant (relates charge in coulombs to concentration in moles)
n = valence (for potassium, valence = 1)
$[K^+]_i$ = concentration of potassium inside cell
$[K^+]_o$ = concentration of potassium outside cell

At physiologic temperatures

$$E_K = 58 \log \frac{[K^+]_o}{[K^+]_i}$$

The equilibrium potential (E_{Na}) for sodium can be found by substituting $[Na^+]_i$ and $[Na^+]_o$ in the Nernst equation; this potential would be found across a membrane that was permeable only to sodium. In reality, most cell membranes are not perfectly selective, ie,

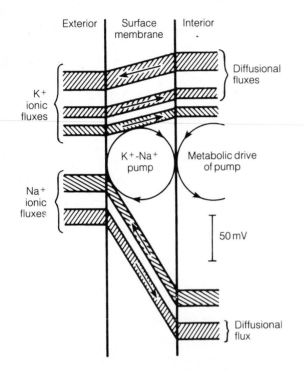

Figure 3–1. Na+ and K+ fluxes through the resting nerve cell membrane. Notice that the Na+-K+ pump (Na+, K+-ATPase) tends to extrude Na+ from the interior of the cell while it carries K+ ions inward. (Reproduced, with permission, from Eccles JC: *The Physiology of Nerve Cells.* Johns Hopkins University Press, 1957.)

Table 3–1. Concentration of some ions inside and outside mammalian spinal motor neurons.*

| ion | Concentration (mmol/L H_2O) | | Equilibrium Potential (mV) |
	Inside Cell	Outside Cell	
Na^+	15.0	150.0	+60
K^+	150.0	5.5	−90
Cl^-	9.0	125.0	−70

Resting membrane potential = −70 mV

* Reproduced with permission, from Ganong WF: *Review of Medical Physiology,* 13th ed. Appleton & Lange, 1987. Data from Mommaerts WFHM, in: *Essentials of Human Physiology.* Ross G (editor). Year Book, 1978.

$$V_m = 58 \log \frac{P_K[K^+]_o + P_{Na}[Na^+]_o}{P_K[K^+]_i + P_{Na}[Na^+]_i}$$

where
[Na]$_i$ = concentration of sodium inside cell
[Na]$_o$ = concentration of sodium outside cell
P_{Na} = membrane permeability to sodium
P_K = membrane permeability to potassium

As seen in this equation, membrane potential is affected by the **relative permeability** to each ion. If permeability to a certain ion increases (eg, by the opening of pores or channels specifically permeable to that ion), membrane potential will move **closer** to the equilibrium potential for that ion. Conversely, if permeability to that ion decreases, eg, by closing of pores or channels permeable to that ion, membrane potential will move **away** from the equilibrium potential for that ion.

In the membrane of resting neurons, K^+ permeability is much higher (~**20**-fold) than Na^+ permeability, ie, the P_K:P_{Na} ratio is approximately 20. Thus, the Goldman-Hodgkin-Katz equation is dominated by K^+ permeability so that membrane potential is close to the equilibrium potential for K (E_K). This accounts for the resting potential of approximately −70 mV.

GENERATOR POTENTIAL

The **generator (receptor) potential** is a local, nonpropagated response that occurs in some sensory receptors (eg, muscle stretch receptors and pacinian corpuscles, which are touch-pressure receptors) where mechanical energy is converted into electric signals. The generator potential is produced in a small area of the sensory cell, the unmyelinated nerve terminal. Most generator potentials are depolarizations, in which membrane potential becomes less negative. In contrast to action potentials (see next section), which are all-or-none responses, generator potentials are **graded**—the larger the stimulus (stretch or pressure), the larger the depolarization, and **additive**—two small stimuli, close together in time, produce a generator potential larger than that made by a single small stimulus. Further increase in stimulation results in larger generator potentials (Fig 3–2). When the magnitude of the generator potential increases to about 10 mV, a propagated action potential (impulse) is generated in the sensory nerve.

they are permeable to *several* ionic species. For these membranes, potential is the *weighted average* of the equilibrium potentials for each permeable ion, with the contribution for each ion weighted to reflect its contribution to total membrane permeability. This is described mathematically, for a membrane that is permeable to Na^+ and K^+, by the Goldman-Hodgkin-Katz equation (also known as the constant field equation):

ACTION POTENTIAL

The sequence of electrical events that occur when an impulse is propagated is called an **action potential.** When a sufficiently strong impulse approaches along a sensory or motor nerve fiber, the membrane begins

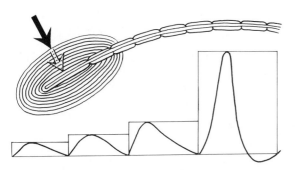

Figure 3–2. Demonstration of a generator potential in a pacinian corpuscle. The electrical responses to a pressure (black arrow) of 1×, 2×, 3×, and 4× are shown. The strongest stimulus produced an action potential in the sensory nerve, originating in the center of the corpuscle (open arrow).

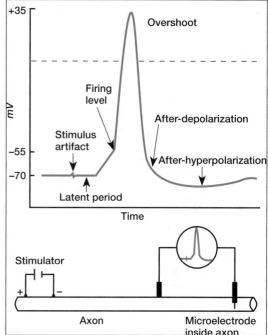

Figure 3–3. Action potential ("spike potential") recorded with one electrode inside cell. In the resting state, the membrane potential (resting potential) is –70 mV. When the axon is stimulated there is a small depolarization. If this depolarization reaches the firing level (threshold), there is an all-or-none depolarization (action potential). The action potential approaches E_{Na} and overshoots the 0 mV level. The action potential ends when the axon repolarizes, again settling at resting potential. (Reproduced, with permission, from Ganong WF: *Review of Medical Physiology,* 14th ed. Appleton & Lange, 1989.)

to **depolarize.** When the initial depolarization reaches about 15 mV, a sufficient number of voltage-sensitive Na^+ channels are activated (opened) and threshold is reached so that the rate of depolarization increases sharply to produce a spike; the **isopotential level (zero potential)** is overshot by about 35 mV as membrane potential approaches E_{Na} (Fig 3–3). As the impulse passes, **repolarization** occurs rapidly at first, then more slowly. Membrane potential thus returns to resting potential; in some fibers, in fact, membrane potential becomes transiently hyperpolarized (the **after-hyperpolarization**) as a result of the opening of the K^+ channels, which tend to drive the membrane toward E_K. In the wake of an action potential, there is a **refractory period** of decreased excitability. This has two phases: The initial **absolute refractory period** during which another action potential cannot be generated, and the **relative refractory period** (lasting up to a few msec) during which a second action potential can be generated but conduction velocity is decreased and threshold is increased (Table 3–2). The refractory period limits the ability of the axon to conduct high-frequency trains of action potentials.

THE NERVE CELL MEMBRANE CONTAINS ION CHANNELS

Voltage-sensitive ion channels are specialized protein molecules that span the cell membrane. These doughnut-shaped molecules contain a **pore** that acts as a tunnel, permitting specific ions (eg, Na^+ or K^+), but not other ions, to permeate. The channel also possesses a **voltage sensor,** which, in response to changes in potential across the membrane, either opens (activates) or closes (inactivates) the channel.

The ability of the neuronal membrane to generate impulses arises from the fact that it contains **voltage-sensitive Na^+ channels,** which are selectively permeable to Na^+ and tend to open when the membrane is de-

polarized. Because these channels open in response to depolarization, and because by opening they drive the membrane closer to Na^+ equilibrium potential (E_{Na}), they tend to further depolarize the membrane (Fig 3–4). If a sufficient number of these channels are opened, there is an explosive, all-or-none response, which is termed the action potential (see Fig 3–3). The degree of depolarization necessary to elicit the action potential is called the **threshold.**

Other voltage-sensitive ion channels (**voltage-sensitive K^+ channels**) open (usually more slowly than Na^+ channels) in response to depolarization and are selectively permeable to K^+. When these channels open, the membrane potential is driven toward the K^+ equilibrium potential (E_K), leading to hyperpolarization.

The behavior of Na^+ and K^+ channels was elegantly inferred by Allen Hodgkin and Andrew Huxley, who subsequently received the Nobel Prize for their important studies, carried out in the 1950s on the squid giant axon. This model system is still used by some neuroscientists because the large diameter of the axons (up to 1 mm) facilitates the insertion of intracellular microelectrodes. Hodgkin and Huxley described the be-

Table 3–2. Nerve fiber types in mammalian nerve.*

Fiber Type		Function	Fiber Diameter (μm)	Conduction Velocity (m/s)	Spike Duration (ms)	Absolute Refractory Period (ms)
A	α	Proprioception; somatic motor	12–20	70–120		
	β	Touch, pressure	5–12	30–70	0.4–0.5	0.4–1
	γ	Motor to muscle spindles	3–6	15–30		
	δ	Pain, temperature, touch	2–5	12–30		
B		Preganglionic autonomic	<3	3–15	1.2	1.2
C	dorsal root	Pain, reflex responses	0.4–1.2	0.5–2	2	2
	sympathetic	Postganglionic sympathetics	0.3–1.3	0.7–2.3	2	2

* Reproduced, with permission, from Ganong WF: *Review of Medical Physiology,* 13th ed. Appleton & Lange, 1987.

havior of these channels in a set of equations, known as the Hodgkin-Huxley equations, which provide a very useful mathematical model of ion channel function.

THE EFFECTS OF MYELINATION

Nonmyelinated axons, in the mammalian PNS and CNS, generally have a small diameter (less than 1 μm in the PNS and less than 0.2 μm in the CNS). The action potential is conducted in a continuous manner along these axons owing to a relatively uniform distribution of voltage-sensitive Na^+ and K^+ channels. As the action potential invades a given region of the axon, it

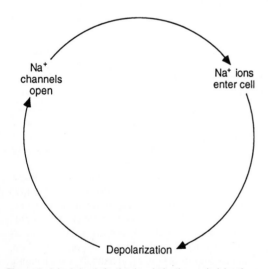

Figure 3–4. Ionic basis for the depolarization underlying the action potential. Voltage-sensitive Na^+ channels open when the membrane is depolarized. This results in increased Na^+ permeability of the membrane, causing further depolarization and the opening of still other Na^+ channels. When a sufficient number of Na^+ channels have opened, the membrane generates an explosive, all-or-none depolarization—the action potential.

depolarizes the region in front of it, so that the impulse crawls continuously along the entire length of the axon (Fig 3–5). In nonmyelinated axons, activation of Na^+ channels accounts for the depolarization phase of the action potential, and activation of K^+ channels produces repolarization.

Myelinated axons, in contrast, are covered by myelin sheaths. The myelin has a high electrical resistance and low capacitance, permitting it to act as an insulator. The myelin sheath is not continuous along the entire length of the axon. On the contrary, it is periodically interrupted by small gaps (approximately 1 μm long) called the **nodes of Ranvier** where the axon is exposed. In mammalian myelinated fibers, the voltage-sensitive Na^+ and K^+ channels are not distributed uniformly. Na^+ channels are clustered in high-density (about 1000 per $μm^2$) in the axon membrane at the node of Ranvier. K^+ channels, on the other hand, tend to be localized in the "internodal" axon membrane, ie, the axon membrane covered by the myelin (Fig 3–6). Because these channels are covered by the insulating myelin sheaths, they are "physiologically masked" and do not contribute to repolarization of the action potential. Repolarization results from the inactivation (closing) of Na^+ channels together with the presence of a "leakage" K^+ conductance.

Because the current flow through the insulating myelin is negligible, the action potential in myelinated axons does not move continuously along the axon; in contrast, it jumps from one node to the next, in a mode of conduction that has been termed **saltatory** (Fig 3–7). There are several important consequences to this saltatory mode of conduction in myelinated fibers. First, the energetic requirement for impulse conduction is lower in myelinated fibers, therefore, the metabolic cost of conduction is lower. Second, myelination results in an **increased conduction velocity.** Figure 3–8 shows conduction velocity, as a function of diameter, for nonmyelinated and myelinated axons. For nonmyelinated axons, conduction velocity is proportional to $(diameter)^{1/2}$. In contrast, conduction velocity in

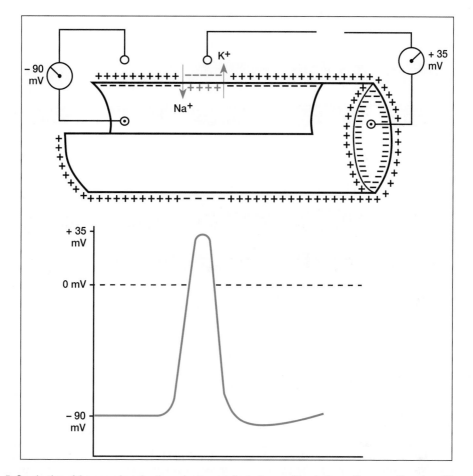

Figure 3–5. Conduction of the nerve impulse through an unmyelinated nerve fiber. In the resting axon, there is a difference of –90 mV between the interior of the axon and the outer surface of its membrane (resting potential). During the conduction of an action potential, Na⁺ passes into the axon interior and subsequently K⁺ migrates in the opposite direction. In consequence, the membrane polarity changes (the membrane becomes relatively positive on its inner surface), and the resting potential is replaced by an action potential (⁺35 mV here). (Reproduced, with permission, from Junqueira LC, Carneiro J, Kelley RO: *Basic Histology*, 6th ed. Appleton & Lange, 1989.)

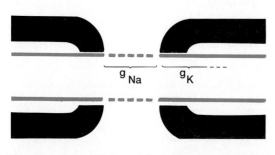

Figure 3–6. Na⁺ and K⁺ channel distributions in myelinated axons are not uniform. Na⁺ channels (g_{Na}) are clustered in high density in the axon membrane at the node of Ranvier where they are available to produce the depolarization needed for the action potential. K⁺ channels (g_K), on the other hand, are located largely in the internodal axon membrane under the myelin, so that they are masked. (Reproduced, with permission, from Waxman SG: Membranes, myelin and the pathophysiology of multiple sclerosis. *New Engl J Med* 1982;**306**:1529.

myelinated axons increases linearly with diameter. Thus, a myelinated axon can conduct impulses at a much higher conduction velocity than a nonmyelinated axon of the same size. In order to conduct as rapidly as a 10-μm myelinated fiber, a nonmyelinated axon would have to have a diameter of over 100 μm. Thus, myelination permits many rapidly conducting axons to fit within a given nerve or tract.

CONDUCTION OF SIGNALS

Types of Fibers

Nerve fibers have been divided into three types according to their diameters, conduction velocities, and physiologic characteristics (Table 3–2). **A fibers** are large and myelinated, conduct rapidly, and conduct

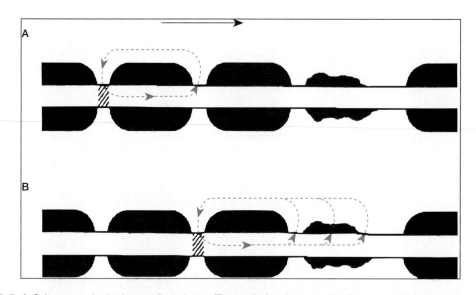

Figure 3–7. *A:* Saltatory conduction in a myelinated axon. The myelin functions as an insulator due to its high resistance and low capacitance. Thus, when the action potential (cross-hatching) is at a given node of Ranvier, the majority of the electrical current is shunted to the next node (along the pathway shown by the broken arrow). Conduction of the action potential proceeds in a discontinuous manner, jumping from node to node with a high conduction velocity. ***B:*** In demyelinated axons there is loss of current through the damaged myelin. As a result, it either takes longer to reach threshold and conduction velocity is reduced, or threshold is not reached and the action potential fails to propagate. (Reproduced, with permission, from Waxman SG: Membranes, myelin and the pathophysiology of multiple sclerosis. *New Engl J Med* 1982;**306**:1529.

various motor or sensory impulses. They are most susceptible to injury by mechanical pressure or lack of oxygen. **B fibers** are smaller myelinated axons that conduct less rapidly than A fibers. These fibers serve autonomic functions. **C fibers** are the smallest and are unmyelinated; they conduct impulses the slowest and serve pain conduction and autonomic functions. An al-

ternative classification, used by some authorities to describe sensory axons in peripheral nerves, is shown in Table 3–3.

The large A fibers are least sensitive to local anesthetics and the small-diameter, poorly myelinated C fibers are most sensitive. Conversely, large-diameter fibers are most easily excited by electrical stimuli (ie, they have the lowest thresholds), and those with small-diameter fibers are least easily excited (ie. they have the highest thresholds).

Physiology

Because fibers with larger diameters have lower thresholds for electrical stimulation, only the large-di-

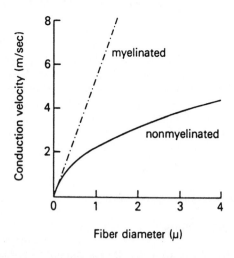

Figure 3–8. Relationship between conduction velocity and diameter in myelinated and nonmyelinated axons. Myelinated axons conduct more rapidly than nonmyelinated axons of the same size.

Table 3–3. Numerical classification sometimes used for sensory neurons.*

Number		Origin	Fiber Type
I	a	Muscle spindle, annulospiral ending	A α
	b	Golgi tendon organ	A α
II		Muscle spindle, flower-spray ending; touch, pressure	A β
III		Pain and temperature receptors; some touch receptors	A δ
IV		Pain and other receptors	C

* Reproduced, with permission, from Ganong WF: *Review of Medical Physiology,* 16th ed. Appleton & Lange, 1993.

ameter fibers (IA) are stimulated when a mixed peripheral nerve (one containing both sensory and motor fibers) is stimulated by a low-intensity electric current. A stimulus of greater intensity affects the smaller efferent as well as the afferent fibers. The nerve itself is most sensitive to stimulation, the myoneural junction is intermediate in sensitivity, and the muscle is least sensitive.

The nerve-conduction velocity is normally 50–60 m/s in ulnar and median nerves and 45–55 m/s in the common peroneal nerve. The conduction velocity of a nerve may be markedly slowed by a decrease in temperature, compression, and other conditions; it may decrease by 2 m/s for each drop of 1 °C (1.8 °F) in temperature.

Clinical Correlations

A. Neuropathy: In peripheral neuropathies—diseases affecting peripheral nerves—the conduction velocity of motor nerves may be reduced, frequently to less than 40 msec. Conduction block, whereby impulses fail to propagate past a point of axonal injury, can also occur. The reduction in conduction velocity can be seen in terms of increased conduction time between nerve stimulation and muscle contraction and in the longer duration of the muscle action potential. Marked slowing in conduction velocity occurs in neuropathies when there is acute demyelination, such as the **Guillian-Barré syndrome,** in some chronic or heredito-familial neuropathies and during nerve regeneration (while myelination is being formed and is not yet mature).

B. Demyelination: Demyelination, or damage to the myelin sheath, is seen in a number of neurologic diseases. The most common is **multiple sclerosis,** in which myelin is damaged as a result of abnormal immune mechanisms. As a result of loss of myelin insulation and exposure of the internodal axon membrane, which contains a low density of Na^+ channels, the conduction of action potentials is slowed or blocked in demyelinated axons (see Fig 3–7). Clinical Illustration 3–1 describes a patient with multiple sclerosis.

CLINICAL ILLUSTRATION 3–1

C.B., an emergency room nurse, was well until she was 23-years-old when she noticed blurred vision in her left eye. Twenty-four hours later, her vision had dimmed, and a day later, she was totally blind in her left eye. A neurologist found a normal neurologic examination. Visual evoked potentials revealed decreased conduction velocity in the left optic nerve (see Chapter 24). A magnetic resonance scan demonstrated several areas of demyelination in the subcortical white matter of both cerebral hemispheres. Despite the persistence of these abnormalities, C.B. recovered full vision in four weeks.

A year later, C.B. developed weakness in her legs, associated with tingling in her right foot. Her physician told her that she probably had multiple sclerosis. She was treated with corticosteroids and recovered three weeks later with only mild residual weakness.

After a symptom-free interval for two years, C.B. noticed the onset, following a cold, of a tremor that was worse when she attempted to perform voluntary actions ("intention tremor") and double vision. On examination, the neurologist found signs suggesting demyelination in the brain stem and cerebellum. Again, she recovered with only mild residua.

C.B.'s history is typical for patients with the relapsing-remitting form of multiple sclerosis. This disorder, which occurs in young adults (20–50 years old), is due to inflammatory destruction of myelin sheaths within the CNS. This demyelination occurs in well-defined lesions ("plaques") that are disseminated both in space and in time (hence, the term "multiple sclerosis"). Remyelination, within the core of the demyelination plaques, occurs sluggishly if at all.

The relapsing-remitting course exemplified by C.B. presents an interesting example of **functional recovery** in a neurologic disorder. Because the myelin does not regenerate and the internodal axon membrane does not contain Na^+ channels, how does recovery occur? Recent studies have demonstrated molecular plasticity of the demyelinated axon membrane, which develops increased numbers of Na^+ channels in regions that were formerly covered by the myelin sheath. This permits impulses to propagate in a continuous, slow manner (similar to nonmyelinated axons) along demyelinated regions of some axons. The slowly-conducted impulses carry enough information to support clinical recovery of some functions, such as vision, even though the axons remain demyelinated. Although neuroscientists have begun to understand this molecular plasticity, they do not yet know how to "turn on" the production of Na^+ channels in demyelinated axons, and cannot, therefore, induce remissions.

SYNAPSES

In the most general sense, there are two broad classes of synapses (Table 3–4). **Electrical** (or **electrotonic**) synapses are characterized by **gap junctions,** which are specialized structures where the pre- and postsynaptic membranes come into close apposition. Gap junctions act as conductive pathways, so electric current can flow directly from the presynaptic axon into the postsynaptic neuron. Transmission at electrical synapses does not involve neurotransmitters.

Table 3–4. Modes of synaptic transmission.

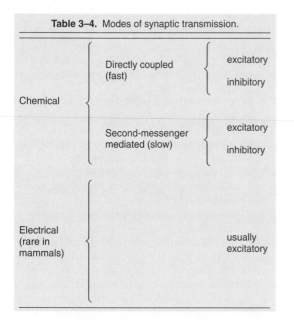

Chemical	Directly coupled (fast)	excitatory
		inhibitory
	Second-messenger mediated (slow)	excitatory
		inhibitory
Electrical (rare in mammals)		usually excitatory

Synaptic delay is much shorter at electrical synapses than at chemical synapses. While electrical synapses occur commonly in the CNS of inframammalian species, they occur only rarely in the mammalian CNS.

The second broad class of synapse, which accounts for the overwhelming majority of synapses in the mammalian brain and spinal cord, is the **chemical synapse.** At chemical synapse, there is distinct cleft (about 30 nm wide), which represents an extension of the extracellular space, separating the pre- and postsynaptic membranes. The pre- and postsynaptic components at chemical synapses communicate via diffusion of **neurotransmitter** molecules; some common transmitters that consist of relatively small molecules are listed with their main areas of concentration in the nervous system

Table 3–5. Areas of concentration of common neurotransmitters.

Neurotransmitter	Areas of concentration
Acetylcholine (ACh)	Neuromuscular junction, autonomic ganglia, parasympathetic neurons, motor nuclei of cranial nerves, caudate nucleus and putamen, basal nucleus of Meynert, portions of the limbic system
Norepinephrine (NC)	Sympathetic nervous system, locus ceruleus, lateral tegmentum
Dopamine (DA)	Hypothalamus, midbrain nigrostriatal system
Serotonin (5-HT)	Parasympathetic neurons in gut, pineal gland, nucleus raphe magnus of pons
Gamma-aminobutyric acid (GABA)	Cerebellum, hippocampus, cerebral cortex, striatonigral system
Glycine	Spinal cord
Glutamic acid	Spinal cord, brain stem, cerebellum, hippocampus, cerebral cortex

in Table 3–5. As a result of depolarization of the presynaptic ending by action potentials, neurotransmitter molecules are released from the presynaptic ending, diffuse across the synaptic cleft, and bind to postsynaptic **receptors.** These receptors are associated with and trigger the opening of (or in some cases closing) of **ligand-gated ion channels.** The opening (or closing) of these channels produces postsynaptic potentials.

Neurotransmitter in presynaptic terminals is contained in membrane-bound packets, termed **presynaptic vesicles.** The morphology of these vesicles varies, depending on the particular transmitter they contain. Release of neurotransmitter occurs when the presynaptic vesicles fuse with the presynaptic membrane, permitting release of their contents by **exocytosis.** Vesicular transmitter release is triggered by an influx of Ca^{2+} into the presynaptic terminal, an event which is mediated by the activation of presynaptic Ca^{2+} channels by the invading action potential. As a result of this activity-induced increase in Ca^{2+} in the presynaptic terminal, there is phosphorylation of proteins called **synapsins,** which appear to cross-link vesicles to the cytoskeleton, thereby preventing their movement. This permits fusion of vesicles with the presynaptic membrane, resulting in release of neurotransmitter. The release process and diffusion across the synaptic cleft accounts for the **synaptic delay** of 0.5 to 1.0 msec at chemical synapses. This sequence is shown in diagrammatic form for a small part of the neuromuscular junction, a prototypic synapse, in Figure 3–9.

SYNAPTIC TRANSMISSION

Directly Linked (Fast)

Transmitter molecules bind at the postsynaptic membrane with either of two types of postsynaptic receptor. The first type of receptor is found exclusively in the nervous system and is **directly linked** to an ion channel (a **ligand-gated ion channel**). By binding to the postsynaptic receptor, the transmitter molecule acts directly on the postsynaptic ion channel. Moreover, the transmitter molecule is rapidly removed. This mode of synaptic transmission takes only a few milliseconds and is rapidly terminated; therefore, it is termed "fast." Depending on the type of ion channel that is open or closed, fast synaptic transmission can be either excitatory or inhibitory (see Table 3–4).

Second-Messenger Mediated (Slow)

A second mode of chemical synaptic transmission, which is closely related to endocrine communication in non-neural cells, utilizes receptors that are not directly linked to ion channels; these receptors open or close ion channels or change the levels of intracellular second messengers via activation of **G-proteins** and production of **second messengers.** When the transmitter is bound

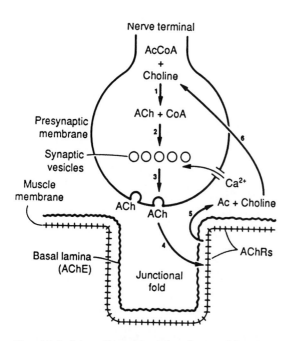

Nerve terminal

AcCoA
+
Choline

ACh + CoA

Presynaptic membrane

Synaptic vesicles

Muscle membrane

Ca^{2+}

ACh   ACh   Ac + Choline

Basal lamina (AChE)

AChRs

Junctional fold

Figure 3–9. Schematic representation of some of the events involved in neurotransmitter synthesis, release, and action at a prototypic synapse, the neuromuscular junction. ACh is the transmitter at this synapse. Part of the nerve terminal is shown, lying in close apposition to a muscle end-plate. Synthesis of ACh occurs locally, in the presynaptic terminal, from acetyl-CoA and choline (1). ACh is then incorporated into membrane-bound synaptic vesicles (2). Release of ACh occurs by exocytosis, which involves fusion of the vesicles with the presynaptic membrane (3). This process is triggered by an influx of Ca^{2+} that occurs in response to propagation of the action potential into the presynaptic axons. The contents of approximately 200 synaptic vesicles are released into the synaptic cleft in response to a single action potential. The released ACh diffuses rapidly across the synaptic cleft (4) and binds to postsynaptic ACh receptors (5) where it triggers a conformational change that leads to an influx of Na^+ ions that depolarizes the membrane. When the channel closes, the ACh dissociates and is hydrolyzed by acetylcholinesterase (6). (Reproduced, with permission, from Murray RK, Granner DK, Mayes PA, Rodwell VW: *Harper's Biochemistry*, 23rd ed. Appleton & Lange, 1993).

to the receptor, the receptor interacts with the G-protein molecule, which binds GTP and is activated. Activation of the G-protein leads to production of cAMP, diacylglycerol (**DAG**) or inositol trisphosphate ($\mathbf{IP_3}$). cAMP, DAG, and IP_3 participate in the phosphorylation of ion channels, thus opening channels that are closed at the resting potential or closing channels that are open at the resting potential. The cascade of molecular events, leading from binding of transmitter at these receptors to opening or closing of channels takes hundreds of milliseconds to seconds and the effects on channels are relatively long-lasting (seconds to minutes). This mode of synaptic transmission has therefore been termed "slow." G-protein coupled receptors have been identified for a broad range of neurotransmitters, including dopamine, acetylcholine (**muscarinic ACh receptor**), and neuropeptides (Tables 3–6 and 3–7).

In contrast to fast synaptic transmission, which is highly-targeted and acts on only a single postsynaptic element, second messenger-linked transmission is slower and may affect a wider range of postsynaptic neurons. Thus, this mode of synaptic transmission serves an important **modulatory** function.

EXCITATORY AND INHIBITORY SYNAPTIC ACTIONS

Excitatory postsynaptic potentials (EPSPs) are produced by the binding of neurotransmitter molecules to receptors that result in the opening of channels (eg, Na^+ or Ca^{2+} channels) or the closing of channels (eg, K^+ channels) that result in depolarization. In general, excitatory synapses tend to be **axodendritic** (see Fig 2–11). In contrast, **inhibitory postsynaptic potentials (IPSPs)** in many cases are caused by a localized increase in membrane permeability to Cl^- or to K^+. This tends to cause **hyperpolarization** and most commonly occurs at **axosomatic** synapses where it is called **postsynaptic inhibitory transmission** (Fig 3–10).

Information processing by neurons involves the **integration** of synaptic inputs from many other neurons. If they occur close enough in time, EPSPs (depolarizations) and IPSPs (hyperpolarizations) tend to sum with each other. As a neuron integrates the incoming synaptic information, depending on whether or not threshold is reached at the impulse initiation zone (usually the axon initial segment), an action potential is either generated or not. If an action potential is initiated, it propagates along the axon to impinge, via synapses, on still other neurons. The **rate** and **pattern** of action potentials carry information.

SYNAPTIC PLASTICITY AND LONG-TERM POTENTIATION

One of the unique properties of the nervous system is that it can **learn.** It has long been suspected that memory has its basis in the strengthening of particular synaptic connections. In the past few years, much progress has been made in understanding synaptic plasticity. One particular phenomenon, called **long-term potentiation (LTP)**, is characterized by the enhanced transmission at synapses that follow high-frequency stimulation. This phenomenon was first observed at synapses in the hippocampus and may play a role in associative learning. LTP depends on the presence of NMDA receptors in the postsynaptic membrane. These specialized glutamate receptors open postsynaptic Ca^{2+} channels in response to binding of the transmitter glutamate, but they do this only if the postsynaptic membrane is depolarized. Depolarization of the postsynaptic element requires the activation of other synapses, and the NMDA receptor-linked Ca^{2+}

Table 3–6. Common neurotransmitters and their actions

Transmitter	Receptor	Second Messenger*	Effect on Channels	Action
Acetylcholine (Ach)	N	—	Opens Na^+ and other small ion channels	Excitatory
	M	cAMP or IP_3, DAG	Opens or closes Ca^{2+} channels	Excitatory or inhibitory
Glutamate	NMDA	—	Opens channels, which permit Ca^{2+} influx if membrane is depolarized	Senses simultaneous activity of 2 synaptic inputs, May trigger molecular changes that strengthen synapse (LTP)
	Kainate	—	Opens Na^+ channels	Excitatory
	AMPA	—	Opens Na^+ channels	Excitatory
	Metabotropic	IP_3, DAG	—	Excitatory, raises intracellular Ca^{2+}
Dopamine	D_1	cAMP	Opens K^+ channels, closes Ca^{2+} channels.	Inhibitory
	D_2	cAMP	Opens K^+ channels, closes Ca^{2+} channels	Inhibitory
γ-aminobutyric acid (GABA)	$GABA_A$	—	Opens Cl^- channels	Inhibitory (postsynaptic)
	$GABA_B$	IP_3, DAG	Closes Ca^{2+} channels, opens K^+ channels	Inhibitory (presynaptic)
Glycine	—	—	Opens Cl^- channels	Inhibitory

* Directly linked receptors do not utilize 2nd messengers.
Modified, with permission, from Ganong, **W.F.**: *Review of Medical Physiology,* 16th ed., Appleton & Lange 1993.

channels open only when both sets of synapses are activated. Thus, these synapses sense the "pairing" of two synaptic inputs in a manner analogous to conditioning to behavioral stimuli. Recent work suggests that as a result of increased Ca^{2+} admitted into postsynaptic cells by this scheme, protein kinases are activated and, via mechanisms that are still poorly understood, alter the synapse so as to strengthen it. These structural changes, triggered by specific patterns of synaptic activity, may provide a basis for memory.

The production of second messengers by synaptic activity may also play a role in **regulation of gene expression** in the postsynaptic cell. Thus, second messengers can activate enzymes that modify **pre-existing proteins** or induce the expression of **new proteins.** This provides a mechanism whereby the synaptic activation of the cell can induce long-term changes. These changes in protein synthesis in the postsynaptic cell may participate in learning and memory and may be important in nervous system development.

PRESYNAPTIC INHIBITION

Presynaptic inhibition is mediated by **axo-axonal synapses** (Fig 3–10). Binding of neurotransmitters to the receptors mediating presynaptic inhibition leads to a reduction in the amount of neurotransmitter secreted by the postsynaptic axon. This is caused by either a decrease in the size of the action potential in the presynaptic terminal as a result of activation of K^+ or Cl^- channels or by reduced opening of Ca^{2+} channels in the presynaptic terminal, thereby decreasing the amount of transmitter release. Presynaptic inhibition, thus, provides a mechanism whereby the "gain" at a particular synaptic input to a neuron can be reduced without reducing the efficacy of other synapses that impinge on that neuron.

THE NEUROMUSCULAR JUNCTION AND THE END-PLATE POTENTIAL

The axons of lower-motor-neurons project through peripheral nerves to muscle cells. These motor axons terminate at a specialized portion of the muscle membrane called the **motor end-plate,** which represents localized specialization of the sarcolemma—the membrane surrounding a striated muscle fiber (Fig 3–11). The nerve impulse is transmitted to the muscle across the **neuromuscular synapse** (also called the **neuromuscular junction**). The end-plate potential is the prolonged depolarizing potential that occurs at the end-plate in response to action potential activity in the motor axon. It is localized to the myoneural junction. The transmitter at the neuromuscular synapse is acetylcholine. Small amounts of acetylcholine are released randomly from the nerve cell membrane at rest; each release produces a minute depolarization, a miniature end-plate potential, about 0.5 mV in amplitude. These miniature end-plate potentials, also called **quanta,** reflect the random discharge of ACh from single synap-

Table 3–7. Mammalian neuropeptides.

Hypothalamic releasing hormones
  Thyrotropin-releasing hormone (TRH)
  Gonadotropin-releasing hormone
  Somatostatin
  Corticotropin-releasing factor (CRF)
  Growth-hormone-releasing hormone
  Luteinizing-hormone-releasing hormone (LHRH)
Pituitary peptides
  Corticotropin (ACTH)
  Growth hormone (GH), somatotropin
  Lipotropin
  Alpha melanocyte-stimulating hormone (alpha MSH)
  Prolactin
  Luteinizing hormone
  Thyrotropin
Neurohypophyseal hormones
  Vasopressin
  Oxytocin
  Neurophysin(s)
Circulating hormones
  Angiotensin
  Calcitonin
  Glucagon
  Insulin
Gut brain peptides
  Vasoactive intestinal peptide (VIP)
  Cholecystokinin (CCK)
  Gastrin
  Motilin
  Pancreatic polypeptide
  Secretin
  Substance P
  Bombesin
  Neurotensin
Opioid peptides
  Dynorphin
  Beta-endorphin
  Met-enkephalin
  Leu-enkephalin
  Kyotorphin
Others
  Bradykinin
  Carnosine
  Neuropeptide Y
  Proctolin
  Substance K
  Epidermal growth factor (EGF)

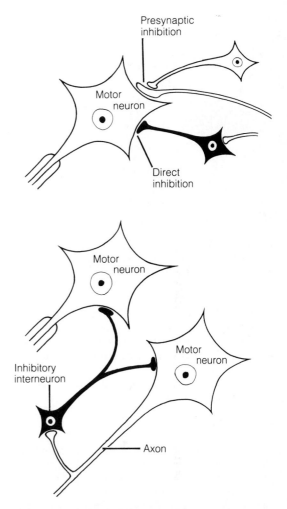

Figure 3–10. ***Top:*** Schematic illustration of two types of inhibition in the spinal cord. In direct inhibition (also called postsynaptic inhibition), a chemical mediator released from an inhibitory neuron causes hyperpolarization (inhibitory postsynaptic potential) of a motor neuron. In presynaptic inhibition, a second chemical mediator released onto the ending (axon) of an excitatory neuron causes a reduction in the size of the postsynaptic excitatory potential. ***Bottom:*** Diagram of a specific inhibitory system involving an inhibitory interneuron (Renshaw cell).

tic vesicles. When a nerve impulse reaches the myoneural junction, however, substantially more transmitter is released as a result of the synchronous discharge of ACh from many synaptic vesicles. This causes a full end-plate potential that exceeds the firing level of the muscle fiber.

NEUROTRANSMITTERS

One of the most exciting areas in the neurosciences focuses on neurotransmitters; the discovery of an increasing number of transmitter agents is drawing a new type of chemical brain map that enriches the traditional pathways map.

A large number of compounds act as neurotransmitters at chemical synapses. Such substances are present in the synaptic terminal, and their action may be blocked by pharmacologic agents. Some presynaptic nerves can release more than one transmitter; differences in the frequency of nerve stimulation probably control which transmitter is released. Common transmitters that consist of relatively small molecules are listed with their main areas of concentration in the nervous system (see Table 3–5).

It has been shown that some neurons in the central nervous system not only make and store the common

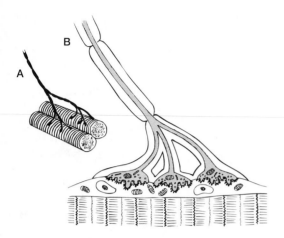

Figure 3–11. Schematic illustrations of a myoneural junction. **A:** Motor fiber supplying several muscle fibers. **B:** Cross section as seen in an electron micrograph.

transmitters but also accumulate a variety of peptides (see Table 3–5). Some of these peptides act much like conventional transmitters; others appear to be hormones. A few are both classic transmitters and hormone-type neuropeptides.

Some relatively well-understood neurotransmitters and their distributions are discussed below.

Acetylcholine

Acetylocholine (ACh) is synthesized by the enzyme choline acetyltransferase and is broken down after release into the synaptic cleft by the enzyme acetylcholinesterase (AChase). These enzymes are synthesized in the neuronal cell body, and they are carried by axonal transport to the presynaptic terminal; synthesis of ACh, *per se,* occurs in the presynaptic terminal.

ACh acts as a transmitter at a variety of sites in the PNS and CNS. ACh, for example, is responsible for excitatory transmission at the neuromuscular junction (N-type, nicotinic ACh receptors). ACh is also the transmitter in autonomic ganglia and is released by preganglionic sympathetic and parasympathetic neurons. Postganglionic parasympathetic neurons, as well as one particular type of postganglionic sympathetic axon (ie, the fibers innervating sweat glands), utilize ACh as their transmitter (M-type, muscarinic receptors).

Within the CNS, several well-defined groups of neurons use ACh as a transmitter. These groups include neurons that project widely from the **basal forebrain nucleus of Meynert** to the cerebral cortex and from the **septal nucleus** to the hippocampus. It appears likely that, in fact, the basal forebrain nucleus is the primary source of cholinergic input to the cerebral cortex. Cholinergic neurons, located in the brain stem tegmentum, project to the hypothalamus and thalamus where they use ACh as a transmitter.

Considerable interest has focused recently on the role of cholinergic CNS neurons in neurodegenerative diseases. Cholinergic neurons in the basal forebrain nucleus degenerate, and their cholinergic terminals in the cortex are lost as part of the pathology in Alzheimer's disease.

Glutamate

The amino acid glutamate has been identified as a major excitatory transmitter in the mammalian brain and spinal cord. Four types of postsynaptic glutamate receptors have been identified. Three of these are **ionotrophic** and are linked to ion channels (these receptors are named for drugs that bind specifically to them). The **kainate** and **AMPA** types of glutamate receptor are linked to Na^+ channels, and when glutamate binds to these receptors produce EPSPs. The **NMDA** receptor is linked to a channel that is permeable to both Ca^{2+} and Na^+. The NMDA-activated channel, however, is blocked (so that influx of these ions cannot occur) unless the postsynaptic membrane is depolarized. Thus, NMDA-type synapses mediate Ca^{2+} influx, but only when activity at these synapses is paired with excitation via other synaptic inputs that depolarize the postsynaptic neuron. The Ca^{2+} influx mediated by these synapses may lead to structural changes that strengthen the synapse. NMDA-type glutamate synapses appear to be designed to detect coincident activity in two different neural pathways and, in response to such paired activity, alter the strength of the synaptic connection; it has been hypothesized that this may provide a basis for memory.

A **metabotropic** type of glutamate receptor has also been identified. When the transmitter glutamate binds to this receptor, there is liberation of the second messengers, IP_3 and DAG. This can lead to increased levels of intracellular Ca^{2+}, which may activate a spectrum of enzymes that alter neuronal function and structure.

It has been suggested that excessive activation of glutamatergic synapses can lead to very large influxes of Ca^{2+} into neurons, which can cause neuronal cell death. Because glutamate is an excitatory transmitter, excessive glutamate release might lead to further excitation of neuronal circuits by positive feedback, resulting in a damaging avalanche of depolarization and calcium influx into neurons. This **excitotoxic** mechanism of neuronal injury may be important in acute neurologic disorders such as stroke and CNS trauma and possibly in some chronic neurodegenerative diseases, such as Alzheimer's.

Catecholamines

The catecholamines **norepinephrine** (noradrenaline), **epinephrine** (adrenaline), and **dopamine** are formed by hydroxylation and decarboxylation of the essential amino acid, phenylalanine. Phenylethanolamine-N-methyl-transferase, the enzyme responsible for converting norepinephrine to epinephrine, is found in high concentration primarily in the adrenal medulla. Epinephrine is found at only a few sites in the CNS.

Dopamine is synthesized, via the intermediate molecule DOPA, from the amino acid tyrosine by tyrosine hydroxylase and DOPA decarboxylase. Norepinephrine, in turn, is produced via hydroxylation of dopamine. Dopamine, like norepinephrine, is inactivated by monoamine oxidase (MAO) and catechol-O-methyltransferase (COMT). The biochemical events that occur in cholinergic and noradrenergic junctions are summarized in Figure 3–12.

Dopamine

Dopaminergic neurons generally have an inhibitory effect. Dopamine-producing neurons project from the **substantia nigra** to the caudate nucleus and putamen (via the **nigrostriatal system**) and from the **ventral tegmental area** to the limbic system and cortex (via the **mesolimbic** and **mesocortical** projections). In **Parkinson's disease,** there is degeneration of the dopaminergic neurons and the substantia nigra. Thus, dopaminergic projections from the substantia nigra to the caudate nucleus and putamen are damaged, and there is impaired inhibition of neurons in caudate nucleus and putamen. The dopaminergic projection from the ventral tegmental area to the limbic system and cortex may be involved in schizophrenia; antipsychotic drugs such as phenothiazines act as dopamine receptor antagonists and can temporarily reduce psychotic behavior in some schizophrenic patients.

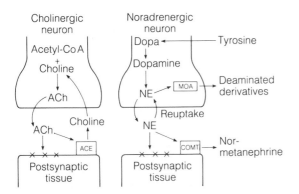

Figure 3–12. Comparison of the biochemical events at cholinergic endings with those at noradrenergic endings. ACh, acetylcholine; ACE, acetylcholinesterase; NE, norepinephrine; X, receptor. Because monoamine oxidase (MAO) is intracellular, some norepinephrine is constantly being deaminated in noradrenergic endings. Catechol-O-methyltransferase (COMT) acts on norepinephrine after it is secreted. (Reproduced, with permission, from Ganong WF: *Review of Medical Physiology,* 14th ed. Appleton & Lange, 1989.)

Dopamine-containing neurons have also been found in the **retina** and the **olfactory system** where they appear to mediate inhibition that filters sensory input.

Norepinephrine

Norepinephrine-containing neurons in the PNS are located in the **sympathetic ganglia** and project to all of the postganglionic sympathetic neurons except those innervating sweat glands, which are innervated by axons that use ACh as a transmitter. Norepinephrine-containing cell bodies in the CNS are located in two areas: the **locus ceruleus** and the **lateral tegmental nuclei.** Although the locus ceruleus is a relatively small nucleus containing only several hundred neurons, it projects widely into the cortex, hippocampus, thalamus, midbrain, cerebellum, pons, medulla, and spinal cord. The noradrenergic projections from these cells branch extensively and are distributed widely. Some of the axons branch and project to both the cerebral cortex and cerebellum. Noradrenergic neurons in the lateral tegmental areas of the brain stem appear to have a complementary projection, projecting axons to regions of the CNS that are not innervated by the locus ceruleus.

The noradrenergic projections from the locus ceruleus and the lateral tegmental area appear to play a modulatory role in the sleep-wake cycle and in cortical activation and may also regulate sensitivity of sensory neurons.

Serotonin

Serotonin (5-hydroxytryptamine) is an important regulatory amine in the CNS. Serotonin-containing neurons are present in the **raphe nuclei** in the pons and medulla. These cells are part of the **reticular formation,** and they project widely to the cortex and hippocampus, basal ganglia, thalamus, cerebellum, and spinal cord. Serotonin-containing neurons can also be found in the mammalian gastrointestinal tract, and serotonin is present in blood platelets.

Serotonin is synthesized from the amino acid tryptophan. It has vasoconstrictor and pressor effects. Some drugs, eg, reserpine, may act by releasing bound serotonin within the brain. In small doses, lysergic acid diethylamide (LSD), a structural analog of serotonin, is capable of evoking mental symptoms similar to those of schizophrenia. The vasoconstrictive action of LSD is inhibited by serotonin.

Serotonin-containing neurons, along with norepinephrine-containing neurons, appear to play an important role in determining the level of arousal. Firing levels of neurons in the raphe nuclei, for example, are correlated with sleep level and show a striking cessation of activity during rapid eye movement (REM) sleep. Lesions of the serotonin-containing neurons in the raphe nuclei can produce insomnia in experimental animals.

Serotonin-containing neurons may also participate in the modulation of sensory input, particularly for pain.

Gamma-aminobutyric Acid

Gamma-aminobutyric acid (GABA) is present in relatively large amounts in the gray matter of the brain and spinal cord. It is an inhibitory substance and probably the mediator responsible for presynaptic inhibition. GABA and glutamic acid decarboxylase (GAD), the enzyme that forms GABA from L-glutamic acid, occur in the CNS and the retina. Two forms of GABA receptor, $GABA_A$ and $GABA_B$ have been identified. Both mediate inhibition, but by different ionic pathways (see Table 3–6). GABA-containing inhibitory interneurons are present in the cerebral cortex, cerebellum, and in many nuclei throughout the brain and spinal cord. The drug **baclofen** acts as an agonist at $GABA_B$ receptors; its inhibitory actions may contribute to its efficacy as an antispasticity agent.

Endorphins

This general term refers to some endogenous morphine-like substances whose activity has been defined by their ability to bind to opiate receptors in the brain. Endorphins (brain polypeptides with actions like opiates) may function as synaptic transmitters or modulators. When injected into animals, endorphins can be analgesic and tranquilizing.

Enkephalins

Two closely related polypeptides (pentapeptides) found in the brain that also bind to opiate receptors are **methionine enkephalin (met-enkephalin)** and **leucine enkephalin (leu-enkephalin).** The amino acid sequence of met-enkephalin has been found in alpha-endorphin and beta-endorphin, and that of beta-endorphin has been found in beta-lipotropin, a polypeptide secreted by the anterior pituitary gland.

Histamine

Histamine in large amounts has been found in the pituitary gland and the adjacent median eminence of the hypothalamus, as well as in mast cells in the blood. In injured tissues, damaged cells release histamine, increasing capillary permeability. Histamine is, therefore, probably responsible for some swelling in certain areas of inflammation.

Substance P

This polypeptide, formed by 11 amino acids, is found in the hypothalamus, substantia nigra, and dorsal roots of the spinal nerves. There is evidence that substance P is a transmitter in primary sensory afferent neurons ending in the dorsal horn of the spinal cord where it can mediate long-lasting excitation. Pain fibers, in particular, appear to utilize substance P as a neurotransmitter.

Other Peptides

Peptides such as cholecystokinin and vasoactive intestinal polypeptide, which were first known as intestinal hormones, have been found in the brain. In some cases, it appears that a peptide may occur together with a classic transmitter in the same neuron. About 30 small peptides have been found in neurons in the mammalian central nervous system.

Clinical Correlations

Myasthenia gravis and the myasthenic syndrome: Mysasthenia gravis is an autoimmune disorder in which antibodies against the acetylcholine receptor, ie, the postsynaptic receptor at the neuromuscular junction, are produced. As a result of this, the responsiveness of muscle to activity in motor nerves and to synaptic activation is reduced. Patients classically complain of fatigue and weakness that involve the limb muscles and, in some patients, bulbar muscles such as those controlling eye movement and swallowing. Upon repetitive electrical stimulation, the involved muscles rapidly show fatigue and finally do not respond at all; excitability usually returns after a rest period.

The **myasthenic syndrome** (also called the **Eaton-Lambert syndrome**), in contrast, is a disorder involving the presynaptic component of the neuromuscular junction. The myasthenic syndrome is a paraneoplastic disorder and often occurs in the context of systemic neoplasms, especially those involving the lung and breast. Antibodies directed against Ca^{2+} channels located in presynaptic terminals at the neuromuscular junction interfere with transmitter release causing weakness.

B. Myotonia: In this class of disorders, affected muscles show a prolonged response to a single stimulus. Some of these disorders involve an abnormality of voltage-sensitive Na^+ channels, which fail to close following an action potential. As a result of this, inappropriate, sustained muscle contraction may occur.

CASE 1

Six months before presentation, a 35-year-old unmarried woman began to complain that she occasionally saw double when watching television. The double vision often disappeared after she had some bed rest. Subsequently, she felt that her eyelids tended to droop during reading, but after a good night's rest she felt normal again. Her physician referred her to a specialty clinic.

At the clinic, the woman said she tired easily and her jaw muscles became fatigued at the end of the meal. No sensory deficits were found. A preliminary diag-

nosis was made and some tests were performed to confirm the diagnosis.

What is the differential diagnosis? Which diagnostic procedures, if any, would be useful? What is the most likely diagnosis?

Cases are discussed further in Chapter 25. Questions and answers pertaining to Section I (Chapters 1–3) can be found in Appendix D.

REFERENCES

Cooper JR, Bloom FE, Roth RH: *The Biochemical Basis of Neuropharmacology,* 6th ed. Oxford, 1991.

DeCamilli P, John R: Pathways to regulated exocytosis in neurons. *Ann Rev Physio* 1990;**52:**624.

Ganong WF: *Review of Medical Physiology,* 15th ed. Appleton & Lange, 1991.

Hille B: *Ionic Channels of Excitable Membranes,* 2nd ed. Sinauer, 1991.

Kandel ER, Schwartz JH: Molecular biology of learning: Modulation of transmitter release. *Science* 1982;**218:**433.

Kandel ER, Schwartz JN, Jessell TM: *Principles of Neural Science*, 3rd Ed. Elsevier, 1991.

Levitan IB, Kaczmarek LK: *The Neuron: Cell and Molecular Biology.* Oxford, 1991.

Llinás R: The intrinsic electrophysiological properties of mammalian neurons: Insights into central nervous system function. *Science* 1988;**242:**1654.

Madison DV, Malenka RC, Nicoll RA: Mechanisms underlying long-term potentiation of synaptic transmission. *Ann Rev Neurosci* 1991;**14:**379.

Shepherd GM: *The Synaptic Organization of the Brain,* 3rd ed. Oxford, 1990.

Waxman SG, Ritchie JM: Molecular dissection of the myelinated axon. *Ann Neurol* 1993;**33:**121.

Introduction to Clinical Thinking: The Relationship Between Neuroanatomy and Neurology

4

Neurology, more than any other specialty, rests on clinico-anatomic correlation. The neurologic clinician attempts, in each patient, to answer two questions: (1) **Where** is (are) the lesion(s)? and (2) **What** is (are) the lesion(s)?

The term **lesion** refers to a zone of localized dysfunction within the CNS or PNS. Lesions can be **anatomic**, with dysfunction resulting from structural damage (examples are provided by stroke, trauma, and brain tumors). Lesions also can be **physiologic,** reflecting physiologic dysfunction in the absence of demonstrable anatomic abnormalities (an example is provided by transient ischemic attacks (TIAs) where there is temporary and reversible loss of function of part of the brain without structural damage to neurons or glial cells, as a result of metabolic changes due to vascular insufficiency).

The answers to the previously mentioned questions permit the clinician to define the disease process in a given patient, thus leading to a **diagnosis.** This sequence of events is crucial for the development of an appropriate **treatment plan.** The diagnosis also suggests the patient's **prognosis.** In addition, by arriving at a correct diagnosis and following the patient, the clinician begins to understand the **natural history** of neurologic disease, both in each single patient and in the population, and can begin to understand the **pathophysiology** of the disorder as well as assess the **efficacy** of various treatments.

This chapter gives a brief overview of clinical thinking in neurology, and emphasizes the relationship between neuroanatomy and neurology. It is not meant as a comprehensive or even introductory primer in neurology (a number of excellent neurology texts are available and are listed in the references at the end of this chapter). On the contrary, it has been included to help the reader to begin to think as the clinician does, and thus, to place neuroanatomy, as outlined in the subsequent chapters, in a patient-oriented framework. Together with the Clinical Illustrations and Cases placed throughout this book, the information in this chapter provides a clinical perspective of neuroanatomy.

SYMPTOMS AND SIGNS OF NEUROLOGIC DISEASES

Neurologic diagnosis depends on a careful **history** obtained from the patient, his family, and colleagues and on the **neurologic examination,** which tests the function of each part of the nervous system. The information obtained is synthesized using a knowledge of the relevant neuroanatomy to arrive at a provisional diagnosis. This diagnosis may be confirmed or refined via a variety of **laboratory tests** and **neuroimaging.**

In taking a history and examining the patient, the neurologic clinician elicits both **symptoms** and **signs**. Symptoms are subjective sensations resulting from the disorder (ie, "I have a headache"; "The vision in my right eye became blurry for two or three days a month ago"). Signs are objective abnormalities detected on examination or via laboratory tests (eg, a hyperactive reflex or abnormal eye movements).

The clinician usually obtains a history first. The history may provide crucial information about diagnosis. For example, a patient was admitted to the hospital in a coma. His wife told the admitting physician: "My husband has high blood pressure, but doesn't like to take his medicine. This morning he complained of the worst headache in his life. Then he passed out." On the basis of this history and a brief (but careful) examination, the physician rapidly reached a tentative diagnosis of subarachnoid hemorrhage (bleeding from an aneurism, ie, a defect in a cerebral artery into the subarachnoid space). He confirmed this diagnostic impression with appropriate (but focused) laboratory tests and instituted appropriate therapy.

The astute clinical observer may be able to detect signs of neurologic disease by carefully observing the patients' spontaneous behavior as they walk into the room and tell their story; thus, for example, even prior to touching the patient, the clinician may observe the "festinating" (shuffling, small-stepped) gait of Parkinson's disease, hemiparesis (weakness of one side of the body) owing to a hemispheric lesion such as a stroke or a third nerve palsy suggesting an intracranial mass.

The **way** patients tell their story also may be informative, eg, it may reveal aphasia (difficulty with language), confusion, or impaired memory. A carefully taken history can provide very important information about the patient's illness and is essential. Details of history-taking and the neurologic examination are included in Appendix A.

In synthesizing the information obtained from the history and examination, the clinician usually keeps asking the questions, "Where is the lesion? What is the lesion?" Several points should be kept in mind while going through the diagnostic process.

Manifestations of Neurologic Disease May be Negative or Positive

Negative manifestations result from **loss of function,** eg, hemiparesis, weakness of an eye muscle, impaired sensation, or loss of memory. Negative manifestations of neurologic disease may reflect damage to neurons (eg, in Parkinson's disease, where there is degeneration of neurons in the substantia nigra) or to glial cells or myelin (eg, in multiple sclerosis where there is inflammatory damage to myelin). **Positive** abnormalities result from inappropriate excitation. These include, for example, seizures (caused by abnormal cortical discharge) and spasticity (from the loss of inhibition of motor neurons). Another example is provided by Lhermitte's phenomenon, in which the patient experiences tingling paresthesias extending into the legs, triggered by flexion of the neck; this phenomenon is seen when there is pathology in or near the cervical spinal cord, and is a result of abnormal mechanosensitivity of sensory axons in the spinal cord.

Lesions of White and Gray Matter Cause Neurologic Dysfunction

Damage to **gray** or **white matter** (or both) interferes with normal neurologic function. Lesions in gray matter interfere with the function of neuronal cell bodies and synapses, thereby leading to negative or positive abnormalities as previously described. Lesions in white matter, on the other hand, interfere with axonal conduction and produce **disconnection syndromes**, which usually cause negative manifestations; examples of these syndromes include optic neuritis (demyelination of the optic nerve), which interferes with vision; and infarction affecting pyramidal tract axons, which descend from the motor cortex in regions such as the internal capsule, which can cause "pure motor stroke" (Fig 4–1).

Some neurologic disorders affect primarily gray matter (eg, amyotrophic lateral sclerosis, a degenerative disease leading to the death of motor neurons in the cerebral cortex and gray matter of the spinal cord). Others affect primarily white matter (eg, multiple scle-

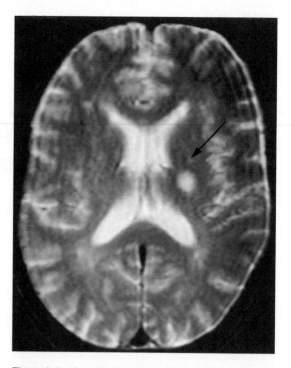

Figure 4–1. Magnetic resonance (MR) scan in a 51-year-old hypertensive accountant. The patient complained of weakness of the right side of the face and the right arm and leg, which had developed over a five-hour period. There was no sensory loss, and there were no problems with language or cognition. The MR scan revealed a small infarction in the internal capsule (arrow), which destroyed axons descending from the motor cortex, thus causing a "pure motor stroke" in this patient.

rosis). Still other disorders affect both gray and white matter, for instance large strokes, which lead to necrosis of the cerebral cortex and underlying white matter.

Neurologic Disease Can Result in Syndromes

A **syndrome** is a constellation of signs and symptoms frequently associated with each other and suggest a common origin. Recognition of a syndrome may point to a specific localization and can suggest a particular diagnosis. An example is **Wallenberg's syndrome,** which is characterized by vertigo, nausea, hoarseness, and dysphagia (difficulty swallowing). Other signs and symptoms include ipsilateral ataxia, ptosis, and meiosis, impairment of all sensory modalities over the ipsilateral face, and loss of pain and temperature sensitivity over the contralateral torso and limbs. This syndrome results from dysfunction of a group of clustered nuclei and tracts in the **lateral medulla** and is usually due to infarction resulting from occlusion of the posterior inferior cerebellar artery, which irrigates these neighboring structures.

Neighborhood Signs May Help to Localize the Lesion

The brain and spinal cord are highly complex structures and contain many tracts and nuclei that are intimately associated with each other. Particularly in the brain stem and spinal cord where there is not much room in the transverse plane, there is crowding of nuclei and fiber tracts. Many pathologic processes result in lesions that are larger than any single nucleus or tract. **Combinations of signs and symptoms** may help to localize the lesion. Figure 4–2 shows a section through the medulla of a patient with multiple sclerosis. The patient had a long-standing history of sensory loss in the legs (impaired touch-pressure sense and position sense) and also had weakness of the tongue. As an alternative to positing the presence of two separate lesions to account for these two abnormalities, the clinician should pose the question "Might a *single* lesion account for both abnormalities?" In this case, knowledge of brain stem neuroanatomy allowed the clinician to predict the presence of a lesion located in the medial part of the medulla, and this was confirmed at postmortem examination.

Dysfunction of the Nervous System Can be Due to Destruction or Compression of Neural Tissue, or Compromise of the Ventricles or Vasculature

Several types of structural pathology can lead to dysfunction of the nervous system (Table 4–1). **Destruction** of neurons (or associated glial cells) accounts for the clinical abnormalities in disorders such as stroke (where neurons are acutely injured as a result of vascular compromise which results in ischemia) and Parkinson's disease (where there is chronic degeneration of neurons in one particular region of the brain stem, the substantia nigra). Destruction of axons secondary to trauma causes much of the dysfunction in spinal cord injury, and destruction of myelin as a result of inflammatory processes leads to the abnormal function in multiple sclerosis.

Compression of the nervous system can also cause dysfunction, without the invasion of the brain and spinal cord *per se.* This occurs, for example, in subdural hematoma, when an expanding blood clot, contained by the skull vault, compresses the adjacent brain, initially causing reversible dysfunction, prior to triggering the death of neural tissue. Early recognition of this disorder and surgical drainage of the clot can lead to full recovery of function.

Finally, **compromise of ventricular pathways** or of the **vasculature** can lead to neurologic signs and symptoms. For example, a small cerebellar astrocytoma, critically located above the fourth ventricle, may compress the ventricle and obstruct the outflow of cerebrospinal fluid. Even if the tumor has not produced symptoms, it may lead to obstructive hydrocephalus with wide-spread destructive effects on both cerebral hemispheres. In this case, a small, critically placed mass produces wide-spread neural dysfunction as a result of its effect on the outflow tracts for cerebrospinal fluid. Critically placed vascular lesions can also produce devastating effects on the nervous system. For example, occlusion of the carotid artery, owing to atherosclerosis in the neck, can lead to infarction in the cerebral hemisphere, which it supplies.

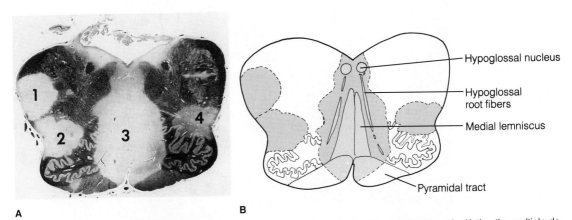

A   **B**

Figure 4–2. *A:* Section through the medulla, stained for myelin, from a patient with multiple sclerosis. Notice the multiple demyelinated plaques (labeled 1–4) that are disseminated throughout the CNS. ***B:*** Even a single lesion can interfere with function in multiple neighboring parts of the CNS. Notice that plaque 3 involves the hypoglossal root (producing weakness of the tongue) and the medial lemnisci (causing an impairment of vibratory and touch pressure sense). Figure 7–7B shows, for comparison, a diagram of the normal medulla at this level.

Table 4–1. Mechanisms leading to dysfunction in typical neurologic diseases.

Mechanism	Disease Example	Target	Comments
Destruction	Stroke	Neurons (often cortical)	Acute destruction, within hours of loss of blood flow
Destruction	Parkinson's disease	Neurons (subcortical)	Chronic degeneration of neurons in substantia nigra
Destruction	Spinal cord injury	Ascending and descending axons	Injury to fiber tracts due to trauma
Destruction	Multiple sclerosis	Myelin	Inflammatory damage to myelin sheaths in CNS
Compression	Subdural hematoma	Cerebral hemisphere	Expanding blood clot injures underlying brain tissue
Compromise of ventricular pathways	Cerebellar tumor	Fourth ventricle	Expanding mass compresses ventricle, impairs CSF outflow

WHERE IS THE LESION?

Processes Causing Neurologic Disease

Focal process: **Focal** pathology causes signs and symptoms on the basis of a single, geographically contiguous lesion. The most common example is stroke, which occurs when ischemia within the territory of a particular artery leads to infarction of neural tissue in a well-defined area (Fig 4–3). Another example is provided by solitary brain tumors. In thinking about the patient, the physician should ask, "Is there a *single* lesion that can account for the signs and symptoms?"

Multi-focal process: **Multi-focal** pathology results in damage to the nervous system at numerous, separate sites. In multiple sclerosis, for example, lesions are disseminated throughout the nervous system in the spatial domain, and they are also disseminated in time (ie, the lesions do not develop at once). Figure 4–2 shows the multi-focal nature of the pathology in a patient with multiple sclerosis. Another example is provided by leptomeningeal seeding of a tumor. As a result of dissemination throughout the subarachnoid space, tumor deposits can affect numerous spinal and cranial nerve roots that are distributed along the entire neuraxis and can also block CSF outflow, thereby producing hydrocephalus.

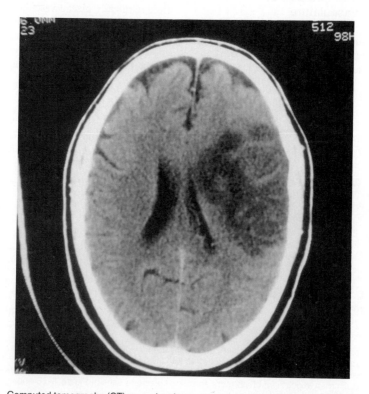

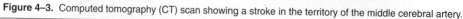

Figure 4–3. Computed tomography (CT) scan showing a stroke in the territory of the middle cerebral artery.

Diffuse process: Diffuse dysfunction of the nervous system can be produced by a number of toxins and metabolic abnormalities. In arriving at a diagnosis, the clinician must ask, "Is there a **systemic** disorder that can account for the patient's signs and symptoms?" Metabolic or toxic coma, for instance, can result in abnormal function of neurons throughout the nervous system.

Rostro-Caudal Localization

In determining the rostro-caudal localization of the lesion, it is important to determine the nuclei and fiber tracts that are affected, and to consider the *constellation* of structures that is involved. Each of the major motor (descending) and sensory (ascending) pathways decussates (ie, crosses from one side of the neuraxis to the other) at a specific level. The levels of decussation of three major pathways are briefly summarized in Figure 4–4 and are discussed in Chapter 5. By examining the constellation of deficits in a given patient, and relating them to appropriate tracts and nuclei, it is often possible to place the lesion at the appropriate level along the rostro-caudal axis.

For example, consider a patient with weakness of the left leg. This could be caused by a lesion involving the nerves innervating the leg or by a lesion affecting the corticospinal pathway at any level from the cortex, through the midbrain, and down to the lumbar spinal cord. If the patient also had loss of vibratory and position sense of the left leg (indicating dysfunction in the dorsal column pathway) and loss of pain and temperature sensation over the *right* leg (indicating impaired function of the spinothalamic pathway), the clinician would then think about dysfunction of the left half of the spinal cord, above the decussation of the spinothalamic fibers (which decussate within the spinal cord, close to the level where they enter the cord) but *below* the medullary-cervical spinal cord junction where the corticospinal tract decussates. Furthermore, if function in the arms and trunk were normal, this would suggest normal function in cervical and thoracic parts of the spinal cord (which carry fibers for the arm and trunk). The combination of deficits could, in fact, be parsimoniously explained by a *single* lesion, located in the left side of the spinal cord.

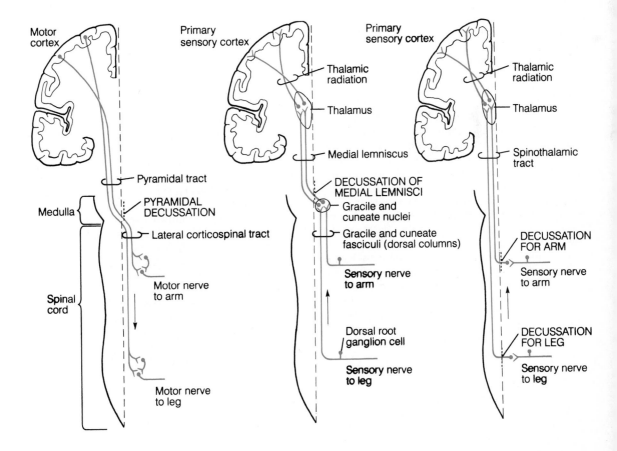

Figure 4–4. *A:* Pyramidal tract. *B:* Dorsal column system. *C:* Spinothalamic system.

Transverse Localization

In localizing the lesion, the clinician must also consider its placement in the transverse plane, ie, within the cross section of the brain or spinal cord. Here again, neighborhood signs are important. In the previously described patient with a spinal cord lesion, the dorsal and lateral white matter columns in the spinal cord must be involved because the dorsal column pathway and corticospinal tract are involved. Moreover, the clinician can predict that the lesion is centered in the left half of the spinal cord because there is no evidence of dysfunction of the corticospinal tract, dorsal column system, or spinothalamic tract on the right in this patient.

By carefully considering the tracts and nuclei involved and their relationships along the rostro-caudal axis and in the transverse plane, it is often possible to identify, with a high degree of probability, the site(s) of the nervous system that are involved in a given patient.

WHAT IS THE LESION?

In considering the pathologic nature of a lesion, the neurologic clinician utilizes information derived from both the examination and the history. The **age** of the patient must be considered. Cerebrovascular disease, for example, is more common in individuals over the age of 50; in contrast, multiple sclerosis is a disease of the second and third decades and rarely presents in elderly individuals.

The **gender** of the patient may provide important information. **Duchenne's muscular dystrophy,** for instance, is a sex-linked disorder and occurs only in males. Carcinoma of the prostate (a male disease) and of the breast (predominantly a female disease) commonly metastasize to the vertebral column, and these metastases can cause spinal cord compression.

The **general medical context** also provides an important cortex: Is the patient a smoker? Has the patient lost weight? Lung and breast tumors, for example, commonly metastasize to the nervous system. The development of hemiparesis in an otherwise healthy, non-smoking 75-year-old is most likely the result of cerebrovascular disease. In a smoker with a lesion on chest X-ray, on the other hand, hemiparesis may result from a metastasis in the brain. The neurologic examination and history *must* be interpreted in the context of a patient's general medical status.

Time-Course of the Illness

The **time-course** of the illness may provide invaluable information about its nature. Brief episodes of dysfunction lasting minutes to hours, occurring throughout the life of the patient, may represent seizures or migraine attacks (Fig 4–5). A **recent-onset**

cluster of brief episodes or a **crescendo pattern** of neurologic dysfunction, on the other hand, may represent nonstable evolving disease. For example, **transient ischemic attacks** (brief episodes of neurologic dysfunction followed by full recovery, resulting from reversible ischemia) are the harbingers of stroke in some patients. A pattern of recent-onset headaches on wakening, increasing in intensity, may be caused by the presence of an expanding brain tumor (Fig 4–5B). A **relapsing-remitting** course, in which the patient experiences bouts of dysfunction lasting days to weeks followed by functional recovery, is characteristic of multiple sclerosis (Fig 4–5C). **Sudden onset** of a fixed deficit is characteristic of cerebrovascular disease, which includes ischemic stroke and intracerebral hemorrhage (Fig 4–5D). **Slowly progressive dysfunction** evolves over years and is suggestive of neurodegenerative diseases such as Alzheimer's and Parkinson's (Fig 4–5E). **Subacutely progressive dysfunction,** which advances over weeks to months, is often seen with brain tumors (Fig 4–5F). Although the time and course of the illness does not permit a definitive diagnosis, it can provide helpful information.

THE ROLE OF NEURO-IMAGING AND LABORATORY INVESTIGATIONS

A careful synthesis of the clinical data permits the clinician to arrive, with a high degree of accuracy, at a differential diagnosis (ie, a list of diagnostic possibilities that fit, in a positive way, with the patient's clinical picture). Armed with a good working knowledge of correlative neuroanatomy, the clinician should not have to blindly "rule out" a multitude of diseases. On the contrary, by focusing on the questions "Where is the lesion?" and "What is the lesion?", it is usually possible to identify a limited field of diagnostic choices that have a high probability of explaining the patient's clinical picture. This field of possibilities can be further delimited, and the diagnosis refined, by the use of neuro-imaging methods. Recent progress in neuro-imaging has provided a number of important new diagnostic techniques that permit rapid, precise, and in many cases, noninvasive visualization of the brain, spinal cord, and surrounding structures such as the skull and vertebral column.

Neuro-imaging investigations include plain x-rays, dye-studies, such as angiography (to visualize cerebral vessels), myelography, which fills and outlines the subarachnoid space surrounding the spinal cord, CT scanning, and MRI scans. Neuro-imaging can provide invaluable information in terms of confirming the location of a lesion within the CSN. In addition, neuro-imaging studies can help define the size of the lesion and sometimes provide information about the nature of the lesion. For example, some brain tumors can be dif-

Time ⟶

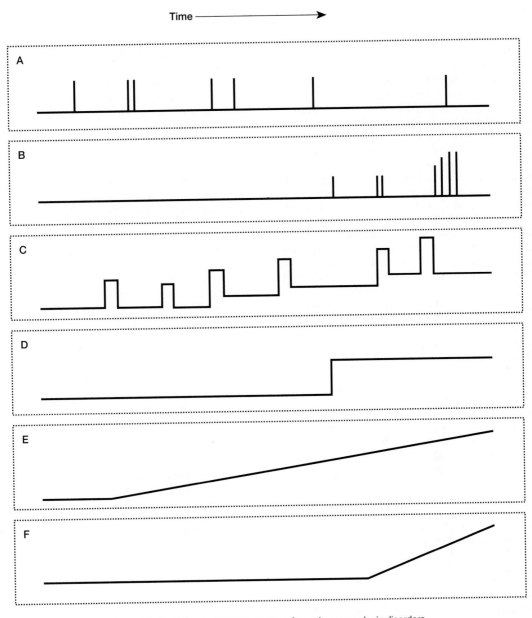

Figure 4–5. Characteristic time-courses for various neurologic disorders.

ferentiated from cerebral abscesses on the basis of their radiographic appearance.

In obtaining neuro-imaging studies, the radiologist is usually guided by clinical information. This helps in choosing the most appropriate imaging procedure and to "target" the imaging studies on the right part of the nervous system.

While neuro-imaging procedures represent an extremely powerful set of tools, they do not always, in themselves, provide the correct diagnosis. The results of neuro-imaging studies must be interpreted in the light of history and clinical examination and interpreted in terms of neuroanatomy. Examples are provided by Clinical Illustrations 4–1 and 4–2.

CLINICAL ILLUSTRATION 4–1

A 52-year-old accountant weighing 320 pounds saw his physician with the complaints of back pain and weakness in his legs. A neurologic consultant found moderate weakness in both legs associated with hyperactive reflexes, Babinski reflexes, and sensory loss below the umbilicus. There was focal tenderness over the spine at the T5 level.

The weakness of the legs, associated with signs of upper-motor-neuron dysfunction (hyperactive reflexes and Babinski responses), suggested the possibility of a lesion affecting the spinal cord and the sensory loss, which extended to the T10 level, indicated that the lesion was located above this level. Because of the patient's focal back pain, the neurologist suspected that there was a mass compressing the spinal cord, close to the T5 level of the spinal column. Because the patient would not fit in the MR scanner at the hospital, he was sent to another clinic, 60 miles away, where an older MR scanner had a wider bore that would accommodate him. The neurologist's report, outlining his findings and requesting an MR scan of the entire spine including thoracic regions, was lost in transit. The radiologist, who had not examined the patient, noted his history of leg weakness and obtained MR scans of the lumbar spinal cord. No lesion was seen.

Despite the report of a "normal" MR scan, the neurologist reasoned there was a lesion, compressing the spinal cord in the midthoracic region. He ordered a myelogram that revealed a meningioma at the T4 level. Following surgery, the patient's strength improved.

This case illustrates several points. First, a careful history and examination, together with knowledge of neuroanatomy, provides crucial information that will guide the neuroradiologist so the proper regions of the nervous system will be examined. In this case, the neurologist's guidance might have focused the radiologist's attention on the appropriate part of the spinal column. Second, clinical intuition can be as good as, or in some cases better than, imaging. "Normal" radiologic results most commonly reflect normal anatomy, but can also result from technical difficulties, improper patient positioning, or imaging methodology. In situations where imaging results are not consistent with the history and examination, a repeat examination, together with a re-examination of the questions, "Where is the lesion? What is the lesion?" can be helpful.

CLINICAL ILLUSTRATION 4–2

A 45-year-old Latin teacher was evaluated by her family doctor after she complained of pain in her left arm. Because of weakness, he suspected a herniated intervertebral disk and ordered cervical spine x-rays that revealed an intervertebral disk protrusion at the C6–7 level, which was confirmed by CT scans. The pain progressed over several weeks, and surgery (excision of the protruded disk) was considered.

As part of her workup, the patient was seen by a neurologist. Careful examination revealed sensory loss in the distribution of the C6, C7, and C8 dermatomes. There was a pattern of weakness that did not conform to any single nerve root, but rather suggested involvement of the lower brachial plexus. Chest x-ray demonstrated a small-cell carcinoma located in the apex of the lung, which had invaded the brachial plexus. The patient was immediately referred for chemotherapy.

This case illustrates that radiographic studies can, in some patients, reveal structural abnormalities that are not relevant to the patient's disease. In this case, the patient's herniated cervical disk had not caused symptoms. The family physician had not appreciated all of these findings and could not correlate the full clinical picture with the radiographic images. Therefore, he ascribed the patient's pain to the wrong lesion (the asymptomatic herniated intervertebral disk), and was lulled into a sense of false security so that he missed the relevant pathology, ie—the patient's tumor.

A more complete examination coupled with the question "Where is the lesion?", would have led to the conclusion that the brachial plexus was involved. Once this localization was appreciated, the radiologist obtained apical views of the lungs, to examine the possibility of a tumor that had spread to the brachial plexus. As illustrated by this case, abnormal neuro-imaging studies do not necessarily lead to a definitive diagnosis. A careful examination of the patient with appropriate emphasis on neuroanatomy must be correlated with the neuro-imaging studies.

A number of other laboratory tests can provide additional information about the patient's illness. The **lumbar puncture** or **spinal tap,** for instance, provides cerebrospinal fluid (CSF). Analysis of the CSF (measurement of its protein, glucose, and immunoglobulin content and its cell count) can provide a definitive diagnosis of infections (such as bacterial meningitis) and can help to confirm the diagnosis in disorders such as multiple sclerosis and brain tumor.

A variety of **electrophysiologic tests** permit the measurement of electrical activity from the brain, spinal cord, and peripheral nerves and can provide important information. These tests include the **electroencephalogram (EEG), evoked potentials, electromyography (EMG),** and **nerve conduction studies.** Like CSF analysis, the results of electrophysiologic studies should be interpreted in the context of the history and physical examination. These tests are discussed further in Chapter 24.

THE TREATMENT OF PATIENTS WITH NEUROLOGIC DISEASE

In collecting a history, performing an examination, and implementing treatment, the clinician is interacting not only as doctor to patient, but as care-giver to another human being. It is essential to remember this, and to keep in mind the important role that sensitivity and caring can have. The effective clinician can play a crucial role in helping the patient cope with neurologic disease. Listening is very important. Neurological clinicians do not just treat cases or diseases; they treat patients. An example is provided in Clinical Illustration 4–3.

CLINICAL ILLUSTRATION 4–3

A neurologic consultant was asked to evaluate a patient who was known to have a malignant melanoma. The patient had been in the hospital for 10 days and the nursing staff noticed that he did not dress himself properly, tended to get lost while walking on the ward, and bumped into things.

Although the patient had no complaints, his wife recalled that, beginning several months earlier, he had developed difficulty putting on his clothes properly. He had been fired after working for 30 years as a truck driver because he had developed difficulty reading a map.

Careful examination revealed a hemi-inattention syndrome. The patient tended to neglect the left half of the world. When asked to draw a clock, he squeezed all of the numbers in the right-hand half. He drew only the right half of a flower, and tended to eat only off the right half of his plate. When asked to put on his hospital robe, he wrapped it around his waist, but was unable to properly put it on. Careful examination of the motor system revealed that, in addition, the patient had a mild left hemiparesis.

"Hemi-inattention" syndrome usually occurs as a result of lesions in the nondominant (right) cerebral hemisphere, most commonly the parietal lobe. Lesions in this area can also cause difficulty dressing ("dressing apraxia"). The presence of a hemi-inattention syndrome and dressing apraxia, together with a mild left hemiparesis, strongly suggested the presence of a lesion in the right cerebral hemisphere, most likely in the right parietal lobe, and the history suggested metastatic melanoma. Subsequent imaging confirmed the diagnosis.

Following the examination, the neurologic consultant asked the patient and his wife whether they had any questions. His wife replied, "We know that my husband has metastatic cancer and that he will die. He has been in the hospital for 10 days, but nobody has explained what will happen. Will my husband have pain? Will he need to be sedated? Will he be able to make out a will? As he gets worse, will he be able to recognize the children?"

In this instance, the patient's physician had correctly diagnosed and managed the primary melanoma. However, he did not have a strong knowledge of neuroanatomy, and during the neurologic examination he had failed to recognize the presence of metastasis in the brain. Equally important, the treating physician had focused his attention on the patient's *disease,* and not met his needs as a *person.* An open, relaxed discussion ("How do you feel about your disease? What frightens you the most? Do you have any questions?") is an essential part of the physician's role.

REFERENCES

Adams RE, Victor M: *Principles of Neurology,* 5th Edition. McGraw-Hill, 1993.

Bradley WG, Daroff RB, Fenichel GM, Marsden CD: *Neurology In Clinical Practice.* Butterworth-Heinemann, 1991.

Brazis PW, Masdeu JC, Biller J: *Localization in Clinical Neurology.* Little Brown and Co., 1990.

Greenberg DA, Aminoff MF, Simon RP: *Clinical Neurology.* Appleton & Lange, 1993.

Haymaker W: *Bing's Local Diagnosis in Neurological Disease.* 15th Edition. Moss B. 1969.

Menkes JH: *Textbook of Child Neurology.* 3rd Edition. Lea & Febiger, 1985.

Plum F, Posner JB: *The Diagnosis of Stupor and Coma.* 3rd Edition. FA Davis, 1980.

Rowland LP: *Merritt's Textbook of Neurology.* 8th Edition. Lea & Febiger, 1989.

Section III.
Spinal Cord & Spine

The Spinal Cord

5

DEVELOPMENT OF THE SPINAL CORD

Differentiation

At about the third week of prenatal development, the ectoderm of the embryonic disk forms the **neural plate,** which folds at the edges into the **neural tube (neuraxis).** A group of cells migrates to form the **neural crest,** which gives rise to dorsal and autonomic ganglia, the adrenal medulla, and other structures (Fig 5–1). The middle portion of the neural tube closes first; the openings at each end close later.

The cells in the wall of the neural tube divide and differentiate, forming an ependymal layer that encircles the central canal and is surrounded by intermediate (mantle) and marginal zones of primitive neurons and glial cells (Figs 5–1 and 5–2). The mantle zone differentiates into two regions: an **alar plate** that contains mostly sensory neurons and a **basal plate** that is mostly motor neurons. These two regions are demarcated by the **sulcus limitans,** a groove on the wall of the central canal. The alar plate differentiates into a dorsal gray column; the basal plate becomes a ventral gray column. The processes of the mantle zone and other cells are contained in the marginal zone, which becomes the white matter of the spinal cord (Fig 5–2).

An investing layer of ectodermal cells around the primitive cord forms the two inner meninges: the arachnoid and pia mater (pia) (Fig 5–2). The thicker outer investment, the dura mater (dura), is formed from mesenchyma.

Clinical Correlations

Failure of the neural tube to close at the cranial end results in **anencephaly,** a type of maldevelopment of the brain and skull that is incompatible with life. Failure of closure at the caudal end results in **spina bifida,** which is associated with maldevelopment of the vertebrae (see Fig 6–9).

Sometimes the meninges balloon out to form a sac, or **meningocele,** associated with a defect in the over-lying vertebra. If such a sac contains nervous tissue, it is a **myelomeningocele** and is associated with severe disturbances of function.

EXTERNAL ANATOMY OF THE SPINAL CORD

The spinal cord is an elongated, cylindrical mass of nerve tissue occupying the upper two-thirds of the adult spinal canal within the vertebral column (Fig 5–3). The cord is normally 42–45 cm long in adults and is continuous with the brain stem at its upper end. The **conus medullaris** is the conical distal (inferior) end of the spinal cord; the **filum terminale** extends from the tip of the conus and attaches to the distal dural sac. The filum terminale consists of pia and glial fibers and often contains a vein.

The **central canal** extends the length of the spinal cord during development. It is lined with ependymal cells and filled with cerebrospinal fluid (CSF). It opens upward into the inferior portion of the fourth ventricle in the lower brain stem. In adults, the canal usually disappears except at cervical levels; nests of ependymal cells are found elsewhere in the cord.

Enlargements

The spinal cord widens laterally in two regions: the **cervical enlargement** and the **lumbar enlargement** (Fig 5–3). The latter tapers off to form the conus medullaris. The enlargements of the cord correspond to the origins of the nerves of the upper and lower extremities. The nerves of the brachial plexus originate at the cervical enlargement; the nerves of the lumbosacral plexus arise from the lumbar enlargement.

Segments

The spinal cord is divided into approximately 30 segments (see Fig 5–3 and Appendix C)—8 **cervical** (C) segments, 12 **thoracic** (T) segments (termed dor-

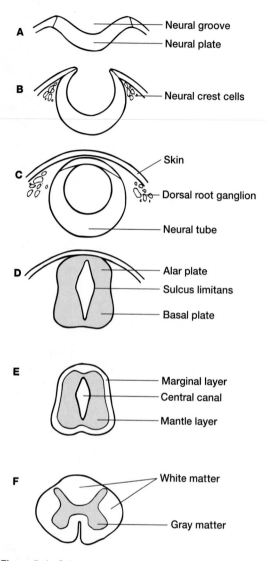

Figure 5–1. Schematic cross sections showing the development of the spinal cord.

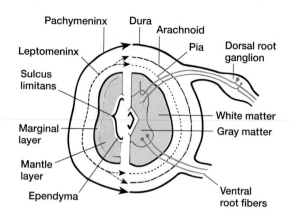

Figure 5–2. Cross section showing two phases in the development of the spinal cord (each half shows one phase). *A:* Early phase. *B:* Later phase with central cavity.

sal in some texts), 5 **lumbar** (L) segments, 5 **sacral** (S) segments, and a few small **coccygeal** (Co) segments—that correspond to attachments of groups of nerve roots (Figs 5–3 and 5–5). Individual segments vary in length; they are about twice as long in the midthoracic region as in the cervical or upper lumbar area. There are no sharp boundaries between segments within the cord itself.

Longitudinal Divisions

A cross section of the spinal cord shows a deep anterior **median fissure** and a shallow **posterior (or dorsal) median sulcus,** which divide the cord into symmetric right and left halves that are joined in the central

midportion (Fig 5–4). The anterior median fissure contains a fold of pia and blood vessels; its floor is the **anterior (or ventral) white commissure** (a misnomer, because no fibers decussate here). The dorsal nerve roots are attached to the spinal cord along a shallow vertical groove, the **posterolateral sulcus,** which lies a short distance anterior to the posterior median sulcus. The ventral nerve roots exit in the **anterolateral sulcus.**

A note on terminology: In descriptions of the spinal cord, the terms *ventral* and *anterior* are used interchangeably. Similarly, *dorsal* and *posterior* have the same meaning.

SPINAL ROOTS & NERVES

Each segment of the spinal cord pertains to four roots: a ventral and a dorsal root of the left half, and a similar pair of the right half (Fig 5–4). The first cervical segment usually lacks dorsal roots.

Each of the 31 pairs of spinal nerves that arise from the spinal cord has a ventral root and a dorsal root; each root is made up of 1–8 rootlets (Fig 5–7). Each root consists of bundles of nerve fibers. In the dorsal root of a typical spinal nerve, close to the junction with the ventral root, lies a **dorsal root (spinal) ganglion,** a swelling that contains nerve cell bodies. The portion of a spinal nerve outside the vertebral column is sometimes referred to as a peripheral nerve. The spinal nerves are divided into groups that correspond to the spinal cord segments (Fig 5–5).

The **vertebral column** surrounds and protects the spinal cord and normally consists of 7 cervical, 12 thoracic, and 5 lumbar vertebra as well as the sacrum, which is usually formed by fusion of five vertebra, and the coccyx. The nerve roots exit from the vertebral column through **intervertebral foramina.** In the cervical spine, the numbered roots exit the vertebral column

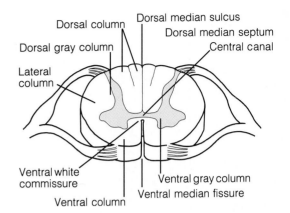

Figure 5–4. Anatomy of the spinal cord shown in cross section. Note that the terms "dorsal" and "posterior" are used interchangeably, and that "ventral" and "anterior" are also used interchangeably to describe the spinal cord.

above the corresponding vertebral body. The C8 root exits between vertebral bodies C7 and T1. In the lower parts of the spine, the numbered roots exit below the correspondingly numbered vertebral body. The anatomy of the vertebral column is discussed further in Chapter 6.

Direction of Roots

Until the third month of fetal life, the spinal cord is as long as the vertebral canal. After that point, the vertebral column elongates faster than the spinal cord, so that at birth the cord extends to about the level of the third lumbar vertebra. In adults, the tip of the cord normally lies at the level of the first or second lumbar vertebra. Because of the different growth rates of the cord and spine, the cord segments are displaced upward from their corresponding vertebrae, with the greatest discrepancy in the lowest cord segments (Fig 5–5). In the lumbosacral region, the nerve roots descend almost vertically below the cord to form the **cauda equina (horse's tail).**

Ventral Root

The ventral roots carry the large-diameter alpha motor neuron axons to the extrafusal striated muscle fibers; the smaller gamma motor neuron axons, which supply the intrafusal muscle of the muscle spindles (Fig 5–6); preganglionic autonomic fibers at the thoracic, upper lumbar, and midsacral levels (see Chapter 20); and a few afferent, small-diameter axons that arise from cells in the dorsal root ganglia and convey sensory information from the thoracic and abdominal viscera.

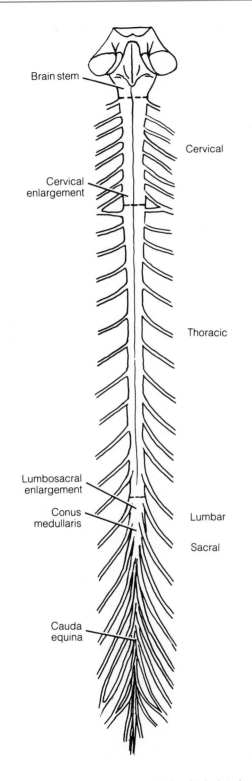

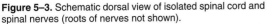

Figure 5–3. Schematic dorsal view of isolated spinal cord and spinal nerves (roots of nerves not shown).

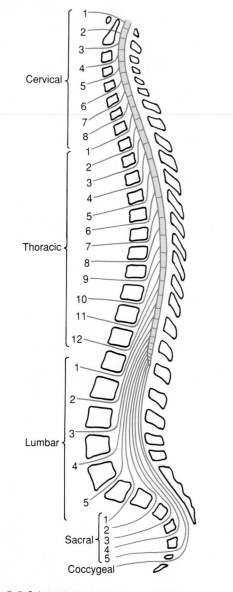

Cervical

Thoracic

Lumbar

Sacral

Coccygeal

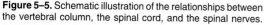

Figure 5–5. Schematic illustration of the relationships between the vertebral column, the spinal cord, and the spinal nerves.

Dorsal Root

Each dorsal nerve root (except usually C1) contains afferent fibers from the nerve cells in its ganglion. The dorsal roots contain a variety of fibers from cutaneous and deep structures (see Table 3–2). The largest fibers (Ia) come from muscle spindles and participate in spinal cord reflexes; the medium-sized fibers (A-beta) convey impulses from mechanoreceptors in skin and joints. Most of the axons in the dorsal nerve roots are small (C, nonmyelinated; A-delta, myelinated) and carry information of noxious (eg, pain) and thermal stimuli.

Branches of Typical Spinal Nerves

A. Posterior Primary Division: This usually consists of a medial branch, which is in most instances largely sensory, and a lateral branch, which is mainly motor.

B. Anterior Primary Division: Usually larger than the posterior primary division, the anterior primary divisions form the cervical, brachial, and lumbosacral plexuses. In the thoracic region they remain segmental, as intercostal nerves.

C. Rami Communicantes: The rami join the spinal nerves to the sympathetic trunk. Only the thoracic and upper lumbar nerves contain a white ramus communicans, but the gray ramus is present in all spinal nerves (Fig 5–7).

D. Meningeal or Recurrent Meningeal Branches: These nerves, also called **sinuvertebral nerves,** are quite small; they carry sensory and vasomotor innervation to the meninges.

Types of Nerve Fibers

Nerve fibers can be classified on a physioanatomic basis (Table 5–1):

A. Somatic Efferent Fibers: These motor fibers innervate the skeletal muscles. They originate in large cells in the anterior gray column of the spinal cord and form the ventral root of the spinal nerve.

B. Somatic Afferent Fibers: These fibers convey sensory information from the skin, joints, and muscles to the central nervous system. Their cell bodies are unipolar cells in the spinal ganglia that are interposed in the course of dorsal roots (dorsal root ganglia). The peripheral branches of these ganglionic cells are distributed to somatic structures; the central branches convey sensory impulses through the dorsal roots to the dorsal gray column and the ascending tracts of the spinal cord.

C. Visceral Efferent Fibers: The **autonomic fibers** are the motor fibers to the viscera. **Sympathetic fibers** from the thoracic segments and L1 and L2 are distributed throughout the body to the viscera, glands, and smooth muscle. **Parasympathetic fibers,** which are present in the middle three sacral nerves, go to the pelvic and lower abdominal viscera (other parasympathetic fibers are carried by cranial nerves III, VII, IX, and X).

D. Visceral Afferent Fibers: These fibers convey sensory information from the viscera. Their cell bodies are in the dorsal root ganglia. Experimental evidence suggests that some visceral afferent fibers enter the cord through the ventral roots.

Dermatomes

The sensory component of each spinal nerve is distributed to a dermatome, ie, a well-defined segmental portion of the skin. The pattern of cutaneous innerva-

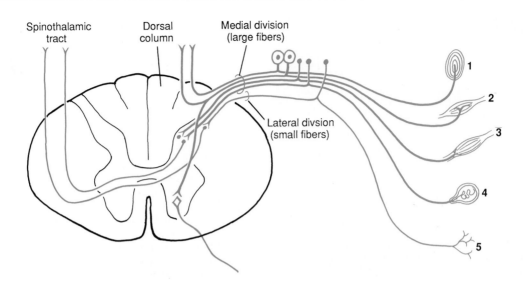

Figure 5–6. Schematic illustration of a cord segment with its dorsal root, ganglion cells, and sensory organs. *1:* Pacinian corpuscle; *2:* muscle spindle; *3:* Golgi tendon organ; *4:* encapsulated ending; *5:* free nerve endings.

tion generally follows the segmental distribution of underlying muscle innervation (Fig 5–8).

- Because, in many patients, there is no C1 dorsal root, there is no C1 dermatome (when a C1 dermatome does exist as an anatomic variant, it covers a small area in the central part of the neck, close to the occiput).
- The dermatomes for C5, C6, C7, C8, and T1 are confined to the arm, and the C4 and T2 dermatomes are contiguous over the anterior trunk.
- The thumb, middle finger, and fifth digit are within the C6, C7, and C8 dermatomes, respectively.
- The nipple is at the level of T4.
- The umbilicus is at the level of T10.

The territories of dermatomes tend to overlap, making it difficult to determine the absence of a single segmental innervation on the basis of sensory testing (Fig 5–9).

Myotomes

The term **myotome** refers to the skeletal musculature innervated by motor axons in a given spinal root. Testing of motor functions (see Appendix B) can be very useful in determining the extent of a lesion in the nerve, spinal cord segment, or tract, especially when combined with a careful sensory examination. Most muscles, as indicated in Appendix B, are innervated by motor axons that arise from several adjacent spinal

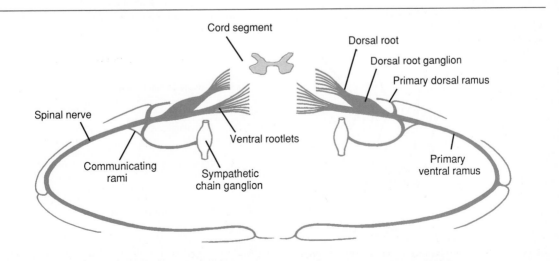

Figure 5–7. Schematic illustration of a cord segment with its roots, ganglia, and branches.

Table 5–1. Anatomic relationships of spinal cord and bony spine in adults.

Cord Segments	Vertebral Bodies	Spinous Processes
C8	Lower C6 and upper C7	C6
T6	Lower T3 and upper T4	T3
T12	T9	T8
L5	T11	T10
S	T12 and L1	T12 and L1

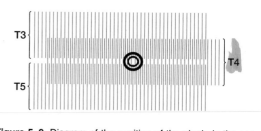

Figure 5–9. Diagram of the position of the nipple in the sensory skin fields of the third, fourth, and fifth thoracic spinal roots showing the overlapping of the cutaneous areas.

roots. Nevertheless, lesions of a single spinal root, in many cases, can cause weakness and atrophy of a muscle. Table 5–2 presents a list of "segment-pointer muscles," whose weakness or atrophy may suggest a lesion involving a single nerve root, or a pair of adjacent nerve roots.

INTERNAL DIVISIONS OF THE SPINAL CORD

Gray Matter

A. Columns: A cross section of the spinal cord shows an H-shaped internal mass of gray matter surrounded by white matter (see Fig 5–4). The gray matter is made up of two symmetrical portions joined across the midline by a transverse connection (commissure) of gray matter that contains the minute central canal or its remnants. The **ventral (or anterior) gray column** (in cross section, called the **anterior,** or **ventral horn**) is in front of the central canal. It contains the cells of origin of the fibers of the ventral roots. The **intermediolateral gray column** (or **horn**) is the portion of gray matter between the dorsal and ventral gray columns; it is a prominent lateral triangular projection in the thoracic and upper lumbar regions, but not in the midsacral region. It contains preganglionic cells for the autonomic nervous system. The **dorsal gray column** (in cross section, the **posterior,** or **dorsal horn**) reaches almost to the posterolateral (dorsolateral) sulcus; a compact bundle of small fibers, the **dorsolateral fasciculus (Lissauer's tract),** part of the pain pathway, lies on the periphery of the spinal cord.

The form and quantity of the gray matter vary at different levels of the spinal cord (Fig 5–10). The proportion of gray to white is greatest in the lumbar and cervical enlargements. In the cervical region, the dorsal gray column is comparatively narrow and the ventral column is broad and expansive, especially in the four lower cervical segments. In the thoracic region, both the dorsal and ventral columns are narrow, and there is a lateral column. In the lumbar region, the dorsal and ventral columns are broad and expanded. In the conus medullaris, the gray matter looks like two oval masses, one in each half of the cord, connected by a wide gray commissure.

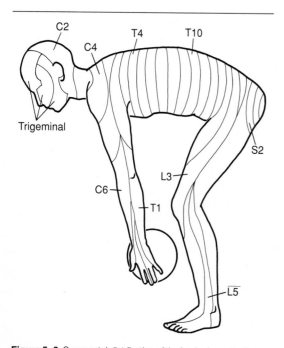

Figure 5–8. Segmental distribution of the body viewed in the approximate quadruped position.

Table 5–2. Segment-pointer muscles.

Root	Muscle	Primary Function
C3, C4	Diaphragm	Respiration
C5	Deltoid	Abduction of arm
C5	Biceps	Flexion of forearm
C6	Brachioradialis	Flexion of forearm
C7	Triceps	Extension of forearm
L3, L4	Quadriceps femoris	Extension of knee
L5	Extensor hallucis longus	Dorsiflexion of great toe
S1	Gastrocnemius	Plantar flexion

(Modified, with permission, from Byrne TN and Waxman SG: *Spinal Cord Compression,* FA Davis, 1990.)

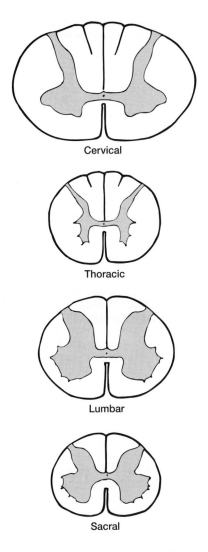

Figure 5–10. Transverse sections of the spinal cord at various levels.

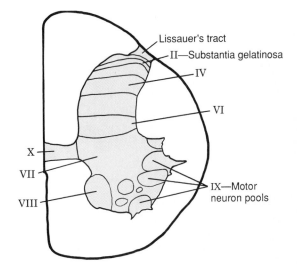

Figure 5–11. Laminas of the gray matter of the spinal cord (only one half shown).

B. Laminas: A cross section of the gray matter of the spinal cord shows a number of laminas (layers of nerve cells), termed **Rexed laminae** after the neuroanatomist who described them (Fig 5–11).

1. Lamina I–This thin marginal layer contains neurons that respond to noxious stimuli and send axons to the contralateral spinothalamic tract.

2. Lamina II–Also known as **substantia gelatinosa,** this lamina is made up of small neurons, some of which respond to noxious stimuli. **Substance P,** a neuropeptide involved in pathways mediating sensibility to pain, is found in high concentrations in laminae I and II.

3. Laminas III and IV–These are referred to together as the **nucleus proprius.** Their main input is from fibers that convey position and light touch sense.

4. Lamina V–This layer contains cells that respond to both noxious and visceral afferent stimuli.

5. Lamina VI–The deepest layer of the dorsal horn and contains neurons that respond to mechanical signals from joints and skin.

6. Lamina VII–This is a large zone that contains the cells of the **dorsal nucleus (Clarke's column)** medially, as well as a large portion of the ventral gray column. Clarke's column contains cells that give rise to the **posterior spinocerebellar tract.** Lamina VII also contains the **intermediolateral nucleus** (or intermediolateral cell column) in thoracic and upper lumbar regions; preganglionic sympathetic fibers project from cells in this nucleus, via the ventral roots and white rami communicantes, to sympathetic ganglia.

7. Laminas VIII and IX–These layers represent motor neuron groups in the medial and lateral portions of the ventral gray column. The medial portion (also termed the **medial motor neuron column**) contains the lower motor neurons that innervate axial musculature (ie, muscles of the trunk and proximal parts of the limbs). The **lateral motor neuron column** contains lower motor neurons for the distal muscles of the arm and leg. In general, flexor muscles are innervated by motor neurons located centrally in the ventral horn, close to the central canal, while extensor muscles are innervated by motor neurons located more peripherally (Fig 5–12).

8. Lamina X–This represents the small neurons around the central canal or its remnants.

White Matter

A. Columns: Each lateral half of the spinal cord has white columns (funiculi)—dorsal (also termed

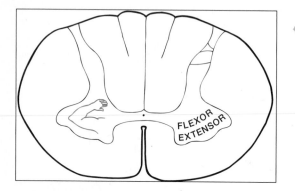

Figure 5–12. Diagram showing the functional localization of motor neuron groups in the ventral gray horn of a lower cervical segment of the spinal cord.

posterior), lateral, and ventral (also termed anterior)—around the spinal gray columns (see Fig 5–4). The dorsal column lies between the posterior median sulcus and the posterolateral sulcus. In the cervical and upper thoracic regions, the dorsal column is divided into a medial portion, the **fasciculus gracilis,** and a lateral portion, the **fasciculus cuneatus.** The lateral column lies between the posterolateral sulcus and the anterolateral sulcus. The ventral column lies between the anterolateral sulcus and the anterior median fissure.

B. Tracts: The white matter of the cord is composed of myelinated and unmyelinated nerve fibers. The fast-conducting myelinated fibers form bundles (fasciculi) that ascend or descend for varying distances. Glial cells (oligodendrocytes, which form myelin, and astrocytes) lie between the fibers. Fiber bundles with a common function are called **tracts.** The lateral and ventral white columns contain tracts that are not well delimited and may overlap in their cross-sectional areas; the dorsal column tracts are sharply defined by glial septa. Slow-conducting unmyelinated fibers form ill-defined bundles at the margin of the white matter. Their function is poorly understood.

PATHWAYS IN WHITE MATTER

Descending Fiber Systems

A. Corticospinal Tract: Arising from the cerebral cortex (primarily the precentral motor cortex, or area 4 and the premotor area, or area 6), is a large bundle of myelinated axons that descends through the brain stem via a tract called the **medullary pyramid,** and then largely crosses over (decussates) to descend downward in the lateral white columns. These tracts contain over 1,000,000 axons; the majority are myelinated. Most of the fibers in this tract are less than 6 μm

in diameter, but there are some very large fibers that arise from the giant Betz cells in the motor cortex.

The corticospinal tracts contain the axons of upper motor neurons, ie, neurons of the cerebrum and subcortical brain stem which descend and provide input to the anterior horn cells of the spinal cord; these latter cells, which project directly to muscle and control muscular contraction, are called lower motor neurons.

The great majority of axons in the corticospinal system decussate in the **pyramidal decussation** within the medulla, and descend within the **lateral corticospinal tract** (Fig 5–13 and Table 5–3). These fibers terminate throughout the ventral gray column and at the base of the dorsal column. Some of the lower motor neurons supplying the muscles of the distal extremities receive direct monosynaptic input from the lateral corticospinal tract; other lower motor neurons are innervated by interneurons (via polysynaptic connection).

The lateral corticospinal tract is relatively new in phylogenetic terms, present only in mammals, and most highly developed in primates. It provides the descending pathway that controls voluntary, highly-skilled, and fractionated movements.

In addition to the lateral corticospinal tract that decussates and is the largest descending motor pathway, there are two smaller descending motor pathways in the spinal cord, which are uncrossed.

About 10% of the corticospinal fibers that descend from the hemisphere do not decussate in the medulla, and descend uncrossed in the **anterior** (or **ventral**) **corticospinal tract**, located in the anterior white matter column of the spinal cord. After descending within the spinal cord, many of these fibers decussate, via the anterior white commissure, and then project to interneurons (which project to lower motor neurons), or directly to lower motor neurons, of the contralateral side.

Finally, a small fraction (0–3%) of the corticospinal axons descend, without decussating, as uncrossed fibers within the lateral corticospinal tract. This small population of axons, which does not decussate, terminates in the base of the posterior horn and the intermediate gray matter of the spinal cord, where it provides synaptic input (probably via polysynaptic circuits) to lower motor neurons controlling axial (ie, trunk and proximal limb) musculature involved in maintaining body posture.

A small percentage of the fibers of the corticospinal tract project to the dorsal gray column and function as modifiers of afferent (sensory) information, allowing the brain to suppress, or filter, certain incoming stimuli and pay attention to others (see Chapter 14); these fibers may also modify local reflex activity within the spinal cord.

B. Vestibulospinal Tracts: There are two major components to the vestibulospinal tracts. Fibers of the **lateral vestibulospinal tract** arise from the lateral vestibular nucleus in the brain stem and course down-

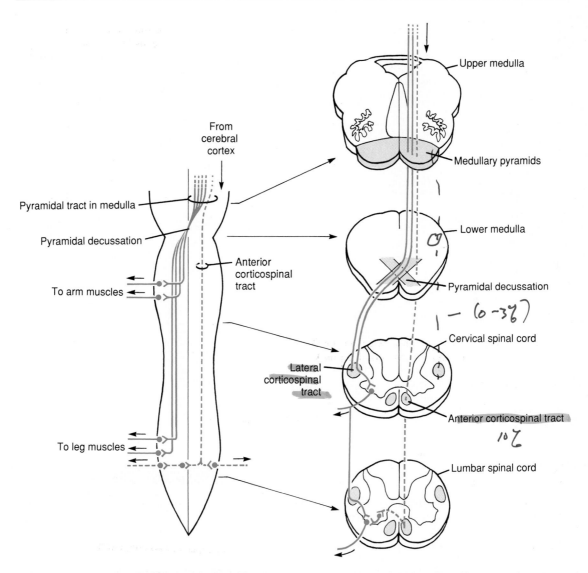

Figure 5–13. Schematic illustration of the course of corticospinal tract fibers in the spinal cord, together with cross sections at representative levels. This and the following schematic illustrations show the cord in an upright position.

ward, uncrossed, in the ventral white column of the spinal cord. Fibers of the **medial vestibulospinal tract** arise in the medial vestibular nucleus in the brain stem and descend within the cervical spinal cord, with both crossed and uncrossed components, to terminate at cervical levels. Fibers of both vestibulospinal tracts provide synaptic inputs to interneurons in Rexed laminae VII and VIII, which project to both alpha and gamma lower motor neurons. Fibers of the vestibulospinal tracts provide excitatory input to the lower motor neurons for extensor muscles. The vestibulospinal system facilitates quick movements in reaction to sudden changes in body position (eg, falling) and provide essential control of anti-gravity muscles.

C. Rubrospinal Tract: This fiber system arises in the contralateral red nucleus in the brain stem and courses in the lateral white column. The tract projects to interneurons in the spinal gray columns and plays a role in motor function (see Chapter 7).

D. Reticulospinal System: This tract arises in the reticular formation of the brain stem and descends in both the ventral and lateral white columns. Both crossed and uncrossed descending fibers are present. The fibers terminating on dorsal gray column neurons may modify the transmission of sensation from the body, especially pain (some of these fibers originate in the brain stem raphe nuclei and are serotoninergic; see Chapter 14). Those that end on ventral gray neurons

Table 5–3. Descending fiber systems in the spinal cord.

System	Function	Origin	Ending	Location in Cord
Lateral corticospinal (pyramidal) tract	Fine motor function (controls distal musculature) Modulation of sensory functions	Motor and premotor cortex	Anterior horn cells (interneurons and lower-motor-neurons)	Lateral column (crosses in medulla at pyramidal decussation)
Anterior corticospinal tract	Gross and postural motor function (proximal and axial musculature)	Motor and premotor cortex	Anterior horn neurons (interneurons and lower-motor-neurons)	Anterior column (uncrossed until after descending, when some fibers decussate)
Vestibulospinal tract	Postural reflexes	Lateral and medial vestibular nucleus	Anterior horn interneurons and motor neurons (for extensors)	Ventral column
Rubrospinal	Motor function	Red nucleus	Ventral horn interneurons	Lateral column
Reticulospinal	Modulation of sensory transmission (especially pain) Modulation of spinal reflexes	Brain stem reticular formation	Dorsal and ventral horn	Anterior column
Descending autonomic	Modulation of autonomic functions	Hypothalamus, brain stem nuclei	Preganglionic autonomic neurons	Lateral columns
Tectospinal	Reflex head turning	Midbrain	Ventral horn interneurons	Ventral column
Medial longitudinal fasciculus	Coordination of head and eye movements	Vestibular nuclei	Cervical gray	Ventral column

influence gamma motor neurons and, thus, various spinal reflexes.

E. Descending Autonomic System: Arising from the hypothalamus and brain stem, this poorly defined fiber system projects to preganglionic sympathetic neurons in the thoracolumbar spinal cord (lateral column) and to preganglionic parasympathetic neurons in sacral segments (see Chapter 20). Descending fibers in this system modulate autonomic functions such as blood pressure, pulse and respiratory rates, sweating, etc.

F. Tectospinal Tract: This tract arises from the superior colliculus in the roof **(tectum)** of the midbrain, then courses in the contralateral ventral white column to provide synaptic input to ventral gray interneurons. It causes head turning in response to sudden visual or auditory stimuli.

G. Medial Longitudinal Fasciculus: This tract arises from vestibular nuclei in the brain stem. As it descends, it runs close to, and intermingles with, the tectospinal tract. Some of its fibers descend into the cervical spinal cord to terminate on ventral gray interneurons. It coordinates head and eye movements. These last two descending fiber systems are present on each side and descend only to the cervical segments of the spinal cord.

Ascending Fiber Systems

All afferent axons in the dorsal roots have their cell bodies in the dorsal root ganglia (Table 5–4). Different ascending systems decussate at different levels. In general, ascending axons synapse within the spinal cord prior to decussating.

A. Dorsal Column Tracts: These tracts, the **medial lemniscal system,** convey well-localized sensations of fine touch, vibration, 2-point discrimination, and proprioception (position sense) from the skin and joints; they ascend, without crossing, in the dorsal white column of the spinal cord to the lower brain stem (Fig 5–14). The **fasciculus gracilis** courses next to the posteromedian septum; it contains input from the lower half of the body, with fibers that arise from the lowest, most medial segments. The **fasciculus cuneatus** lies between the fasciculus gracilis and the dorsal gray column; it contains input from the upper half of the body, with fibers from the lower (thoracic) segments more medial than the higher (cervical) ones. Thus, one dorsal column contains fibers from all segments of the ipsilateral half of the body arranged in an orderly fashion from medial to lateral; such an arrangement is called **somatotopic organization** (Fig 5–15). Ascending fibers in the gracile and cuneate fasciculi terminate

Table 5–4. Ascending fiber systems in the spinal cord.

Name	Function	Origin	Ending	Location in Cord
Dorsal column system	Fine touch, proprioception, 2-point discrimination	Skin, joints, tendons	Dorsal column nuclei. Second-order neurons project to contralateral thalamus (cross in medulla at lemniscal decussation)	Dorsal column
Spinothalamic tracts	Sharp pain, temperature, crude touch	Skin	Dorsal horn. Second-order neurons project to contralateral thalamus (cross in spinal cord close to level of entry)	Ventrolateral column
Dorsal spinocerebellar tract	Movement and position mechanisms	Muscle spindles, Golgi tendon organs, touch and pressure receptors	Cerebellar paleocortex (via ipsilateral inferior cerebellar peduncle)	Lateral column
Ventral spinocerebellar	Movement and position mechanisms	Muscle spindles, Golgi tendon organs, touch and pressure receptors	Cerebellar paleocortex (via contralateral and ipsilateral superior cerebellar peduncle)	Lateral column
Spinoreticular pathway	Deep and chronic pain	Deep somatic structures	Reticular formation of brain stem	Polysynaptic, diffuse pathway in ventrolateral column

on neurons in the **gracile** and **cuneate nuclei (dorsal column nuclei)** in the lower medulla; these second-order neurons send their axons, in turn, across the midline via the **lemniscal decussation** (also called the **internal arcuate tract**) and the **medial lemniscus** to the **thalamus.** From the **ventral posterolateral (VPL) thalamic nuclei,** sensory information is relayed upward to the **somatosensory cortex.**

B. Spinothalamic Tracts: Small-diameter sensory axons conveying the sensations of sharp (noxious) pain, temperature, and crudely localized touch course upward, after entering the spinal cord via the dorsal root, for one or two segments at the periphery of the dorsal horn. These short, ascending stretches of incoming fibers that are termed the **dorsolateral fasciculus** or **Lissauer's tract**, then synapse with dorsal column neurons, especially in laminae I, II, and V (Fig 5–11 and Fig 5–16). After one or more synapses, subsequent fibers cross to the opposite side of the spinal cord, and then ascend within the spinothalamic tracts, also called the **ventrolateral (or anterior)** system. These spinothalamic tracts actually consist of two adjacent pathways: The **anterior spinothalamic tract** carries information about light touch. The **lateral spinothalamic tract** conveys pain and temperature sensibility upward.

The spinothalamic tracts, like the dorsal column system, show somatotopic organization (Fig 5–15). In particular, sensation from sacral parts of the body is carried in lateral parts of the spinothalamic tracts, while impulses originating in cervical regions are carried by fibers in medial parts of the spinothalamic tracts. Axons of the spinothalamic tracts project rostrally after sending branches to the reticular formation in the brain stem and project to the thalamus (VPL, intralaminar thalamic nuclei).

C. Clinical Correlations: It should be emphasized that the second-order neurons of both the dorsal column system and spinothalamic tracts decussate. However, the pattern of decussation is different: The axons of second-order neurons of the dorsal column system cross, in the lemniscal decussation, in the medulla; these second-order sensory axons are called **internal arcuate fibers** where they cross. In contrast, the axons of second-order neurons in the spinothalamic tracts cross at every segmental level in the spinal cord. This fact aids in determining whether a lesion is in the brain or the spinal cord. With lesions in the brain stem or higher, deficits of pain perception, touch sensation, and proprioception are all contralateral to the lesion. However, with spinal cord lesions, the deficit in pain perception is contralateral to the lesion while the other deficits are ipsilateral. Clinical Illustration 5–1 provides an example.

Segregation of second-order sensory axons carrying pain sensibility within the lateral spinothalamic tract is of considerable clinical importance. As might be expected, unilateral interruption of the lateral spinothalamic tract causes a loss of sensibility for pain and temperature, beginning about a segment below the level corresponding to the lesion, on the opposite side of the body. This fact is occasionally used by neurosurgeons who may perform an anterolateral cordotomy in patients with intractable pain syndrome.

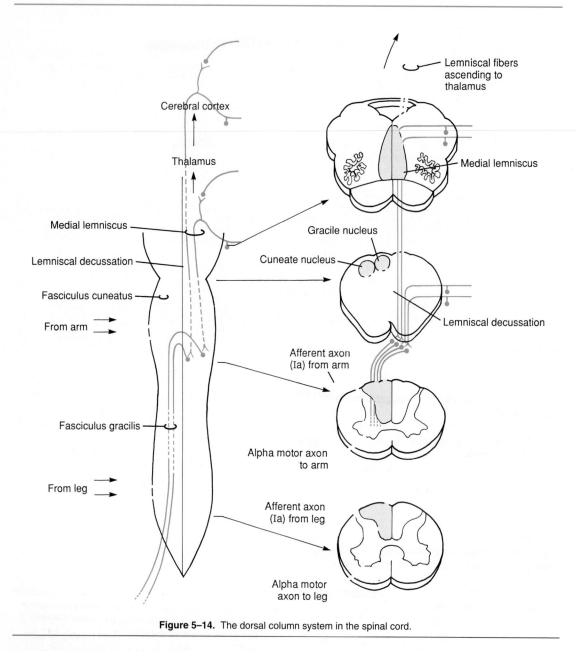

Figure 5–14. The dorsal column system in the spinal cord.

CLINICAL ILLUSTRATION 5–1

A 27-year-old electrician became involved in a bar room brawl and was stabbed in the back, close to the midline in the midthoracic level. On examination in the hospital, he was unable to move his right leg, and there was moderate weakness of finger flexion, abduction, and adduction on the right. There was loss of position sense in the right leg, and he could not appreciate a vibrating tuning fork that was placed on his toes, or bony prominences at the right ankle, knee, or iliac crest. There was loss of pain and temperature sensibility below the T2 level on the left.

Following an MRI scan that showed a hemorrhagic lesion involving the spinal cord at the C8-T1 level, the patient was taken to the operating room. A blood clot, partially compressing the cord, was removed and several bone fragments were retrieved from the spinal canal. The surgeon observed that the spinal cord had been partially severed, on the right side, at the C8 level. The patient remained stable, but his deficits did not improve over the ensuing two years.

This case provides an example of the **Brown-Sequard syndrome.** This syndrome is due to unilateral lesions or transections of the spinal cord and occurs most commonly in the context of stab injuries

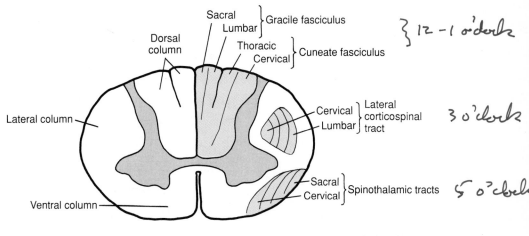

Figure 5–15. Somatotopic organization (segmental arrangement) in the spinal cord.

or gunshot wounds. There is ipsilateral weakness and loss of position and vibration sense below the lesion as a result of transsection of the lateral corticospinal tract and dorsal columns. There is usually a loss of pain and temperature that manifests a few segments below the level of the lesion because the decussating fibers enter the spinothalamic tract a few segments rostral to the level of entry of the nerve root. The absence of function recovery in this patient graphically illustrates the inability of CNS neurons to regenerate following injury in man.

D. Spinoreticular Pathway: The ill-defined spinoreticular tract courses within the ventrolateral portion of the spinal cord, arising from cord neurons and ending (without crossing) in the reticular formation of the brain stem. This tract plays an important role in the sensation of pain, especially deep, chronic pain (see Chapter 14).

E. Spinocerebellar Tracts: Two ascending pathways (of lesser importance in human neurology) provide input from the spinal cord to the cerebellum (Fig 5–17 and Table 5–4).

1. Dorsal spinocerebellar tract–Afferent fibers from muscle and skin (which convey information from muscle spindles, Golgi tendon organs, touch and pressure receptors) enter the spinal cord via dorsal roots at levels T1-L2 and synapse on second-order neurons of the **nucleus dorsalis (Clarke's column).** Afferent fibers originating in sacral and lower lumber levels ascend within the spinal cord (within the dorsal columns) to reach the lower portion of the nucleus dorsalis.

The dorsal nucleus of Clarke is not present above C8; it is replaced, for the upper extremity, by a homologous nucleus called the **accessory cuneate nucleus.** Dorsal root fibers originating at cervical levels synapse with second-order neurons in the accessory cuneate nucleus.

The second-order neurons from the dorsal nucleus of Clark form the dorsal spinocerebellar tract; second-order neurons from the lateral cuneate nucleus form the **cuneocerebellar tract.** Both tracts remain on the ipsilateral side of the spinal cord, ascending via the inferior cerebellar peduncle to terminate in the paleocerebellar cortex.

2. Ventral spinocerebellar tract–This system is involved with movement control. Second-order neurons, located in Rexed laminae V, VI, and VII in lumbar and sacral segments of the spinal cord, send axons that ascend through the superior cerebellar peduncle to the paleocerebellar cortex. The axons of the second-order neurons are largely, but not entirely crossed, and this tract is of little value in localizing lesions in the spinal cord.

REFLEXES

Reflexes are subconscious stimulus-response mechanisms. The instinctive behavior of lower animals is governed largely by reflexes; in humans, behavior is more a matter of conditioning, and reflexes act as basic defense mechanisms. The reflexes are, however, extremely important in the diagnosis and localization of neurologic lesions (see Appendix B).

Simple Reflex Arc

Several structures are involved in the reflex arc (Fig 5–18): **a receptor,** eg, a special sense organ, cutaneous end organ, or muscle spindle, whose stimulation initiates an impulse; the **afferent neuron,** which transmits the impulse through a peripheral nerve to the central nervous system, where the nerve synapses with a lower motor neuron or an intercalated neuron; one or more **intercalated neurons (interneurons),** which relay the

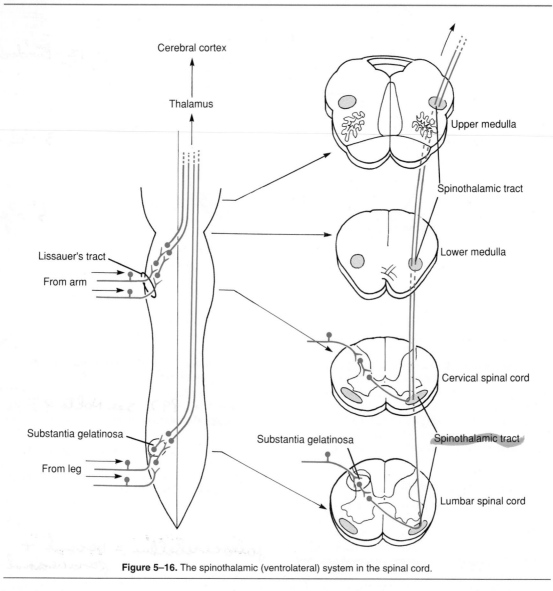

Figure 5–16. The spinothalamic (ventrolateral) system in the spinal cord.

impulse to the efferent nerve; the **efferent neuron,** which passes outward in the nerve and delivers the impulse to an effector; and an **effector,** eg, the muscle or gland that produces the response.

Notice that interruption of this simple reflex arc at any point will abolish the response.

Types of Reflexes

The reflexes of importance to the clinical neurologist may be divided into four groups: superficial (skin and mucous membrane) reflexes, deep tendon (myotatic) reflexes, visceral (organic) reflexes, and pathologic (abnormal) reflexes (Table 5–5).

Reflexes can also be classified according to the level of their central representation, eg, as spinal, bulbar (postural and righting reflexes), midbrain, or cerebellar reflexes.

Spinal Reflexes

The segmental spinal reflex involves the afferent neuron and a motor unit at the same level (Fig 5–18). Simple reflex reactions involve patterns of movement rather than specific muscle contractions. The delay between stimulation and effect is caused by the time needed for propagation of the impulse along the nerve fibers concerned and the synaptic delay (1 msec at each synapse).

A. Stretch Reflexes and Their Anatomic Substrates: Stretch reflexes (also called **deep tendon reflexes or myotatic reflexes)** provide a feedback mechanism for maintaining appropriate muscle tone (Fig 5–18). The stretch reflex depends on specialized sensory receptors (muscle spindles), afferent nerve fibers (primarily Ia fibers) extending from these re-

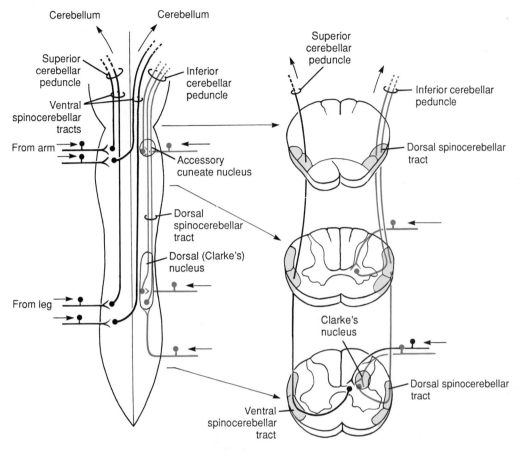

Figure 5–17. The spinocerebellar systems in the spiral cord.

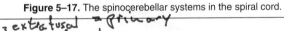

ceptors via the dorsal roots to the spinal cord, two types of lower motor neurons **(alpha and gamma motor neurons)** that project back to muscle, and specialized inhibitory interneurons **(Renshaw cells)**.

B. Muscle Spindles: These specialized mechanoreceptors are located within muscles and provide information about the length and rate of changes in length of the muscle. The muscle spindles contain specialized **intrafusal muscle fibers**, which are surrounded by a connective tissue capsule (these intrafusal muscle fibers should not be confused with **extrafusal fibers** or primary muscle cells, which are the regular contractile units that provide the force underlying muscle contraction).

Two types of intrafusal fibers **(nuclear bag fibers** and **nuclear chain fibers)** are anchored to the connective tissue septae, which run longitudinally within the muscle, and are arranged in parallel with the extrafusal muscle fibers. Two types of afferent axons, **Ia** and **II** fibers, arise from **primary** (or **annulospinal**) endings and **secondary** (or **flower-spray**) endings on the intrafusal fibers of the muscle spindle. These afferent axons carry impulses from the muscle spindle to the spinal cord via the dorsal roots. The muscle spindle and

its afferent fibers provide information about both **muscle length** (the **static response**), and the **rate of change** in muscle length (the **dynamic response**). The static response is generated by nuclear chain fibers; the dynamic response is generated by nuclear bag fibers. After entering the spinal gray matter, Ia afferents from the muscle spindle make monosynaptic, excitatory connections with alpha motor neurons.

The muscle spindles are distributed in parallel with the extrafusal muscle fibers. Lengthening or stretching the muscle distorts the sensory endings in the spindle and generates a receptor potential. This causes the afferent axons from the muscle spindle (Ia afferents) to fire, with a frequency that is proportionate to the degree of stretch (Fig 5–19). Conversely, contraction of the muscle shortens the spindles and leads to a decrease in their firing rate.

Deep tendon reflexes are concerned with resisting inappropriate stretch on muscles, and thus contribute to the maintenance of body posture. The Ia fibers from a muscle spindle end monosynaptically on, and produce EPSPs in, motor neurons supplying extrafusal muscle fibers in the same muscle. Lengthening of a muscle stretches the muscle spindle, thereby causing a

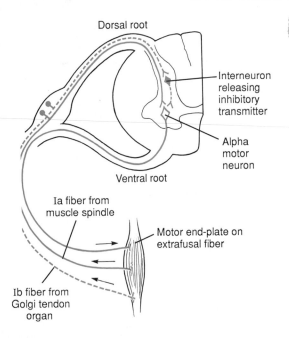

Dorsal root

Interneuron releasing inhibitory transmitter

Alpha motor neuron

Ventral root

Ia fiber from muscle spindle

Motor end-plate on extrafusal fiber

Ib fiber from Golgi tendon organ

Figure 5–18. Diagram illustrating the pathways responsible for the stretch reflex and the inverse stretch reflex. Stretch stimulates the muscle spindle, and impulses pass up the Ia fiber to excite the lower (alpha) motor neuron. Stretch also stimulates the Golgi tendon organ, which is arranged in series with the muscle, and impulses passing up the Ib fiber activate the inhibitory interneuron. With strong stretch, the resulting hyperpolarization of the motor neuron is so great that it stops discharging. (Reproduced, with permission, from Ganong WF: *Review of Medical Physiology*, 16th ed. Appleton & Lange, 1993.)

discharge of an afferent Ia fiber in the dorsal root. This, in turn, activates alpha motor neurons running to the muscle, causing the extrafusal muscle fibers to contract so that the muscle with shorten.

In addition to monosynaptically exciting the alpha motor neurons involved in the stretch reflex, Ia afferents project, via inhibitory interneurons, to antagonistic muscle groups. This provides for **reciprocal inhibition**, whereby flexors are excited and extensors are inhibited (or vice versa) in a coordinated manner.

C. Alpha Motor Neurons: Extrafusal muscle fibers, responsible for muscle contraction, are innervated by large anterior horn neurons termed **alpha motor neurons.** When alpha motor neurons fire, action potentials in their axons propagate, via axons in the ventral roots and peripheral nerves, to the motor endplate, where they have an excitatory effect and produce muscle contraction.

D. Gamma Motor Neurons: Each muscle spindle contains, within its capsule, 2–10 small intrafusal fibers. Intrafusal muscle fibers receive their own innervation from **gamma motor neurons**, which are small, specialized motor neurons whose cell bodies are located in the ventral horn (Fig 5–20). Gamma motor neurons have relatively small axons (in the Aγ groups,

3–6 μm in diameter) that make up about 25–30% of the fibers in the ventral root. Firing in gamma motor neurons excites the intrafusal muscle fibers so they contract. This does not lead directly to detectable muscle contraction because the intrafusal fibers are small. However, firing gamma motor neurons does increase tension on the muscle spindle; this increases its sensitivity to overall muscle stretch. Thus, the gamma motor neuron/intrafusal muscle fiber system sets the "gain" on the muscle spindle. The firing rates of gamma motor neurons are regulated by descending activity from a number of areas in the brain. By modulating the thresholds for stretch reflexes, descending influences regulate postural tone.

E. Renshaw Cells: These interneurons, located in the ventral horn, project to alpha motor neurons and are inhibitory. Renshaw cells receive excitatory synaptic input via collaterals, which branch from alpha motor neurons. These cells appear to be part of local feedback circuits that prevent overactivity in alpha motor neurons.

F. Golgi Tendon Organs: A second set of receptors, the Golgi tendon organs, are present within muscle tendons. These stretch receptors are arranged in series with extrafusal muscle fibers and are activated by either stretching or contracting the muscle. Group Ib afferent fibers run from the tendon organs via the dorsal roots to the spinal gray matter. Here, they end on interneurons that inhibit the alpha motor neuron innervating the agonist muscle, thus, mediating the **inverse stretch reflex** (Fig 5–18). As a result of this feedback arrangement, these specialized receptors prevent overactivity of alpha motor neurons.

G. Flexor Reflex: The flexor reflex represents a withdrawal mechanism that removes an extremity from a harmful stimulus. Much experimental work has been done in vertebrate animals, ie, severing the spinal cord from the brain stem. As a result of the loss of descending influences (which normally inhibit flexor reflexes) animals subsequently exhibit prominent flexion responses that involve several segments. A single afferent nerve can stimulate many motor units; smaller nerve branches to the skin are usually more effective than deep sensory nerves in exciting flexor motor units. The postures seen in some form of prolonged pathologic irritation are probably caused by flexor reflexes. A patient with peritonitis assumes a doubled-up attitude, for example, and stiffness and retraction of the neck occur in irritation of the meninges by infection, blood, or tumor cells.

H. Clinical Correlations: If the alpha motor neuron fibers in a ventral root or peripheral nerve are cut, the muscle's resistance to stretching is reduced. The muscle becomes flaccid and has little tone.

The large extensor muscles that support the body are kept constantly active by coactivation of alpha and gamma motor neurons. Transection of the spinal cord acutely reduces muscle tone, indicating that supraspinal descending axons modulate the alpha and gamma mo-

Table 5–5. Summary of reflexes.

Reflexes	Afferent Nerve	Center	Efferent Nerve
Superficial reflexes			
Corneal	Cranial V	Pons	Cranial VII
Nasal (sneeze)	Cranial V	Brain stem and upper cord	Cranials V, VII, IX, X, and spinal nerves of expiration
Pharyngeal and uvular	Cranial IX	Medulla	Cranial X
Upper abdominal	T7, 8, 9, 10	T7, 8, 9, 10	T7, 8, 9, 10
Lower abdominal	T10, 11, 12	T10, 11, 12	T10, 11, 12
Cremasteric	Femoral	L1	Genitofemoral
Plantar	Tibial	S1, 2	Tibial
Anal	Pudendal	S4, 5	Pudendal
Deep reflexes			
Jaw	Cranial V	Pons	Cranial V
Biceps	Musculocutaneous	C5, 6	Musculocutaneous
Triceps	Radial	C7, 8	Radial
Brachioradialis	Radial	C 5, 6	Radial
Patellar	Femoral	L3, 4	Femoral
Achilles	Tibial	S1, 2	Tibial
Visceral reflexes			
Light	Cranial II	Midbrain	Cranial III
Accommodation	Cranial II	Occipital cortex	Cranial III
Ciliospinal	A sensory nerve	T1, 2	Cervical sympathetics
Oculocardiac	Cranial V	Medulla	Cranial X
Carotid sinus	Cranial IX	Medulla	Cranial X
Bulbocavernosus	Pudendal	S2, 3, 4	Pelvic autonomic
Bladder and rectal	Pudendal	S2, 3, 4	Pudendal and autonomics
Abnormal reflexes			
Extensor plantar (Babinski)	Plantar	L3-L5, S1	Extensor hallucis longus

tor neurons. In the *chronic* phase after transection of the spinal cord, there is hyperactivity of stretch reflexes below the level of the lesion, producing a state of **spasticity.** This appears to be a result of the loss of descending, modulatory influences. Spasticity can be disabling and is often treated with baclofen, a GABA agonist. In some patients, however, the increased extension tone in spastic lower extremities is useful, providing at least a stiff-legged spastic gait after damage to the corticospinal system (eg, after a stroke).

Experimental interruption of both corticospinal and rubrospinal tracts results in a state of extreme extensor rigidity. This type of extensor rigidity has been called **gamma rigidity** because it disappears if the dorsal roots (in which Ia fibers course) are subsequently cut. If the anterior portion of the cerebellum is then removed, the rigidity returns; this is termed as **alpha rigidity** and it occurs when the gamma loop is bypassed and the alpha motor neurons are excited directly.

I.   Polysynaptic Reflexes: In contrast to the extensor stretch reflex (eg, patellar, Achilles tendon), polysynaptic, crossed extensor reflexes are not limited to one muscle; they usually involve many muscles on the same or opposite side of the body (Fig 5–21). These reflexes have several physiologic characteristics:

1. Reciprocal action of antagonists–Flexors are excited and extensors inhibited on one side of the body; the opposite occurs on the opposite side of the body.
2. Divergence–Stimuli from a few receptors are distributed to many motor neurons in the cord.
3. Summation–Consecutive or simultaneous subthreshold stimuli may combine to initiate the reflex.
4. Hierarchy–When two antagonistic reflexes are elicited simultaneously, one will override the other.

Propriospinal axons, located on the periphery of the spinal gray matter, are the axons of local circuit neurons that convey impulses upwards or downwards, for several segments, to coordinate reflexes involving several segments. Some authors refer to these axons as the **propriospinal tract (tractus proprius).**

STOP HERE

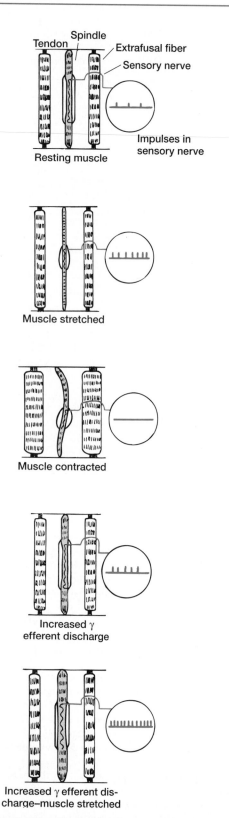

Figure 5–19. Effect of various conditions on muscle spindle discharge. (Reproduced, with permission, from Ganong WF: *Review of Medical Physiology,* 16th ed. Appleton & Lange, 1993.)

Labels in figure:
- Tendon
- Spindle
- Extrafusal fiber
- Sensory nerve
- Impulses in sensory nerve
- Resting muscle
- Muscle stretched
- Muscle contracted
- Increased γ efferent discharge
- Increased γ efferent discharge–muscle stretched

LESIONS IN THE MOTOR PATHWAYS

Lesions in the motor pathways, the muscle, or its myoneural junction, or the peripheral nerve all result in disturbances of motor function (Fig 5–20; see also Chapter 13). Two main types of lesions–of the upper and lower motor neurons–are distinguished in spinal cord disorders (Table 5–6).

Lower-Motor-Neuron Lesions

A lower motor neuron (LMN), the motor cell concerned with striated skeletal muscle activity, consists of a cell body (located in the anterior gray column of the spinal cord or brain stem) and its axon, which passes to the motor end-plates of the muscle by way of the peripheral or cranial nerves (Fig 5–22).

Lower motor neurons, are the last neurons in line prior to the muscle cell. LMN are considered the final common pathway because many neural impulses funnel through them to the muscle; ie, they are acted upon by the corticospinal, rubrospinal, olivospinal, vestibulospinal, reticulospinal, and tectospinal tracts as well as by inter- and intrasegmental reflex neurons.

Lesions of the lower motor neurons may be located in the cells of the ventral gray column of the spinal cord or brain stem or in their axons, which constitute the ventral roots of the spinal or cranial nerves. Lesions can result from trauma, toxins, infections (eg, poliomyelitis, which can affect purely lower motor neurons), vascular disorders, degenerative processes, neoplasms, or congenital malformations affecting lower motor neurons in the brain stem or spinal cord. Compression of ventral root axons (ie, the axons of lower motor neurons in the spinal cord) by herniated intervertebral disks is a common cause of lower motor neuron dysfunction. Signs of lower-motor-neuron lesions include **flaccid paralysis** of the involved muscles (Table 8–6); muscle **atrophy** with degeneration of muscle fibers after some time has elapsed; electrical manifestations of a typical reaction of degeneration (10–14 days after injury; see Electromyography, Chapter 24); **diminished or absent deep tendon reflexes** (hyporeflexia or areflexia) of the involved muscle; and the absence of pathologic reflexes (see next paragraph). Fasciculations and fabrillations may be present.

Upper-Motor-Neuron Lesions

Damage to the cerebral hemispheres or lateral white column of the spinal cord can produce signs of upper-motor-neuron (UMN) lesions. These signs include **spastic paralysis or paresis** (weakness) of the involved muscles (Table 5–6), **little or no muscle atrophy** (merely the atrophy of disuse), **hyperactive deep tendon reflexes,** diminished or absent superficial reflexes, and pathologic reflexes and signs, especially the extensor plantar reflex **(Babinski's sign)** (Fig 5–23).

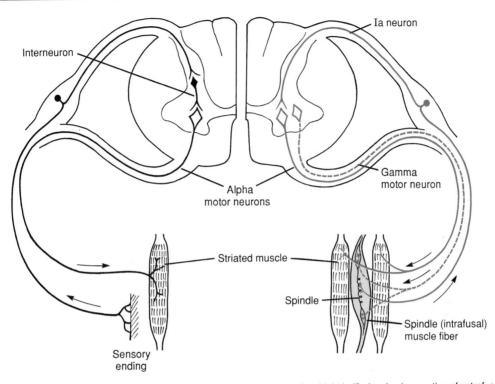

Figure 5–20. Schematic illustration of the neurons involved in the stretch reflex (right half) showing innervation of extrafusal (striated muscle) fibers by alpha motor neurons, and of intrafusal fibers (within muscle spindle) by gamma motor neurons. The left half of the diagram shows an inhibitory reflex arc, which includes an intercalated inhibitory interneuron.

Upper-motor-neuron lesions are commonly seen as a result of strokes, which can damage upper-motor-neurons in the cortex, and infections, or tumors which injure upper-motor-neurons either in the brain or as they descend in the spinal cord. The corticospinal, rubrospinal, and reticulospinal tracts lie close together or overlap within the lateral white column; interruption of the corticospinal tract is usually accompanied by interruption of the other two tracts, resulting in spasticity and hyperreflexia. Isolated lesions of the corticospinal tract are rare; when these lesions occur, they cause loss of fine motor control (eg, loss of dexterity of the individual fingers) but tend to spare axial muscle groups (ie, those located proximally in the limbs) that control gross trunk and limb movement.

Disorders of Muscle Tissue or Neuromuscular Endings

Abnormal muscle tissue may be unable to react normally to stimuli conveyed to it by the lower-motor-neurons. This may manifest as weakness, paralysis, or tetanic contraction caused by disturbances in the mus-

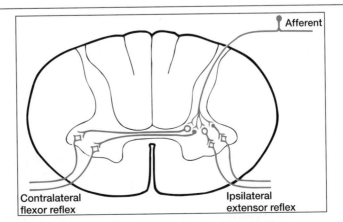

Figure 5–21. Schematic illustration of ipsilateral and crossed polysynaptic reflexes.

Table 5–6. Lower-versus upper-motor-neuron lesions.

	Lower-Motor-Neuron Lesion	Upper-Motor-Neuron Lesion
Weakness	Flaccid paralysis	Spastic paralysis
Deep tendon reflexes	Decreased or absent	Increased
Babinski reflex	Absent	Present
Atrophy	May be marked	Absent or due to disuse
Fasciculations and fibrillations	May be present	Absent

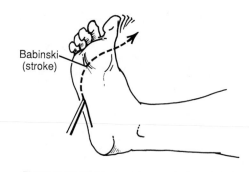

Figure 5–23. Testing for extensor plantar reflexes.

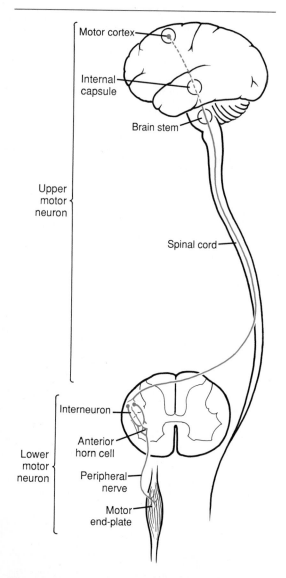

Figure 5–22. Motor pathways divided into upper- and lower-motor-neuron regions.

cle itself or at the neuromuscular junction. **Myasthenia gravis** and the myasthenic syndrome (Eaton-Lambert myasthenic syndrome) are disorders of the neuromuscular juntion that present with weakness. The **muscular dystrophies** and **inflammatory myopathies** (such a polymyositis) are typical disorders of muscle, characterized by muscular dysfunction, ie, weakness in the presence of apparently normal nerve tissue.

Localization of Spinal Cord Lesions

In localizing spinal cord lesions, the student should ask the following questions:

1. Which tracts are involved?
2. On which side?
3. At what level does the abnormality begin (ie, is there a **sensory level,** below which sensation is impaired)? Is motor function impaired below a specific myotomal level?
4. What sensory modalities are involved (all modalities, suggesting involvement of the lateral and dorsal columns; vibration and position sense, suggesting dorsal column dysfunction; or dissociated loss of sensibility for pain and temperature, suggesting a lesion involving the spinothalamic fibers, possibly in the central part of the cord where they cross)?

A **segmental lesion** (ie, a lesion involving only some segments of the spinal cord) will injure motor neurons at the site of injury (causing lower-motor-neuron dysfunction at that level) and will also injure descending tracts (producing upper-motor-neuron dysfunction below the site of injury).

There are several typical sites of pathology in the spinal cord that produce characteristic syndromes:

Types of Spinal Cord Lesions:

1. **A small central lesion** can affect the decussating fibers of the spinothalamic tract from both sides, without affecting other ascending or descending tracts. As a result, these lesions can produce dissociated sensory abnormalities with loss of pain and temperature sensibility in appropriate dermatomes,

but with preserved vibration and position sense. This occurs, for example, in syringomyelia (see below) (Fig 5–24A).

2. A **large central lesion** involves, in addition to the pain and temperature pathways, portions of adjacent tracts, adjacent gray matter, or both. Thus, there can be lower-motor-neuron weakness in the segments involved, together with upper-motor-neuron dysfunction and, in some cases, loss of vibratory and position sense, at levels below the lesion (Fig 5–24B).

3. A **dorsal column lesion** affects the dorsal columns, leaving other parts of the spinal cord intact. Thus, proprioceptive and vibratory sensation are involved, but other functions are normal. Isolated involvement of the dorsal columns occurs in **tabes dorsalis,** a form of tertiary syphillis (see below), which is fortunately rare at present because of the availability of antibiotics (Fig 5–24C).

4. An **irregular peripheral lesion** (eg, stab wound or compression of the cord) involves long pathways and gray matter; functions below the level of the lesion are abolished. In practice, many penetrating wounds of the spinal cord (stab wounds, gunshot wounds) cause irregular lesions (Fig 5–24D).

5. **Complete hemisection** of the cord produces a **Brown-Sequard syndrom**e (see below and Figs 5–24E, 5–25).

   Lesions outside the cord (extramedullary lesions) may affect the function of the cord itself as a result of direct mechanical injury or secondary ischemic injury resulting from the compromise of the vascular structures or vasospasm.

6. A **tumor of the dorsal root**, eg, a neurofibroma or schwannoma, involves the first-order sensory neurons of a segment and can produce pain as well as sensory loss. Deep tendon reflexes at the appropriate level may be lost due to damage to Ia fibers (Fig 5–24F).

7. A **tumor of the meninges** or the bone may compress the spinal cord against a vertebra, causing dysfunction of ascending and descending fiber systems (Fig 5–24G).

EXAMPLES OF SPECIFIC SPINAL CORD DISORDERS

Syringomyelia

Syringomyelia is characterized by loss of pain and temperature sensation at several segmental levels, although the patient usually retains touch and pressure sense as well as vibration and position sense (**dissociated anesthesia**) (Fig 5–26). Because the lesion usually involves the central part of the spinal cord and is confined to a limited number of segments, it affects desussating spinothalamic tracts only in these segments and results in a pattern of **segmental** loss of pain

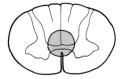

A. Small central lesion

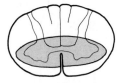

B. Large central lesion

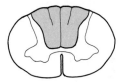

C. Dorsal column lesion

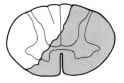

D. Irregular lesion

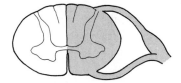

E. Complete hemisection

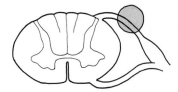

F. Dorsal root tumor

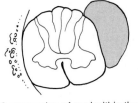

G. Compression of cord within the vertebra by extramedullary mass

Figure 5–24. Schematic illustrations of various types of spinal cord lesions.

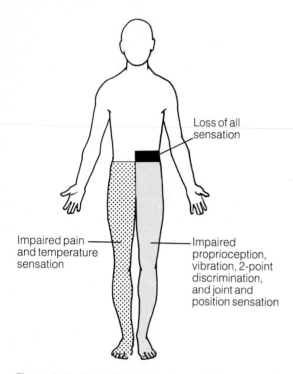

Loss of all sensation

Impaired pain and temperature sensation

Impaired proprioception, vibration, 2-point discrimination, and joint and position sensation

Figure 5–25. Brown-Sequard syndrome with lesion at left tenth thoracic level (motor deficits not shown).

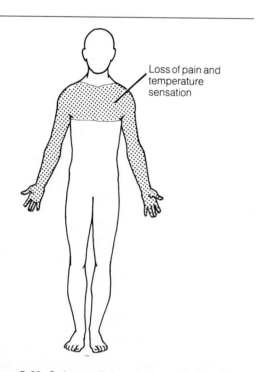

Loss of pain and temperature sensation

Figure 5–26. Syringomyelia involving the cervicothoracic portion of the spinal cord.

and temperature sense. When this occurs in the cervical region, there is a cape-like pattern of sensory loss.

The lesion may also involve the ventral gray matter, resulting in lower-motor-neuron lesions (Fig 5–27). A **cleft (syrinx)** located within the spinal cord itself is often present, although the syndrome may also be caused by abnormal enlargement of the central canal (**hydromyelia**).

Tabes dorsalis

Tabes dorsalis, a form of tertiary neurosyphilis, is characterized by damage to the dorsal roots and dorsal columns. As a result of this, there is impairment of proprioception and vibratory sensation, together with loss of deep tendon reflexes, which cannot be elicited because the Ia afferent pathway has been damaged. Patients exhibit "sensory ataxia." **Romberg's sign** (inability to maintain a steady posture with the feet close together, after the eyes are closed because of loss of proprioceptive input) is usually present. **Charcot's joints** (destruction of articular surfaces as a result of repeated injury of insensitive joints) are sometimes present. Subjective sensory disturbances known as tabetic crises consist of severe cramping pains in the stomach, larynx, or other viscera.

Brown-Sequard Syndrome

This syndrome is caused by hemisection of the spinal cord as a result of bullet or stab wounds, syringomyelia, spinal cord tumor, hematomyelia, etc. Signs and symptoms include ipsilateral lower-motor-neuron paralysis in the segment of the lesion (due to damage of lower-motor-neurons) (Fig 5–25); ipsilateral upper-motor-neuron paralysis below the level of the lesion (due to damage of the lateral corticospinal tract); an ipsilateral zone of cutaneous anesthesia in the segment of the lesion (due to damage of afferent fibers that have entered the cord and have not yet crossed); and ipsilateral loss of proprioceptive, vibratory, and two-point discrimination sense below the level of the lesion (due to damage of the dorsal columns). There is

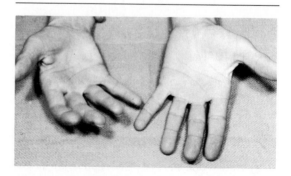

Figure 5–27. Wasting of the small muscles of the hands in a woman with syringomyelia.

also a contralateral loss of pain and temperature sense below the lesion (due to damage of the spinothalamic tracts, which have already decussated below the lesion). Hyperesthesia may be present in the segment of the lesion or below the level of the lesion, ipsilaterally, or on both sides. In practice, "pure" Brown-Sequard syndromes are rare, because most lesions of the spinal cord are irregular.

Subacute Combined Degeneration (Posterolateral Sclerosis)

Extreme deficiency in intake (or utilization) of vitamin B12 (cyanocobalamin) may result in degeneration in the dorsal and lateral white columns. There is a loss of position sense, 2-point discrimination, and vibratory sensation. Ataxic gait, muscle weakness, hyperactive deep muscle reflexes, spasticity of the extremities, and a positive Babinski sign are seen.

Spinal Shock

This syndrome results from acute transection of, or severe injury to, the spinal cord from sudden loss of stimulation from higher levels or from an overdose of spinal anesthetic. All body segments below the level of the injury become paralyzed and have no sensation; all reflexes, including autonomic reflexes, are suppressed. Spinal shock is usually transient; it may disappear in 3–6 weeks and is followed by a period of increased reflex response.

CASE 2

A 15-year-old girl was referred for evaluation of a weakness of the legs that had progressed for two weeks. Two years earlier, she had begun to have pain between the shoulder blades. The pain, which radiated into the left arm and into the middle finger of the left hand, could be accentuated by coughing, sneezing, or laughing. She had seen a chiropractor, who had manipulated the spine; however, mild pain persisted high in the back. The left leg and, more recently, the right leg had become weak and numb. In the last few days, the patient had found it difficult to start micturation.

Neurologic examination showed a minimal degree of weakness in the left upper extremity and wrist. Voluntary movement was markedly decreased in the left leg, less so in the right leg. The joints of the left leg showed increased resistance to passive motion and spasticity was present. The biceps and radial reflexes were decreased on the left but normal on the right side; knee jerk and ankle jerk reflexes were increased bilaterally. Both plantar responses were extensor. Abdominal reflexes were absent bilaterally. Pain sensation was decreased to the level of C8 bilaterally; light touch sensation was decreased to the level of C7.

Where is the lesion? What is the differential diagnosis? Which neuroradiologic procedures would be most informative? What is the most likely diagnosis?

CASE 3

A 66-year-old photographer was referred for evaluation of progressive weakness of both legs, which had started some nine months earlier. Two months previously, his arms had become weak, but to a lesser degree. The patient had recently begun to have difficulty swallowing solid food, and his friends had noted that his speech had become "thick," as though his tongue did not move. He had also lost almost 14 kg (30 lbs) during the nine-month period.

Neurologic examination showed loss of function in the muscles of facial expression, poor elevation of the uvula, a hoarse voice, and loss of mobility of the tongue. Widespread muscular atrophy was noted about the shoulders, in the intrinsic hand muscles, and in the proximal leg muscles—slightly more pronounced on the left than on the right. All four extremities showed fasciculations at rest. Strength in all extremities was poor. Cerebellar tests were normal. All reflexes were reduced and some were absent; both plantar responses were extensor. All sensory modalities were intact everywhere.

Muscle biopsy revealed various stages of denervation atrophy. What is the most likely diagnosis?

Cases are discussed further in Chapter 25.

REFERENCES

Brown AG: *Organization in the Spinal Cord.* Springer-Verlag, 1981.
Byrne TN, Waxman SG: *Spinal Cord Compression.* FA Davis, 1990.
Davidoff RA (editor): *Handbook of the Spinal Cord,* vol 1–3. Marcel Dekker, 1984.
DeMyer W: Anatomy and clinical neurology of the spinal cord. In: *Clinical Neurology,* vol 3. Baker AB, Baker LH (editors). Harper and Row, 1981.
Kuypers, HGJM: The anatomical and functional organization of the motor system. In: *Scientific Basis of Clinical Neurology.* Swash M, Kennard C (editors). Churchill Livingstone, 1985.

Rexed BA: Cytoarchitectonic atlas of the spinal cord. *J Comp Neurol* 1954;**100**:297.

Thach WT, Montgomery EB: Motor system. In: *Neurobiology of Disease.* Pearlman AL, Collins RC (editors). Oxford, 1990.

Williams PL, Warwick R: *Functional Neuroanatomy of Man.* Saunders, 1975.

Willis WD, Coggeshall RE: *Sensory Mechanisms of the Spinal Cord.* Plenum, 1978.

The Spinal Cord in Situ; Imaging

6

INVESTING MEMBRANES

Three membranes surround the spinal cord: The outermost is the dura mater (dura), the next is the arachnoid, and the innermost is the pia mater (pia) (Figs 6–1 and 6–2). The dura is also called the **pachymeninx,** and the arachnoid and pia are called the **leptomeninges.**

Dura Mater

The dura is a tough, fibrous, tubular sheath that extends from the foramen magnum to the level of the second sacral vertebra, where it ends as a blind sac (Fig 6–1). The dura of the spinal cord is continuous with the cranial dura. The epidural, or extradural, space separates the dura from the bony vertebral column; it contains loose areolar tissue and a venous plexus. The subdural space is a narrow space between the dura and the underlying arachnoid.

Arachnoid

The arachnoid is a thin, transparent sheath separated from the underlying pia by the subarachnoid space, which contains cerebrospinal fluid.

Pia Mater

The pia closely surrounds the spinal cord and sends septa into its substance. The pia also contributes to the formation of the **filum terminale internum,** a whitish fibrous filament that extends from the conus medullaris to the tip of the dural sac. The filum is surrounded by the cauda equina and both are bathed in cerebrospinal fluid. Its extradural continuation, the **filum terminale externum,** attaches at the tip of the dural sac and extends to the coccyx. The filum terminale stabilizes the cord and dura lengthwise.

Dentate Ligament

The dentate ligament is a long flange of whitish, mostly pial tissue that runs along both lateral margins of the spinal cord, between the dorsal and ventral rootlets (Fig 6–2). Its medial edge is continuous with the pia at the side of the spinal cord, and its lateral edge pierces the arachnoid at intervals (21 on each side) to attach to the inside of the dura. The dentate ligament helps to stabilize the cord from side to side. It is also an important landmark in neurosurgery.

Spinal Nerves

There are eight pairs of cervical nerves. The first seven emerge above each respective cervical vertebra; the eighth (C8) lies below vertebra C7 and above the first thoracic vertebra (Fig 6–1). Each of the other spinal nerves (T1–12, L1–5, S1–5 and—normally— two coccygeal nerves, Co1 and Co2) emerges from the intervertebral foramen below the vertebra of its type and number. The cauda equina is made up of dorsal and ventral roots from both sides of the lower cord. The composition of a typical spinal nerve (eg, a thoracic nerve) is discussed in Chapter 5.

Investment & Support of Spinal Nerves

As the ventral and dorsal roots (on each side) at each segmental level converge to become a spinal nerve, they are enclosed in sleeves of arachnoidal and dural tissue (Fig 6–2). The dorsal root sleeve contains the dorsal root ganglion near the point at which both sleeves merge to become the connective tissue sheath **(perineurium)** of a spinal nerve. The dorsal root (with its ganglion) and the ventral root of the nerve (surrounded by fat and blood vessels) course through the intervertebral foramen—except in the sacral segments, where the dorsal root ganglia lie within the sacrum itself.

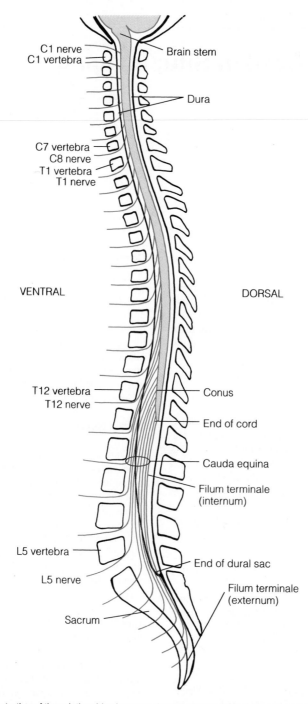

Figure 6–1. Schematic illustration of the relationships between the spinal cord, spinal nerves, and vertebral column (lateral view), showing the termination of the dura (dura mater spinalis) and its continuation as the filum terminale externum. (Compare with Fig 5–5.)

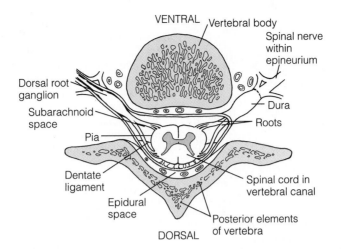

Figure 6–2. Drawing of a horizontal section through a vertebra and the spinal cord, meninges, and roots. Veins (not labeled) are shown in cross section. The vertebra and its contents are positioned as they customarily would be with CT and MR imaging procedures.

Clinical Correlations

Abnormal masses (tumor, infections, hematomas) may occur in any location in or around the spinal cord. Tumors (eg, meningiomas, neurofibromas) are often located in the intradural extramedullary compartment. Epidural masses, including bone tumors or metastases, displace the dura locally (Fig 6–3). Intradural extramedullary masses, most often in the subarachnoid space, may push the spinal cord away from the lesion and may even compress the cord against the dura, epidural space, and vertebra. Intramedullary, and therefore intradural, masses expand the spinal cord itself (see Fig 5–24). An epidural mass is usually the least difficult to remove neurosurgically; however, re-

section of an intramedullary mass is a very difficult and delicate procedure. Clinical Illustration 6–1 describes a patient with an epidural abscess.

CLINICAL ILLUSTRATION 6–1

A 61-year-old former house painter with a history of alcoholism was admitted to the medical service after being found in a hotel room in a confused state that was attributed to alcohol withdrawal syndrome. The patient did not complain of pain, but said he was weak and could not get out of bed. He had a fever. Initial neurologic examination by the intern did not reveal any focal neurologic signs. The lumbar puncture yielded CSF containing a moderate number of white blood cells and protein of about 100 mg/dl (elevated) with normal CSF glucose. Despite treatment with antibiotics the patient did not improve and neurologic consultation was obtained.

On examination by the consultant, the patient was confused and uncooperative. He stated he was weak and could not walk. Motor examination revealed flaccid paraparesis. Deep tendon reflexes were absent in the legs, and the plantar responses were extensor. The patient was not cooperative for vibratory or position sense testing. He denied feeling a pin as painful over any part of the body, but when the examiner watched for a facial wince on pinprick, a sensory level T5–T6 could be demonstrated. On gentle percussion of the spinal column, there was tenderness at T9–T10.

Imaging of the spinal column revealed an epidural mass. The patient was taken to surgery, and an epidural abscess, extending over five vertebral segments, was found. The spinal cord under the abscess was compressed and pale, probably as a result

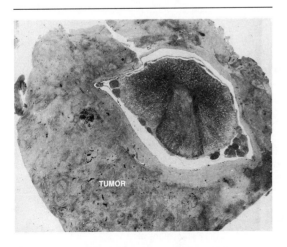

Figure 6–3. Epidural tumor in Hodgkin's disease, showing compression of the thoracic spinal cord (Weil stain). The illustration is positioned to conform with customary CT and MR imaging procedures.

of ischemia (vasospasm leading to inadequate perfusion with blood).

The motor status of this patient suggested a spinal cord lesion and this was confirmed on sensory examination. Percussion tenderness over the spine, which is often seen with epidural abscesses or tumors, provided additional evidence for disease of the spinal column. Epidural spinal cord compression is especially common in the context of neoplasms (eg, breast, prostate) that metastasize to the spine. The possibility of spinal cord compression should be considered, and the vertebral column gently percussed in any patient with a known malignancy and recent-onset or worsening back pain. Epidural spinal cord compression can be effectively treated in many patients if recognized early in its course, but if it is not diagnosed and rapidly treated, it can progress to cause irreversible paraplegia or quadriplegia. Any patient with suspected spinal cord compression, therefore, must be evaluated on an *urgent* basis.

SPINAL CORD CIRCULATION

Arteries

A. Anterior Spinal Artery: This artery is formed by the midline union of paired branches of the vertebral arteries (Figs 6–4 and 6–5). It descends along the ventral surface of the cervical spinal cord, narrowing somewhat near T4.

B. Anterior Medial Spinal Artery: This is the prolongation of the anterior spinal artery below T4.

C. Posterolateral Spinal Arteries: These arise from the vertebral arteries and course downward to the lower cervical and upper thoracic segments.

D. Radicular Arteries: Some (but not all) of the intercostal arteries from the aorta supply **segmental (radicular)** branches to the spinal cord from T1 to L1. The largest of these branches, the **great ventral radicular artery,** also known as the **arteria radicularis magna,** or **artery of Adamkiewicz,** enters the spinal cord between segments T8 and L4 (Fig 6–5). This artery usually arises on the left, and in most individuals, supplies most of the arterial blood supply for the lower half of the spinal cord. Although occlusion in this artery is rare, it results in major neurologic deficits (eg, paraplegia, loss of sensation in the legs, urinary incontinence). Some radicular arteries derived from the lumbar, iliolumbar, and lateral sacral arteries are present in the lumbosacral area. The largest of these vessels appears to enter the intervertebral foramen at vertebra L2 to form the lowermost portion of the anterior spinal artery—the terminal artery—which runs along the filum terminale.

E. Posterior Spinal Arteries: These paired arteries are much smaller than the single large anterior spinal artery; they branch at various levels to form the posterolateral arterial plexus. The posterior spinal arteries supply the dorsal white columns and the posterior portion of the dorsal gray columns.

F. Sulcal Arteries: In each segment, the branches of the radicular arteries that enter the intervertebral foramens accompany the dorsal and ventral nerve roots. These branches unite directly with the posterior and anterior spinal arteries to form an irregular ring of arteries (an **arterial corona**) with vertical connections. Sulcal arteries branch from the coronal arteries at most levels. Anterior sulcal arteries arise at various levels along the cervical and thoracic cord within the ventral sulcus (Fig 6–4); they supply the ventral and lateral columns on either side of the spinal cord.

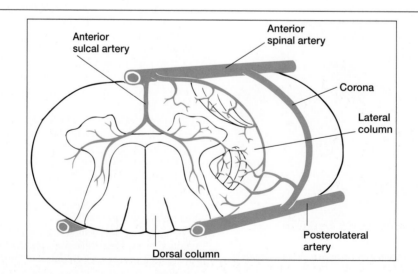

Figure 6–4. Cross section of the cervical spinal cord. The diagram shows the anterior and posterior spinal arteries with their branches and territories. There are numerous variations in the vascular supply.

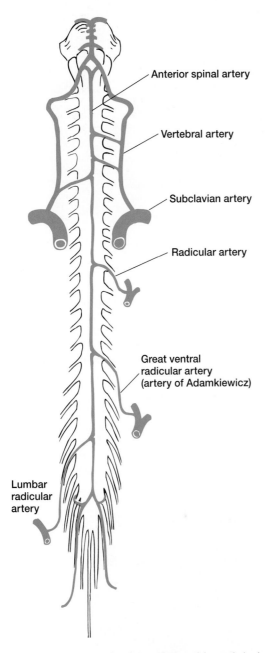

Figure 6–5. Vascularization of the spinal cord (ventral view).

- Anterior spinal artery
- Vertebral artery
- Subclavian artery
- Radicular artery
- Great ventral radicular artery (artery of Adamkiewicz)
- Lumbar radicular artery

Veins

An irregular external venous plexus lies in the epidural space; it communicates with segmental veins, basivertebral veins from the vertebral column, the basilar plexus in the head, and—by way of the pedicular veins—a smaller internal venous plexus that lies in the subarachnoid space. All venous drainage is ultimately into the venae cavae. Both plexuses extend the length of the cord.

THE VERTEBRAL COLUMN

The vertebral column consists of 33 vertebrae joined by ligaments and cartilage. The upper 24 vertebrae are separate and movable, but the lower nine are fixed: five are fused to form the sacrum, and the last four are usually fused to form the coccyx. The vertebral column consists of seven cervical (C1–7), 12 thoracic (T1–12), five lumbar (L1–5), five sacral (S1–5), and four coccygeal (Co1–4) vertebrae. In some individuals, vertebra L5 is partly or completely fused with the sacrum.

The vertebral column is slightly S-shaped when seen from the side (Fig 6–6). The cervical spine is ventrally convex, the thoracic spine ventrally concave, and the lumbar spine ventrally convex, with its curve ending at the lumbosacral angle. Ventral convexity is sometimes referred to as normal lordosis and dorsal convexity as normal kyphosis. The pelvic curve (sacrum plus coccyx) is concave downward and ventrally from the lumbosacral angle to the tip of the coccyx. The spinal column in an adult is often slightly twisted along its long axis; this is called normal scoliosis.

Clinical Correlations

Abnormal curvatures of the spine can be caused by congenital malformations (eg, congenital scoliosis) or by large intra-abdominal or intrathoracic masses. Abnormal angles may be caused by the collapse of one or more vertebral bodies as a result of trauma, infection, or tumors. Lumbar lordosis is more pronounced in late pregnancy. Thoracic kyphosis may be severe, especially in old age (this is often called dowager's hump).

Vertebrae

A typical vertebra (not C1, however) has a body and a vertebral (neural) arch that together surround the vertebral (spinal) canal (Fig 6–7). The neural arch is composed of a pedicle on each side supporting a lamina that extends posteriorly to the spinous process (spine). The pedicle has both superior and inferior notches that form the **intervertebral foramen.** Each vertebra has lateral **transverse processes** and superior and inferior **articular processes** with facets. The ventral portion of the neural arch is formed by the ventral body.

Articulation of a pair of vertebrae is body-to-body, with an intervening intervertebral disk and at the superior and inferior articular facets on both sides. The intervertebral disks help absorb stress and strain transmitted to the vertebral column. They are thicker in the more mobile cervical and lumbar areas than in the thoracic region.

Each disk contains a core of primitive gelatinous large-celled tissue, the **nucleus pulposus,** surrounded

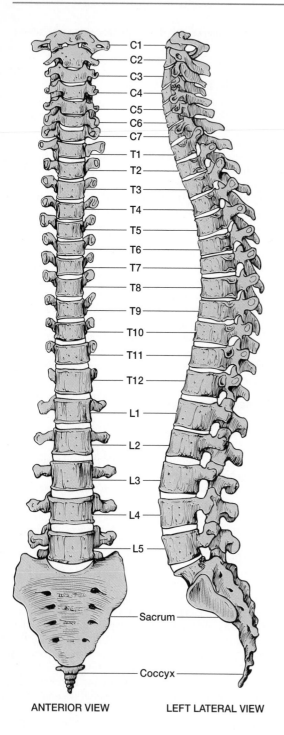

C1
C2
C3
C4
C5
C6
C7
T1
T2
T3
T4
T5
T6
T7
T8
T9
T10
T11
T12
L1
L2
L3
L4
L5

Sacrum

Coccyx

ANTERIOR VIEW   LEFT LATERAL VIEW

Figure 6–6. The vertebral column.

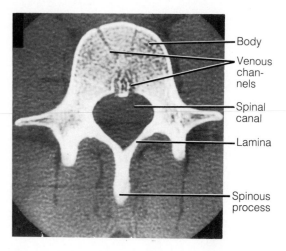

Body

Venous channels

Spinal canal

Lamina

Spinous process

Figure 6–7. CT image of a horizontal section at midlevel of vertebra L4.

by a thick **annulous fibrosus** (Fig 6–8). The disks are intimately attached to the hyaline cartilage, which covers the superior and inferior surfaces of the vertebral bodies. The water content of the disks normally decreases with age resulting in a loss of height in older individuals.

Clinical Correlations

Spina bifida results from the failure of the vertebral canal to close normally because of a defect in vertebral development. There may be associated abnormalities that are caused by defective development of the spinal

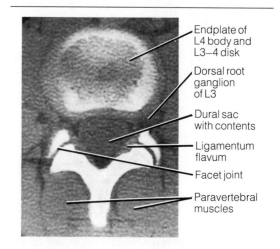

Endplate of L4 body and L3–4 disk

Dorsal root ganglion of L3

Dural sac with contents

Ligamentum flavum

Facet joint

Paravertebral muscles

Figure 6–8. CT image of a horizontal section through L4 at the level of the L3-4 intervertebral disk. (Reproduced, with permission, from deGroot J: *Correlative Neuroanatomy of Computed Tomography and Magnetic Resonance Imaging.* Lea & Febiger, 1984.)

cord, brain stem, cerebrum, or cerebellum; there may also be other developmental defects such as meningoceles, meningomyeloceles, congenital tumors, or hydrocephalus. Because the bony spinal column closes by the twelfth week of intrauterine life, these defects must originate in early intrauterine life.

There are two main types of spina bifida: spina bifida occulta, in which there is a simple defect in the closure of the vertebra, and spina bifida with meningocele or meningomyelocele, in which the defect is associated with saclike protrusions of the overlying meninges and skin that may contain portions of the spinal cord or nerve roots. Simple failure of closure of one or more vertebral arches in the lumbosacral region is a common finding on routine examination of the spine by radiography or at autopsy.

Spina bifida occulta is relatively common and is sometimes noticed as an incidental finding on roentgenographic examination of the vertebral column (Fig 6–9). The palpable bony defect, usually in the lumbar or sacral spine, is because of the failure of the laminas of the affected vertebrae to close. There may

be associated abnormalities such as fat deposits, hypertrichosis (excessive hair) over the affected area, and dimpling of the overlying skin. Symptoms may be caused by intraspinal lipomas, adhesions, bony spicules, or maldevelopment of the spinal cord.

Meningocele is herniation of the meningeal membranes through the vertebral defect. It usually causes a soft, cystic, translucent tumor to appear low in the midline of the back.

In **meningomyelocele,** nerve roots and the spinal cord protrude through the vertebral defect and usually adhere to the inner wall of the meningeal sac. If the meningomyelocele is high in the vertebral column, the clinical picture may resemble that of complete or incomplete transection of the cord, or the symptoms of combined root and spinal cord defects may resemble those of syringomyelia.

Prophylactic repair of the sac and supportive closure of the tissues over the bony defect may be performed early in life. Excision of spinal sacs containing neural elements usually produces poor results. Closure of a sac, particularly a large one, may be followed by progressive hydrocephalus (see Chapter 11).

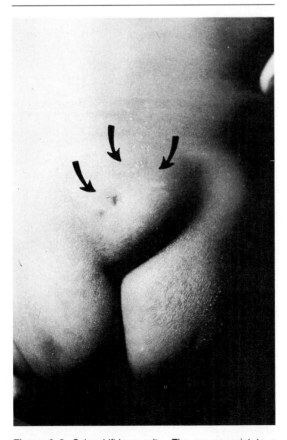

Figure 6–9. Spina bifida occulta. The arrows point to a swelling above the buttocks.

LUMBAR PUNCTURE

Location

Because the spinal cord in adults ends at the level of L1-2, a spinal (lumbar) puncture can be performed below that level—and above the sacrum—without injuring the cord.

Indications

Lumbar puncture is indicated when there is a need for chemical analysis or cytologic examination of the cerebrospinal fluid, injection of a contrast medium for radiologic examination, injection of therapeutic agents (eg, for treatment of cancer or meningitis), or injection of anesthetics. The availability of new neuroradiologic techniques (CT scanning and MR imaging) has reduced (but not eliminated) the need for lumbar puncture.

Selective sacral anesthesia (as used in obstetrics) can be achieved by injecting anesthetic into the epidural space within the sacral canal (see Fig 6–11).

Contraindications

There are few contraindications to lumbar puncture. When there is increased cranial pressure—especially when a tumor lies in the posterior fossa—spinal puncture should be done carefully or not at all, because life-threatening herniation of the cerebellum and medullary compression may follow the removal of cerebrospinal fluid. Suspected epidural abscess at the lumbar puncture site is a contraindication because the needle can introduce infection into the subarachnoid space.

Technique

Lumbar puncture is usually performed with the patient in the lateral decubitus position with legs drawn up (Fig 6–10); in this position, the manometric pressure of cerebrospinal fluid is normally 70–200 mm of water (average is 125 mm). If the puncture is done with the patient sitting upright, the fluid in the manometer normally rises to about the level of the midcervical spine (Fig 6–11). Inadvertent coughing, sneezing, or straining usually causes a prompt rise in pressure from the congestion of the spinal veins and the resultant increased pressure on the contents of the subarachnoid and epidural spaces. The pressure subsequently falls to its previous level.

After the initial pressure has been determined, 3–4 samples of 2–3 mL each are withdrawn into sterile tubes for laboratory examination. Routine examination usually includes cell counts and measurement of total protein. Cultures and special tests, such as those for sugar and chlorides, are done when indicated. The pressure is also routinely measured after the fluid is removed. In cases of spinal subarachnoid block above the puncture site, the pressure will be normal initially but will fall precipitously *after* the removal of 7–10 mL of fluid.

Other sites that reach the subarachnoid space are in the cisterna magna above the atlas or in the C1–2 space. While the latter is easily done with radiographic guidance, cisternal puncture carries a risk of injury to the brain stem.

Complications

Despite hydration of the patient before and after lumbar puncture, a severe headache may follow. The headache may be caused by the loss of fluid or leakage of fluid through the puncture site; it is characteristically relieved by lying down and exacerbated upon raising the head. Injection of the patient's own blood in the epidural space at the puncture site (blood patch) may

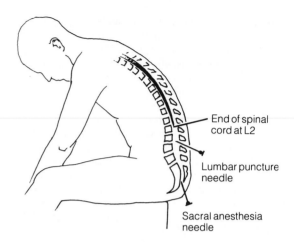

Figure 6–11. Lumbar puncture site with the patient in sitting position. The approach to the sacral hiatus for saddle-block anesthesia is also indicated.

give partial or complete relief. Serious complications, such as infection, epidural hematoma, uncal herniation, or cerebellar tonsil prolapse are very rare.

Queckenstedt's Test

Queckenstedt's test can be used to demonstrate a block in the spinal fluid compartment. The test involves compressing the jugular veins during lumbar puncture. This normally produces a prompt rise in cerebrospinal fluid pressure that lasts as long as the compression is maintained, then promptly returns to its earlier level. A moderate rise in pressure occurs when one jugular vein is compressed, and a further rise occurs when the second jugular vein is compressed. If the cerebrospinal fluid pressure fails to rise and fall promptly, it is presumed there is a block in the system

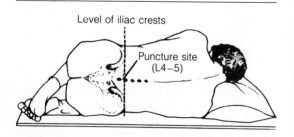

Figure 6–10. Decubitus position for lumbar puncture. (Reproduced, with permission, from Krupp MA et al: *Physician's Handbook*, 21st ed. Lange, 1985.)

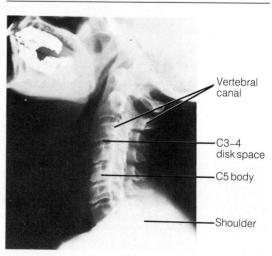

Figure 6–12. Roentgenograms through the neck (lateral view).

between the site of the puncture and the jugular vein compression. The pressure can fail to rise on compression of one jugular because of thrombosis of the lateral sinus on the same side. The absence of a rise in pressure—or a slow rise and slow fall—upon compression of both veins implies a complete or partial block in the spinal subarachnoid compartment.

Queckenstedt's test is contraindicated if intracranial bleeding or an intracranial tumor is present or suspected; the test may abruptly precipitate further bleeding or cause herniation of the cerebellar tonsils with medullary compression.

IMAGING OF THE SPINE & SPINAL CORD

The imaging methods that have been developed, particularly in the past few years, have great value in determining the precise site and extent of the involve-ment of pathologic processes in the spine and neighboring structures. (The methods themselves are discussed in detail in Chapter 23)

Roentgenography

Because roentgenograms (plain films) demonstrate the presence of calcium, various projections (antero-posterior, lateral, and oblique) of the affected area show the skeletal components of the spine and fora-mens (Figs 6–12 and 6–13). Fractures or erosions of the vertebral column's bony elements are often easily seen, but the films provide little or no information about the spinal cord or other soft tissues.

Myelography

Roentgenography after injection of a radiopaque fluid into the subarachnoid shows the contours of the vertebral canal and the size of the spinal cord and roots.

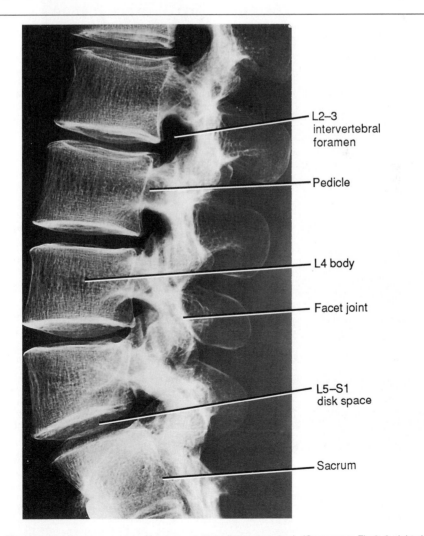

L2–3 intervertebral foramen

Pedicle

L4 body

Facet joint

L5–S1 disk space

Sacrum

Figure 6–13. Roentgenogram of lumbar vertebrae (left lateral view). (Compare to Fig 6–6, right side).

The contrast medium is usually injected via lumbar puncture but can be injected via a C1–2 puncture or a cisternal puncture (above the posterior arch of C1). Myelograms can show the defect caused by an extradural mass, eg, a herniated disk, an intradural extramedullary mass, eg, tumor, within the subarachnoid space, or an enlargement of the cord (intramedullary mass) and roots (Figs 6–14 and 6–15).

Computed Tomography (CT)

Information about the position, shape, and size of all the elements of the spine, cord, roots, ligaments, and surrounding soft tissue can be obtained by a series of thin (0.15–1 cm) transverse (axial) CT images (or scans) with or without contrast medium injected into the subarachnoid space (Figs 6–7 and 6–16). A series of transverse images can be reformed in other planes (sagittal, coronal, or oblique) to provide additional information (Fig 6–17).

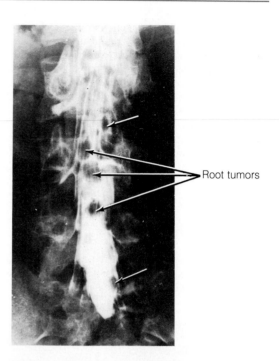

Figure 6–15. Myelogram (anteroposterior view) showing multiple root tumors (arrows) of the cauda equina in a patient with neurofibromatosis (von Recklinghausen's disease).

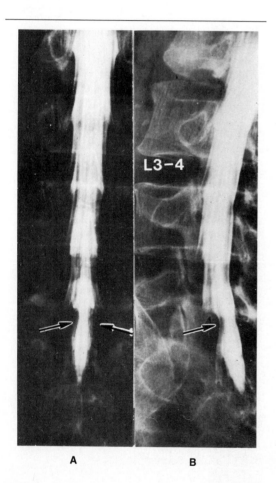

A   **B**

Figure 6–14. Myelograms of an extradural defect representing a herniated L4-5 disk. **A:** anteroposterior view. **B:** oblique view. Note amputation of L5 nerve, best seen in B.

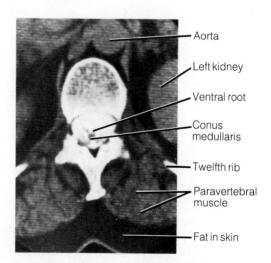

Figure 6–16. CT image of a horizontal section at the level of vertebra T12 in a 3-year-old child. The subarachnoid space was injected with contrast medium.

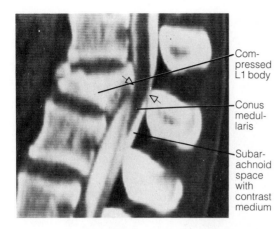

Compressed L1 body

Conus medullaris

Subarachnoid space with contrast medium

Figure 6–17. Reformatted CT image of midsagittal section of the lumbar spine of a patient who fell from a third-floor window. There is a compression fracture in the body of L1, and the lower cord is compressed between bony elements of L1 (arrows). The subarachnoid space was injected with contrast medium. (Reproduced, with permission, from Federle MP, Brant-Zawadski M [editors]. *Computed Tomography in the Evaluation of Trauma.* Williams & Wilkins, 1982.)

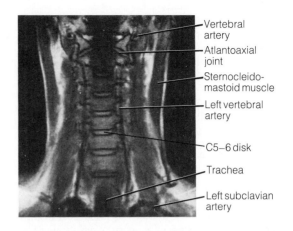

Vertebral artery

Atlantoaxial joint

Sternocleido-mastoid muscle

Left vertebral artery

C5–6 disk

Trachea

Left subclavian artery

Figure 6–19. MR image of a coronal section through the neck at the level of the cervical vertebrae. Because of the curvature of the neck, only five vertebral bodies are seen in this plane. (Reproduced, with permission, from Mills CM, de Groot J, Posin J: *Magnetic Resonance Imaging Atlas of the Head, Neck, and Spine.* Lea & Febiger, 1988.)

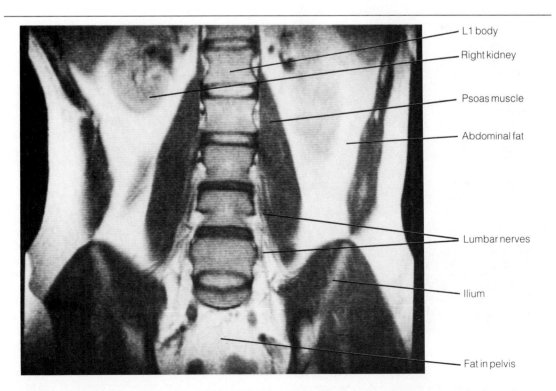

L1 body

Right kidney

Psoas muscle

Abdominal fat

Lumbar nerves

Ilium

Fat in pelvis

Figure 6–18. MR image of a coronal section through the body and (curved) lumbar spine. (Reproduced, with permission, from de-Groot J: *Correlative Neuroanatomy of Computed Tomography and Magnetic Resonance Imaging.* Lea & Febiger, 1984.)

Magnetic Resonance Imaging

Magnetic resonance imaging (MRI) can be used in any plane. It has been used, especially with sagittal images, to demonstrate the anatomy or pathology of the spinal cord and surrounding spaces and structures (Figs 6–18 to 6–21). Because the calcium of bone does not yield an MR signal, MRI is especially useful in showing suspected lesions of the soft tissues in and around the vertebral column (Figs 6–19 and 6–22).

CASE 4

A 49-year-old dock worker was reasonably healthy until he had an accident at work. A heavy piece of equipment fell high on his back, knocking him down— but not unconscious. He was unable to move his arms and legs and complained of vague shooting pains in both arms and some tingling in his right side below the axilla.

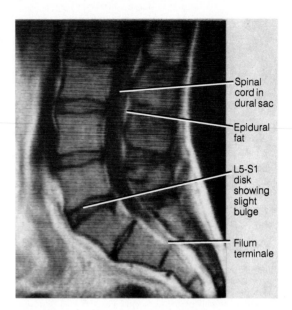

Figure 6–21. MR image of a midsagittal section through the lumbosacral vertebrae and dural sac. Note that the dural sac terminates at the level of S2. The epidural fat is clearly visible. The L5-S1 disk has degenerated and shows a slight posterior bulge.

Spinal cord in dural sac

Epidural fat

L5-S1 disk showing slight bulge

Filum terminale

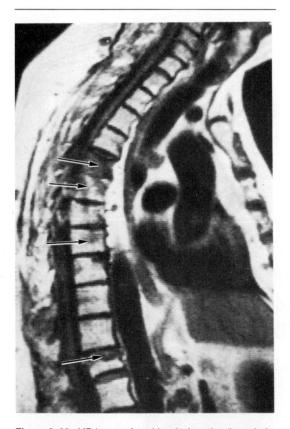

Figure 6–20. MR image of a midsagittal section through the lower neck and upper thorax of a patient with AIDS. Multiple masses are seen in the vertebral bodies at several levels (arrows): pathologic examination showed these to be malignant lymphomas.

He was transported to the emergency room, where the following neurologic abnormalities were recorded: flaccid left hemiplegia, right triceps weakness, and left extensor plantar response. Pain sensation was lost on the right side from the shoulder down, including the axilla and hand, but not the thumb.

What is the tentative diagnosis? What neuroradiologic procedure would you request to localize the lesion?

The patient underwent back surgery to correct the problem. A few days postoperatively, he regained strength in his right arm and left leg, but the left arm continued to be weak. Pain sensation was not tested at this time.

Neurologic examination three weeks later disclosed fasciculations in the left deltoid, marked weakness in the left arm, more pronounced distally, mild spasticity of the left elbow, and minimal spasticity in the left knee on passive motion. Some deep tendon reflexes—all on the left side—were increased: biceps, triceps, quadriceps, and Achilles tendon. There was a left extensor plantar response. Position and vibration senses were intact, and pain sensation was absent on the right half of the body up to the level of the clavicle.

What is the sequence of pathologic events? Where is the lesion and which neural structures are involved? Which syndrome is incompletely represented in this case? Which components of the complete syndrome are not present?

CASE 5

Two months before presentation, a 40-year-old camp counselor playing baseball sustained a minor injury, feeling a stab of pain to his lower back when he slid feet first into third base. Shortly after the incident, he noticed dull pains in the same region in the mornings; these pains seemed to subside during the day. Three weeks before presentation, he began to feel electric-shock-like pain shooting down the back of his right leg to his toes. The pain seemed to start in the right buttock and could be precipitated by coughing, sneezing, straining, or bending backward. The patient had also noticed occasional tingling of his right calf and some spasms of the back and right leg muscles.

Neurologic examination showed no impairment of muscle strength, and there were normal deep tendon reflexes in the upper extremities. The Achilles tendon reflex was absent on the right and normal on the left, and there were flexor plantar responses on both sides. All sensory modalities were intact. There was marked spasm of the right paravertebral muscles and local tenderness on palpation of the spine at L5–S1 and at the sciatic nerve in the right buttock. Straight leg raising was limited to 30 degrees on the right but normal on the left. Radiographs of the lumbar spine were normal. The patient had a 12-day period of complete bed rest, but the symptoms persisted.

What is the most likely diagnosis?

Cases are discussed further in Chapter 25. Questions and answers pertaining to Chapters 5 and 6 are found in Appendix D.

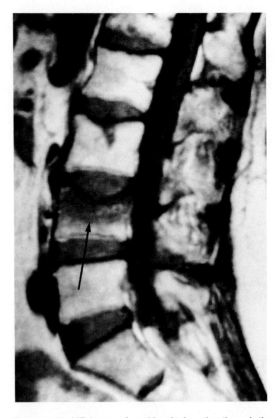

Figure 6–22. MR image of a midsagittal section through the lumbosacral spine. The mass visible in the body of L4 represents a metastasis of a colon carcinoma (arrow).

REFERENCES

Cervical Spine Research Society: *The Cervical Spine,* 2nd ed. Lippincott, 1989.

Crock HV, Yoshizawa H: *The Blood Supply of the Vertebral Column and Spinal Cord in Man.* Springer-Verlag, 1977.

Dorwart RH et al: Lumbosacral spine computed tomography. In: *Diagnostic Radiology.* Margulis AR, Gooding CA (editors). Univ of Calif Press, 1981.

Kricun ME: *Imaging Modalities in Spinal Disorders.* Saunders, 1988.

Newton TH, Potts DG (editors): *Computed Tomography of the Spine and Spinal Cord.* Clavadel Press, 1983.

Norman D, Kjos BO: MR of the spine. In: *Magnetic Resonance Imaging of the Central Nervous System.* Raven, 1987.

Rothman RH, Simeone FA: *The Spine.* Saunders, 1975.

White AA, Paujabi MM: *Clinical Biomechanics of the Spine.* Lippincott, 1978.

The Brain Stem & Cerebellum

7

DEVELOPMENT OF THE BRAIN STEM & CRANIAL NERVES

The lower part of the cranial portion of the **neural tube** (neuraxis) gives rise to the brain stem, which is divided into **mesencephalon** and **rhombencephalon** (Fig 7–1).

The primitive central canal widens into a four-sided pyramid-shape with a rhomboid floor (Fig 7–2); this becomes the **fourth ventricle,** which extends over the future pons and the medulla.

The neural tube undergoes local enlargement and shows two permanent flexures: the **cephalic flexure** at the upper end and the varying **cervical flexure** at the lower end. The cephalic flexure in an adult brain is the angle between the brain stem and the horizontal plane of the brain (see Fig 1–6).

The curved central canal in the rostral brain stem becomes the **cerebral aqueduct**. The fourth ventricle and the cerebral aqueduct contain cerebrospinal fluid and are lined by ependyma. The roof of the rostral fourth ventricle undergoes intense cellular proliferation, and this lip produces the neurons and glia that will populate both the cerebellum and the **inferior olivary nucleus.**

The quadrigeminal plate, the midbrain tegmentum, and the cerebral peduncles develop from the **mesencephalon** (midbrain; Fig 7–1), and the cerebral aqueduct courses through it. The **rhombencephalon** (Fig 7–1A) gives rise to the metencephalon and the myelencephalon. The **metencephalon** forms the cerebellum and pons; it contains part of the fourth ventricle. The **myelencephalon** forms the medulla oblongata; the lower part of the fourth ventricle lies within this portion of the brain stem.

As in the spinal cord, the embryonic brain stem has a central gray core with an **alar plate** (consisting mostly of sensory components) and a **basal plate** (mostly motor components). The gray columns are not continuous in the brain stem, however, and the development of the fourth ventricle causes wide lateral displacement of the alar plate in the lower brain stem. The basal plate takes the shape of a hinge (Fig 7–2). The process is reversed at the other end, resulting in the rhomboid shape of the floor of the fourth ventricle. In addition, long tracts, short neuronal connections, and nuclei become apposed to the brain stem. The cranial nerves, like the spinal nerves, take their origin from the basal plate cells (motor nerves) or from synapses in the alar plate cell groups (sensory nerves). Unlike spinal nerves, however, most cranial nerves emerge as one or more bundles of fibers from the basal or basilateral aspect of the brain stem (Figs 7–1 and 7–3). In addition, not all cranial nerves are mixed; ie, some have only sensory components and others have only motor components (see Chapter 8).

ORGANIZATION OF THE BRAIN STEM

Main Divisions & External Landmarks

Three major external divisions of the brain stem are recognizable: the medulla (medulla oblongata or myelencephalon), a transition to the spinal cord; the pons (metencephalon together with the cerebellum); and the midbrain (mesencephalon) (Figs 7–3 and 7–4). The three internal longitudinal divisions of the brain stem are the **tectum** (mainly in the midbrain), **tegmentum,** and **basis** (Fig 7–4). The main external structures, seen from the dorsal aspect, are shown in Figure 7–5. The superior portion of the rhomboid fossa (which forms the floor of the fourth ventricle) extends over the pons, while the inferior portion covers the open portion of the medulla. The closed medulla forms the transition to the spinal cord.

Three pairs of **cerebellar peduncles** (inferior, middle, and superior) form connections with the cerebellum. The dorsal aspect of the midbrain shows four hillocks: the two **superior** and the two **inferior colliculi,** together called the **corpora quadrigemina.**

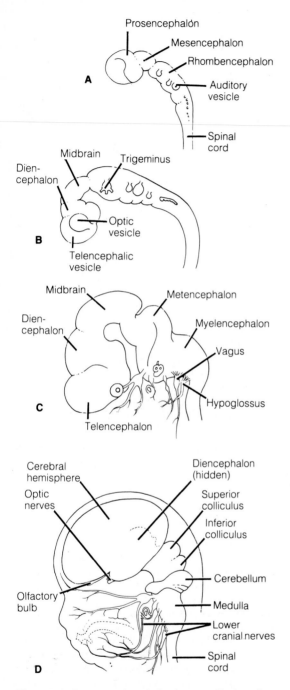

Figure 7–1. Four stages in early development of brain and cranial nerves (times are approximate). *A:* 3½ weeks, *B:* 4½ weeks, *C:* 7 weeks, *D:* 11 weeks.

Internal Structural Components

Although the brain stem is a relatively small structure, it contains much that is essential for normal brain function—indeed for normal body function. Internal structural components include the following:

A. Descending and Ascending Tracts: All descending tracts that terminate in the spinal cord, eg, the corticospinal tract (see Chapter 5) pass through the brain stem; in addition, several descending fiber systems terminate or originate in the brain stem. Similarly, all ascending tracts, eg, the spinothalamic tracts, that reach the brain stem or the cerebral cortex pass through part or all of this region; other ascending tracts originate in the brain stem. The brain stem is, therefore, an important conduit or relay station for many longitudinal pathways, both descending and ascending (Table 7–1).

B. Cranial Nerve Nuclei: Almost all the cranial nerve nuclei are located in the brain stem (the exceptions are the first two nuclei, which are evaginations of the brain itself). Portions of the cranial nerves also pass through the brain stem.

C. Cerebellar Peduncles: The pathways to and from the cerebellum pass through three pairs of cerebellar peduncles as described in the section on the cerebellum (see below).

D. Descending Autonomic System Pathways: These paths to the spinal cord pass through the brain stem (see also Chapter 20).

E. Reticular Formation: Several of these areas in the tegmentum of the brain stem are vitally involved in the control of respiration, cardiovascular system functions, and states of consciousness, sleep, and alertness (see also Chapter 18).

F. Monoaminergic Pathways: These paths can be divided into three systems: the **serotoninergic** pathways from the raphe nuclei (see also Chapter 3); the **noradrenergic** pathways in the lateral reticular formation and the extensive efferents from the locus ceruleus; and the **dopaminergic** pathway from the basal midbrain to the basal ganglia and others.

G. Cerebrospinal Fluid Pathway: This passes through the brain stem and reaches the subarachnoid space through openings in the fourth ventricle (see also Chapter 11).

CRANIAL NERVE NUCLEI IN THE BRAIN STEM

The functional composition of the lower 10 cranial nerves can best be analyzed by referring to the development of their nuclei (Fig 7–6). The nerves are usually referred to by name or by roman numeral (Table 7–2).

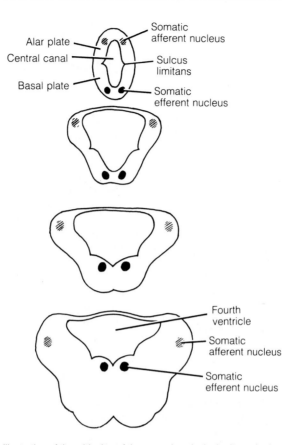

Figure 7–2. Schematic illustration of the widening of the central cavity in the lower brain stem during development.

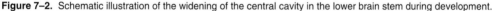

Motor Components

Three types of basal plate derivatives (motor nuclei) can be found in the brain stem (Table 7–2).

General somatic efferent (SE or GSE) components innervate striated muscles that are derived from somites and are involved with movements of the tongue and eyeballs such as the hypoglossal nucleus of XII, oculomotor nucleus of III, trochlear nucleus of IV, and abducens nucleus of VI.

Branchial efferent (BE) components, sometimes referred to as **special visceral efferents (SVE),** innervate muscles that are derived from the branchial arches and are involved in chewing, making facial expressions, swallowing, producing vocal sounds, and turning the head, for example, the masticatory nucleus of V; facial nucleus of VII; ambiguous nucleus of IX, X, and XI; and spinal accessory nucleus of XI located in the cord.

General visceral efferent (VE or GVE) components are parasympathetic preganglionic components that provide autonomic innervation of smooth muscles and the glands in the head, neck, and torso, eg, the Edinger-Westphal nucleus of III, superior salivatory nucleus of VII, inferior salivatory nucleus of IX, and dorsal motor nucleus of X.

Sensory Components

Two types of alar-plate derivatives can be distinguished in the brain stem and are comparable to similar cell groups in the spinal cord (Table 7–2).

General somatic afferent (SA or GSA) components receive and relay sensory stimuli from the skin and mucosa of most of the head: main sensory, descending, and mesencephalic nuclei of V.

General visceral afferent (VA or GVA) components relay sensory stimuli from the viscera and more specialized taste stimuli from the tongue and epiglottis: solitary nucleus for visceral input from IX and X and gustatory nucleus for special visceral taste fibers from VII, IX, and X.

Six **special sensory (SS) nuclei** can also be distinguished: the four vestibular and two cochlear nuclei that receive stimuli via vestibulocochlear nerve VIII.

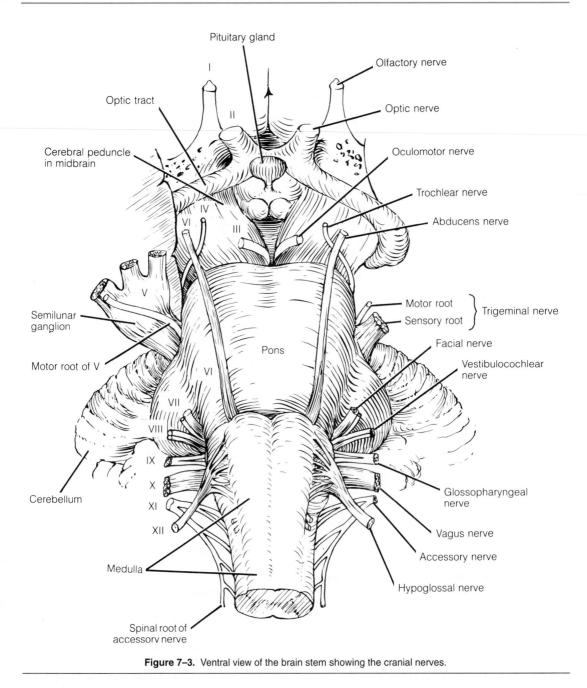

Figure 7–3. Ventral view of the brain stem showing the cranial nerves.

These nuclei are derived from the primitive auditory placode in the rhombencephalon (Fig 7–1A).

Differences between Typical Spinal & Cranial Nerves

It is apparent that the simple and regular pattern of functional fiber components in spinal nerves is not found in cranial nerves. A single cranial nerve may contain one or more functional components; conversely, a single nucleus may contribute to the forma-tion of one or more cranial nerves. Although some cranial nerves are solely efferent, most are mixed, and some contain many visceral components. The cranial nerves are described in detail in Chapter 8.

MEDULLA

The medulla (medulla oblongata) can be divided into a caudal (closed; Fig 7–7B) portion and a rostral

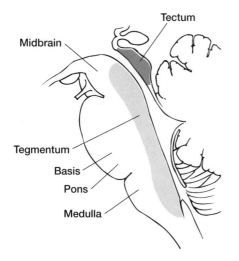

Figure 7–4. Drawing of the divisions of the brain stem in a mid-sagittal plane. The major internal longitudinal divisions are the tectum, tegmentum, and basis. The major external divisions are the midbrain, pons, and medulla.

Table 7–1. Major ascending and descending pathways in the brain stem.

Ascending	Descending
Medial lemniscus	Corticospinal tract
Spinothalamic tract	Corticonuclear tract
Trigeminal lemniscus	Corticopontine fibers
Lateral lemniscus	Rubrospinal tract
Reticular system fibers	Tectospinal tract
Medial longitudinal fasciculus	Medial longitudinal fasciculus
Inferior cerebellar peduncle	Vestibulospinal tract
Superior cerebellar peduncle	Reticulospinal tract
Secondary vestibulary fibers	Central tegmental tract
Secondary gustatory fibers	Descending tract of nerve V

(open; Fig 7–7C) portion, based on the absence or presence of the lower fourth ventricle.

Ascending Tracts

In the closed medulla, the relay nuclei of the dorsal column pathway (nucleus gracilis and nucleus cunea-

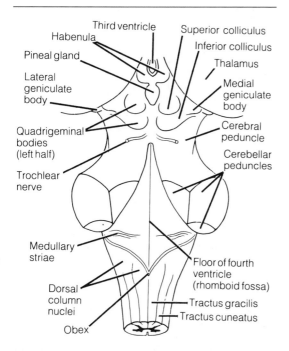

Figure 7–5. Dorsolateral aspect of the brain stem (cerebellum removed).

tus) give rise to a crossed fiber bundle, the **medial lemniscus.** The lower part of the body is represented in the ventral portion of the lemniscus and the upper part of the body in the dorsal. The **spinothalamic tract** (which crossed at spinal cord levels) continues upward throughout the medulla, as do the **spinoreticular tract** and the **ventral spinocerebellar pathway.** The **dorsal spinocerebellar tract** and the **cuneocerebellar tract** continue into the inferior cerebellar peduncle.

Descending Tracts

The **corticospinal tract** in the pyramid begins to cross at the transition between medulla and spinal cord; this decussation takes place over several millimeters. Most of the axons in this tract arise in the motor cortex. Some fibers from the corticospinal tract, which originate in the sensory cerebral cortex, end in the dorsal column nuclei and may modify their function. The **descending spinal tract of V** has its cell bodies, representing all three divisions of this tract, in the trigeminal ganglion. The fibers of the tract convey pain, temperature, and crude touch sensations from the face to the first relay station, the **spinal nucleus of V,** or pars caudalis. The mandibular division is represented dorsally in the nucleus, and the ophthalmic division is represented ventrally. A second-order pathway arises from the cells in the spinal nucleus and then crosses and ascends in a diffuse bundle to end in the thalamus.

The **medial longitudinal fasciculus** is an important pathway involved with control of gaze and head movements. It descends into the cervical cord. The medial longitudinal fasciculus arises in the vestibular nuclei and carries vestibular influences downward (see Fig 17–2). More rostrally in the pons, the medial longitudinal fasciculus carries projections rostrally from the vestibular nuclei to the abducens, trochlear, and oculomotor nuclei, and from the lateral gaze center in the pons to the oculomotor nuclei (see Fig 8–7).

The **tectospinal tract carries** descending axons from the superior colliculus in the midbrain to the cer-

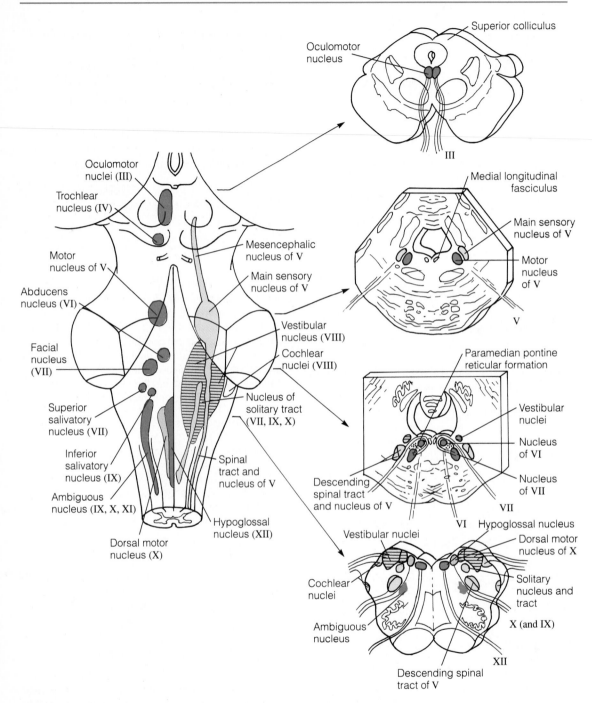

Figure 7–6. Cranial nerve nuclei. *Left:* Dorsal view of the human brain stem with the positions of the cranial nerve nuclei projected upon the surface. Motor nuclei are on the left; sensory nuclei are on the right. *Right:* Transverse sections at the levels indicated by the arrows.

Table 7–2. Cranial nerves and nuclei in the brain stem.

Name	Nerve	Nuclei
Oculomotor	III	Oculomotor, Edinger-Westphal
Trochlear	IV	Trochlear
Trigeminal	V	Main sensory, spinal (descending), mesencephalic, motor (masticatory)
Abducens	VI	Abducens
Facial	VII	Facial, superior salivatory, gustatory (solitary)*
Vestibulocochlear	VIII	Cochlear (2 nuclei), vestibular (4 nuclei)
Glossopharyngeus	IX	Ambiguous,† inferior salivatory, solitary*
Vagus	X	Dorsal motor, ambiguous,† solitary*
Accessory	XI	Spinal accessory (C1-C5), ambiguous†
Hypoglossal	XII	Hypoglossal

* The solitary nucleus is shared by nerves VII, IX, and X.
† The ambiguous nucleus is shared by nerves IX, X, and XI.

vical spinal cord. It presumably relays impulses controlling neck and trunk movements in response to visual stimuli.

Cranial Nerve Nuclei

The hypoglossal nucleus, the dorsal motor nucleus of the vagus, and the solitary tract and nucleus are found in the medulla, grouped around the central canal; in the open medulla, these nuclei lie below the fourth ventricle (Fig 7–7C). The **hypoglossal nucleus,** which is homologous to the anterior horn nucleus in the cord, sends its fibers ventrally between the pyramid and inferior olivary nucleus to exit as nerve XII. This nerve innervates all the tongue muscles.

The **dorsal motor nucleus of X** is a preganglionic parasympathetic nucleus that sends its fibers laterally into nerves IX and X. It controls parasympathetic tone in the heart, lungs, and the abdominal viscera. The **superior salivatory nucleus,** located just rostral to the dorsal motor nucleus, gives rise to parasympathetic axons that project in nerve VII, via the submandibular and pterygopalative ganglia, to the submandibular and sublingual glands and the lacrimal apparatus. This nucleus controls salivary secretion and lacrimation.

The ill-defined **nucleus ambiguous** gives rise to the branchial efferent axons in nerves IX and X and controls swallowing and vocalization.

The **solitary nucleus** is an elongated sensory nucleus in the medulla that receives axons from nerves VII, IX, and X. It is located adjacent to the **solitary tract,** which contains the terminating axons of these nerves. The ros-

tral part of the solitary nucleus is sometimes referred to as the **gustatory nucleus.** The solitary nucleus conveys information about taste and visceral sensations. Secondary fibers ascend from the solitary nucleus to the VPM nucleus in the thalamus, which projects, in turn, to the cortical area for taste (area 43, located near the operculum).

The four **vestibular nuclei**—superior, inferior (or spinal), medial, and lateral—are found under the floor of the fourth ventricle, partly in the open medulla and partly in the pons. The ventral and dorsal **cochlear nuclei** are relay nuclei for fibers that arise in the spiral ganglion of the cochlea. The pathways of the vestibular and cochlear nuclei are discussed in Chapters 16 and 17.

Inferior Cerebellar Peduncle

The neuroanatomic definition of **peduncle** is a visibly well-defined, stalk-like bundle of nerve fibers containing one or more axon tracts.

The inferior cerebellar peduncle is formed in the open medulla from several components: the cuneocerebellar and the dorsal spinocerebellar tracts, fibers from the lateral reticular nucleus, olivocerebellar fibers from the contralateral inferior olivary nucleus, fibers from the vestibular division of nerve VIII, and fibers that arise in the vestibular nuclei. All fibers are afferent to the cerebellum.

PONS

Many pathways to and from the medulla and several spinal cord tracts are identifiable in cross sections of the pons (Figs 7–7D, E).

Basis Pontis

The base of the pons (basis pontis) contains three components: fiber bundles of the corticospinal tracts, **pontine nuclei** that have received input from the cerebral cortex by way of the corticopontine pathway, and pontocerebellar fibers from the pontine nuclei, which cross to most of the neocerebellum by way of the large middle cerebellar peduncle. Along the midline of the pons and part of the medulla lie the **raphe nuclei.** Serotonin-containing neurons in these nuclei project widely to the cortex and hippocampus, basal ganglia, thalamus, cerebellum, and spinal cord. These cells are important in controlling the level of arousal and modulate sleep/wakefulness. They also modulate sensory input, particularly for pain.

Tegmentum

The tegmentum of the pons is more complex than the base. The lower pons contains the nucleus of nerve VI (abducens nucleus) and the nuclei of nerve VII (the facial, superior salivatory, and gustatory nuclei). The

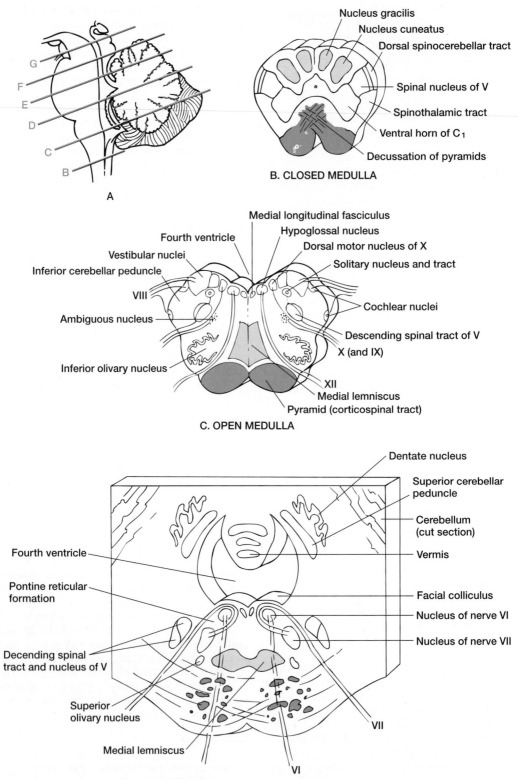

B. CLOSED MEDULLA

- Nucleus gracilis
- Nucleus cuneatus
- Dorsal spinocerebellar tract
- Spinal nucleus of V
- Spinothalamic tract
- Ventral horn of C₁
- Decussation of pyramids

C. OPEN MEDULLA

- Medial longitudinal fasciculus
- Hypoglossal nucleus
- Dorsal motor nucleus of X
- Solitary nucleus and tract
- Fourth ventricle
- Vestibular nuclei
- Inferior cerebellar peduncle
- VIII
- Ambiguous nucleus
- Cochlear nuclei
- Descending spinal tract of V
- X (and IX)
- Inferior olivary nucleus
- XII
- Medial lemniscus
- Pyramid (corticospinal tract)

D. LOWER PONS; level of nerves VI and VII

- Dentate nucleus
- Superior cerebellar peduncle
- Cerebellum (cut section)
- Vermis
- Fourth ventricle
- Pontine reticular formation
- Facial colliculus
- Nucleus of nerve VI
- Nucleus of nerve VII
- Decending spinal tract and nucleus of V
- Superior olivary nucleus
- VII
- Medial lemniscus
- VI

Figure 7–7. A: Key to levels of sections. **B–G:** Schematic transverse sections through the brain stem. The corticospinal tracts and the dorsal column nuclei/medial lemnisci are shown in color so they can be followed as they course through the brain stem.

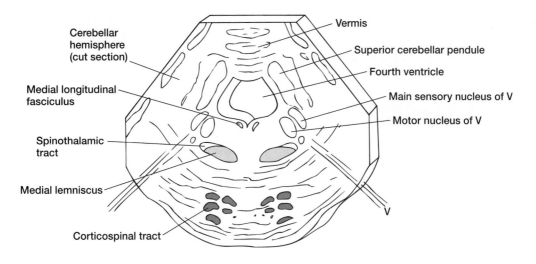

E. MIDDLE PONS; level of nerve V

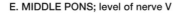

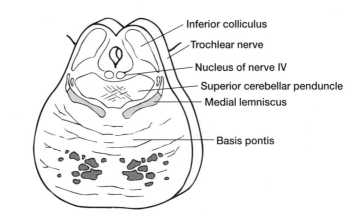

F. PONS/MIDBRAIN; level of nucleus VI

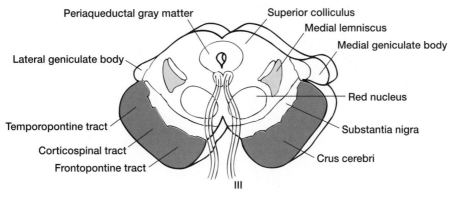

G. UPPER MIDBRAIN; level of nerve III

Figure 7–7 (continued)

branchial motor component of the facial nerve loops medially around the nucleus of nerve VI. The upper half of the pons harbors the main sensory nuclei of nerve V (Figs 7–7E and 7–8). The medial lemniscus assumes a different position (lower body, medial; upper body, lateral), and the spinothalamic tract courses even more laterally.

The **central tegmental tract** (which contains descending fibers from the midbrain to the inferior olivary nucleus and ascending fibers that run from the brain stem reticular formation to the thalamus) runs dorsolateral to the medial lemniscus. The **tectospinal tract** (from midbrain to cervical cord) and the **medial longitudinal fasciculus** are additional components of the pontine tegmentum.

Middle Cerebellar Peduncle

The middle cerebellar peduncle is the largest of the three cerebellar peduncles on each side of the brain stem. It contains numerous fibers that arise from the contralateral basis of the pons and end in the cerebellar hemisphere.

Auditory Pathways

The auditory system from the cochlear nuclei in the pontomedullary junction consists of fibers that ascend ipsilaterally in the lateral lemniscus (see also Chapter 16). It also includes crossing fibers (the trapezoid body) that ascend in the opposite lateral lemniscus. A small **superior olivary nucleus** sends fibers into the cochlear division of nerve VIII as the olivocochlear bundle (Fig 7–7D); this pathway modifies the input from the organ of Corti in the cochlea.

Trigeminal System

The three divisions of the **trigeminal nerve** (nerve V; Figs 7–7D, E, and Fig 7–8) all project to the brain

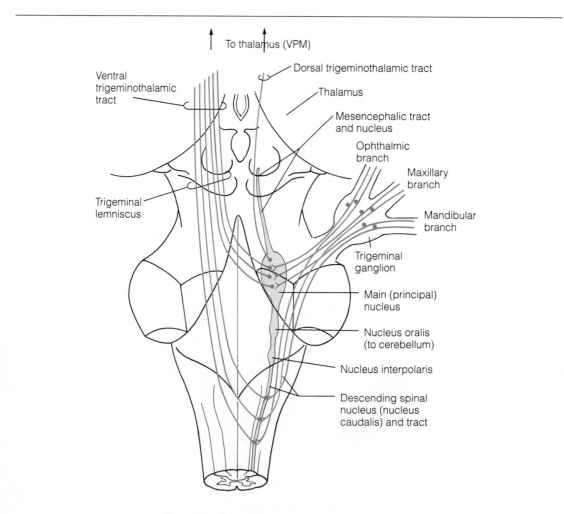

Figure 7–8. Schematic drawing of the trigeminal system.

stem: Fine touch function is relayed by the **main sensory nucleus;** pain and temperature are relayed into the **descending spinal tract of V;** and proprioceptive fibers form a **mesencephalic tract and nucleus** in the midbrain. Some first-order nuclei of this system are found within the brain stem rather than in the trigeminal ganglion itself. The second-order neurons from the main sensory nucleus cross and ascend to the thalamus. The descending spinal tract of V sends fibers to the pars caudalis (the spinal nucleus in the medulla), the pars interpolaris (a link between trigeminal afferent components and the cerebellum), and the pars oralis. The **masticatory nucleus,** which is medial to the main sensory nucleus, sends branchial efferent fibers into the mandibular division of nerve V to innervate most of the muscles of mastication and the tensor tympani of the middle ear.

MIDBRAIN

The midbrain forms a transition (and fiber conduit) to the cerebrum (Figs 1–2, 1–3, and 7–10).

Basis

The base of the midbrain contains the **crus cerebri,** a massive fiber bundle that includes corticospinal, corticobulbar, and corticopontine pathways (Figs 7–7G and 7–9). The base also contains the **substantia nigra.** The substantia nigra (whose cells contain neuromelanin) receives afferent fibers from the cerebral cortex and the striatum; it sends dopaminergic efferent fibers

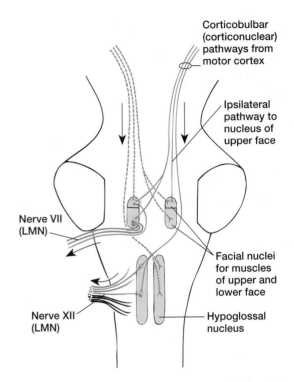

Figure 7–10. Corticobulbar pathways to the nuclei of cranial nerves VII and XII. Notice that the facial nucleus for muscles of the upper face receives descending input from the motor cortex on both sides, whereas the facial nucleus for lower facial muscles receives input from only the contralateral cortex.

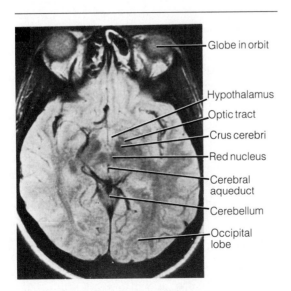

Figure 7–9. Magnetic resonance image of a horizontal section through the head at the level of the midbrain. Note that the position of the midbrain is reversed from that in Fig 7–7G.

to the striatum. The substantia nigra plays a key role in motor control. Degeneration of the substantia nigra occurs in Parkinson's disease (see Chapter 21). The external aspect of the basis of the midbrain is called the **cerebral peduncle.**

The **corticobulbar fibers** from the motor cortex to interneurons of the efferent nuclei of cranial nerves are homologous with the corticospinal fibers (Fig 7–10). The corticobulbar fibers to the lower portion of the facial nucleus and the hypoglossal nucleus are crossed (from the opposite cerebral cortex). All other corticobulbar projections are bilaterally crossed (from both cortices).

Between the cerebral peduncles, in the **interpeduncular fossa,** exit the fibers of the oculomotor (III) nerve. On the other side of the midbrain, the tegmentum, exit the fibers of the trochear (IV) nerve.

Tegmentum

The tegmentum of the midbrain contains all the ascending tracts from the spinal cord or lower brain stem and many of the descending systems. A large and richly vascularized **red nucleus** receives crossed efferent fibers from the cerebellum and sends fibers to the thalamus and the contralateral spinal cord via the rubrospinal tract. The red nucleus is an important component of motor coordination.

Two contiguous somatic efferent nuclear groups lie in the upper tegmentum: the **trochlear nucleus** (which forms contralateral nerve IV) and the **oculomotor nuclei** (which have efferent fibers in nerve III). Each eye muscle innervated by the oculomotor nerve has its own subgroup of innervating cells; the subgroup for the superior rectus muscle is contralateral while the others are ipsilateral to the innervated muscle. The preganglionic parasympathetic system destined for the eye (a synapse in the ciliary ganglion) has its origin in or near the Edinger-Westphal nucleus.

Close to the periventricular gray lie the bilateral **locus ceruleus** nuclei. Neurons in these nuclei contain norepinephrine and project widely to the cortex, hippocampus, thalamus, midbrain, cerebellum, pons, medulla, and spinal cord. The axons of these neurons branch widely and, thus, constitute a diffuse projection. These neurons regulate the sleep/wake cycle and control arousal; they may also modulate the sensitivity of sensory nuclei.

Tectum

The tectum, or roof, of the midbrain is formed by two pairs of colliculi and the **corpora quadrigemina.** The **superior colliculi** contain neurons that receive visual as well as other input and serve ocular reflexes; the **inferior colliculi** are involved in auditory reflexes and in determining the side on which a sound originates. The inferior colliculi receive input from both ears, and they project to the medial geniculate nucleus of the thalamus by way of the **inferior quadrigeminal brachium.** The **superior quadrigeminal brachium** links the lateral geniculate nucleus and the superior colliculus. The colliculi contribute to the formation of the crossed tectospinal tracts, which are involved in blinking and head-turning reflexes following sudden sounds or visual images.

Periaqueductal Gray Matter

The periaqueductal gray matter contains descending autonomic tracts as well as endorphin-producing cells that suppress pain. This region has been used as the target for brain-stimulating implants used in patients suffering from chronic pain.

Superior Cerebellar Peduncle

The superior cerebellar peduncle contains efferent fibers from the dentate nucleus of the cerebellum to the opposite red nucleus (the dentato-rubro-thalamic sys-

tem) and the ventral spinocerebellar tracts. The cerebellar fibers decussate just below the red nuclei.

VASCULARIZATION

The vessels that supply the brain stem are branches of the vertebrobasilar system (Fig 7–11; see also Chapter 12). Those classified as **circumferential vessels** are the posterior inferior cerebellar artery, the anterior inferior cerebellar artery, the superior cerebellar artery, the posterior cerebral artery, and the pontine artery. Each of these vessels sends small branches (a few or many) into the underlying brain stem structures along its course. Other vessels are classified as **median (paramedian) perforators,** because they penetrate the brain stem from the basilar artery. The small medullary and spinal branches of the vertebral artery make up a third group of vessels.

Lesions of the Brain Stem

The brain stem is an anatomically compact, functionally diverse, and clinically important structure. Even a single, relatively small lesion nearly always damages several nuclei, reflex centers, tracts, or pathways. Such lesions are often vascular in nature (eg, infarct or hemorrhage), but tumors, trauma, and degenerative or demyelinating processes can also injure the brain stem. The following are typical syndromes

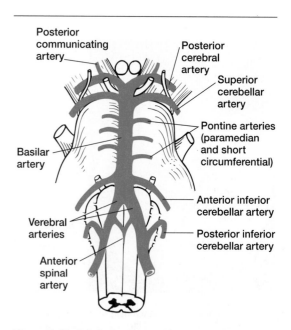

Figure 7–11. Principal arteries of the brain stem (ventral view).

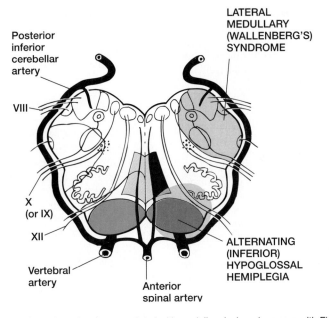

Figure 7–12. Clinical syndromes associated with medullary lesions (compare with Fig 7–7C).

caused by intrinsic (intra-axial) lesions of the brain stem.

Medial (basal) medullary syndrome usually involves the pyramid, part or all of the medial lemniscus, and nerve XII. If it is unilateral, it is also known as **alternating hypoglossal hemiplegia** (Fig 7–12); the term refers to the finding that the cranial-nerve weakness is on the same side as the lesion, while the body paralysis is on the opposite side. Larger lesions can result in bilateral defects. The area involved is supplied by the anterior spinal artery or by medial branches of the vertebral artery.

Lateral medullary, or **Wallenberg's syndrome,** involves some (or all) of the following structures in the open medulla on the dorsolateral side (Fig 7–12): inferior cerebellar peduncle, vestibular nuclei, fibers or nuclei of nerve IX or X, spinal nucleus and tract of V, spinothalamic tract, and sympathetic pathways. (Involvement of the sympathetic pathways may lead to Horner's syndrome). The affected area is supplied by branches of the vertebral artery or, most commonly, the posterior inferior cerebellar artery. An example is provided in Clinical Illustration 7–1.

CLINICAL ILLUSTRATION 7–1

A 49-year-old landscape artist, who had visited many countries in Europe, Asia, and Africa, was admitted to the hospital because of a sudden onset of facial numbness, ataxia, vertigo, nausea, and vomiting. Examination revealed impaired sensation over the left half of the face. The arm and leg on the left side were clumsy, and there was an intention tremor on the left. A left-sided Horner's syndrome [myosis (a constricted pupil), ptosis (a weak, droopy eyelid), and decreased sweating over the forehead] was apparent. There was subjective numbness of the right arm, although no abnormalities could be detected on examination. Over the ensuing 12 hours, he developed difficulty swallowing and complained of intractable hiccups. Vibratory and position sense were now impaired in the left arm, the vocal cord was paralyzed, and the gag reflex was diminished. On the right side, there was impaired pain and temperature sensibility. MRI demonstrated an abnormality, presumably infarction, in the lateral medulla on the left side, and a presumptive diagnosis of Wallenberg's syndrome (lateral medullary syndrome) on the basis of occlusion of the posterior inferior cerebellar artery was made.

Arteriography, carried out on an emergency basis, revealed occlusion of the posterior inferior cerebellar artery with "beading" (evidence of inflammation) of vertebral arteries and anterior inferior cerebellar arteries. Lumbar puncture revealed 40 white blood cells (mostly lymphocytes) per cc of CSF. Serologic testing of the CSF and serum was positive for syphilis. The patient was treated with intravenous penicillin. Over the ensuing six months, many of his deficits resolved, and he resumed his activities including his painting.

This case illustrates the development of the lateral medullary syndrome (Wallenberg's syndrome) as a result of occlusion of the posterior inferior cerebellar artery. Because so many structures are packed closely together in the relatively small brain stem, occlusion of even relatively small arteries, such as the posterior inferior cerebellar arteries, can have profound effects.

In this case, examination of CSF revealed that vascular occlusion was due to syphilitic arteritis, a form of tertiary neurosyphilis. Although neurosyphilis is now rare as a result of the availability of antibiotics, meningovascular syphilis was a common cause of brain stem strokes in the pre-antibiotic era. In evaluating strokes, particularly in young patients, it is essential to consider *all* of the disorders that can lead to cerebrovascular compromise. In this case, treatment with penicillin arrested the patient's neurosyphilis and may have prevented further cerebrovascular events. A significant degree of functional recovery, as seen in this patient, is often observed after brain stem strokes and presumably reflects reorganization of neural circuits controlling swallowing as well as related activities.

Basal pontine syndromes can involve both the corticospinal tract and a cranial nerve (VI, VII, or V) in the affected region, depending on the extent and level of the lesion (Fig 7–13). The syndrome is called **alternating abducens (VI),** facial (V), or trigeminal hemiplegia (V). If the lesion is large, it may include the medial lemniscus. The vascular supply comes from the perforators, or pontine branches, of the anterior inferior cerebellar artery.

The **locked-in syndrome** results from large lesions of the basal pons which interrupt the corticobulbar and corticospinal pathways bilaterally, thus interfering with speech, facial expression, and the capacity to activate most muscles. These large lesions are usually due to infarcts or hemorrhages. Somatosensory pathways and the reticular system are usually spared so that the patient remains awake and aware of his surroundings. Eye movements are often spared. Patients often, therefore, can communicate via a crude code in this tragic syndrome and can survive in this state for years. An example is provided in Clinical Illustration 7–2.

CLINICAL ILLUSTRATION 7–2

A 53-year-old architect led a productive life until he developed, over several hours, weakness in his arms and legs together with double vision and difficulty swallowing. He was taken to the hospital where examination revealed weakness and hyperreflexia of the arms and legs, bilateral Babinski responses, facial weakness on both sides, and dysphagia. Lateral gaze was limited and nystagmus was present. A provisional diagnosis of basilar artery thrombosis was made. Arteriography confirmed this diagnosis.

Over the next two days, despite aggressive treatment, the patient's deficits progressed. He developed total paralysis of all extremities and marked weakness of the face. As a result of weakness of the bulbar musculature, swallowing was impaired, and the patient could not protrude his tongue. Lateral eye movements were impaired, but vertical eye movements were maintained. The patient remained awake, with apparently preserved mentation. He was able to communicate using eye blinks and vertical eye movements. Sensation, tested via simple yes-no questions answered with eye blinks, appeared to be intact. MRI demonstrated a large infarct involving the base of the pons. The patient remained in this state, apparently alert and communicating with friends and family via eye blinks, for the next five months. He died following a cardiopulmonary arrest.

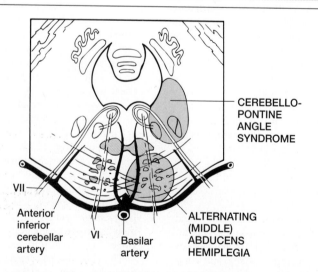

Figure **7–13.** Clinical syndromes associated with pontine lesions (compare with Fig 7–7D).

This tragic patient provides a graphic illustration of the locked-in syndrome. The infarction, in the base of the pons, destroyed the corticospinal and corticobulbar tracts and, thus, produced paralysis of the limbs and bulbar musculature. Preservation of the oculomotor and trochlear nuclei and of their nerves, permitted some limited eye movement that was used for communication. Sensation appeared to be preserved, probably because the infarction did not involve the medial lemniscus and spinothalamic tracts, which are located dorsally within the pons.

This case also illustrates that consciousness can be maintained even when there is significant structural damage in the brain stem if the reticular system is spared. In patients with larger infarcts, there may be coma as a result of ischemia of the reticular system in the brain stem.

Dorsal pons syndrome affects nerve VI or VII or their respective nuclei, with or without involvement of the medial lemniscus, spinothalamic tract, or lateral lemniscus. The "lateral gaze center" is often involved (see also Chapter 15). At a more rostral level, nerve V and its nuclei may no longer be functioning. The affected area is supplied by various perforators (pontine branches) of the circumferential arteries.

Peduncular syndrome, also called **alternating oculomotor hemiplegia** and **Weber's syndrome** in the basal midbrain involves nerve III and portions of the cerebral peduncle (Fig 7–14). There is a nerve III palsy on the side of the lesion and a contralateral hemiparesis (because the lesion is above the pyramidal decussation). The arterial supply is by the posterior perforators and branches of the posterior cerebral artery.

Benedikt's syndrome situated in the tegmentum of the midbrain, may damage the medial lemniscus, the red nucleus, and nerve III and its nucleus and associated tracts (Fig 7–14). This area is supplied by perforators and branches of circumferential arteries.

Lesions near the Brain Stem

Space-occupying processes (eg, tumors, aneurysms, brain herniation) in the area surrounding the brain stem can affect the brain stem indirectly. The following disorders are typically caused by extrinsic (extra-axial) lesions:

Cerebellopontine angle syndrome may involve nerve VIII or VII or deeper structures. It is most often caused by a tumor that begins by affecting the Schwann cells of a cranial nerve in that region, eg, a tumor at nerve VIII (see Fig 7–3).

A tumor in the **pineal region** may compress the upper quadrigeminal plate and cause vertical gaze palsy, loss of pupillary reflexes, and other ocular manifestations. There may be accompanying obstructive hydrocephalus.

Vertical gaze palsy (an inability to move the eyes up or down), also called **Parinaud's syndrome,** is caused by compression of the tectum and adjacent areas (eg, by a tumor of the pineal gland) (Fig 7–14).

Other tumors near the brain stem include medulloblastoma, ependymoma of the fourth ventricle, glioma, meningioma, and congenital cysts. **Medulloblastoma,** a cerebellar tumor (usually of the vermis) that occurs in childhood, may fill the fourth ventricle and block the cerebrospinal fluid pathway. Although compression of the brain stem is rare, the tumor has a tendency to seed to the subarachnoid space of the spinal cord and the brain.

CEREBELLUM

Gross Structure

The cerebellum is located behind the dorsal aspect of the pons and the medulla. It is separated from the occipital lobe by the **tentorium** and fills most of the posterior fossa. A midline portion, the **vermis,** separates two lateral lobes or cerebellar hemispheres (Fig 7–15). The external surface of the cerebellum displays a large number of narrow, ridge-like folds termed **folia,** most of which are oriented transversely.

The cerebellum consists of the **cerebellar cortex** and the underlying **cerebellar white matter** (see section, "Cerebellar Cortex"). Four paired **deep cerebellar nuclei** are located within the white matter of the cerebellum, above the fourth ventricle (because they lie in the roof of the ventricle, they are sometimes referred to as **roof nuclei**). These nuclei are termed (from medial to lateral) the **fastigial, globose, emboliform,** and **dentate.**

The location of the fourth ventricle, ventral to the cerebellum, is anatomically and clinically important. Mass lesions located in the cerebellum, or swelling of the cerebellum (eg, because of edema following an infarct) can compress the fourth ventricle causing obstructive hydrocephalus.

Divisions

The cerebellum is divided into two symmetric hemispheres; they are connected by the **vermis,** which can be further subdivided (Fig 7–15). The phylogenetically old **archicerebellum** consists of the flocculus, the nodulus (nodule of the vermis), and interconnections (**flocculonodular system**); it is concerned with equilibrium and connects with the vestibular system (Fig 7–16). The **paleocerebellum** consists of the anterior portions of the hemispheres and the anterior and posterior vermis and is involved with propulsive, stereotyped movements such as swimming and walking (Fig 7–17). The remainder of the cerebellum is considered the **neocerebellum** and is concerned with the coordination of fine movement.

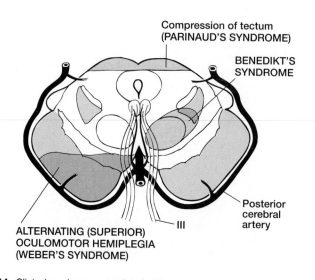

Figure 7–14. Clinical syndromes associated with midbrain lesions (compare with Fig 7–7G).

Functions

The cerebellum has two main functions: coordinating skilled voluntary movements by influencing muscle activity and controlling equilibrium and muscle tone through connections with the vestibular system and the spinal cord and its gamma motor neurons. There is a somatotropic organization of body parts within the cerebellar cortex (Fig 7–18). In addition, the cerebellum receives collateral input from the sensory and special sensory systems. Recent work suggests that the cerebellum is also involved in the mechanism of memory for motor activities, eg, piano playing.

Peduncles

Three pairs of peduncles, located above and around the fourth ventricle, attach the cerebellum to the brain

stem and contain pathways to and from the brain stem (see Figs 7–5 and 7–16 and Table 7–3). The **inferior cerebellar peduncle** contains many fiber systems from the spinal cord (including fibers from the dorsal spinocerebellar tracts and cuneocerebellar tract; see Fig 5–17) and lower brain stem (including the olivocerebellar fibers from the inferior olivary nuclei, which give rise to the climbing fibers within the cerebellar cortex). The inferior cerebellar peduncle also contains inputs from the vestibular nuclei and nerve and efferents to the vestibular nuclei.

The **middle cerebellar peduncle** consists of fibers from the contralateral pontine nuclei, which receive input from many areas of the cerebral cortex.

The **superior cerebellar peduncle**, composed mostly of efferent fibers, sends impulses to both the thalamus and spinal cord, with relays in the red nuclei

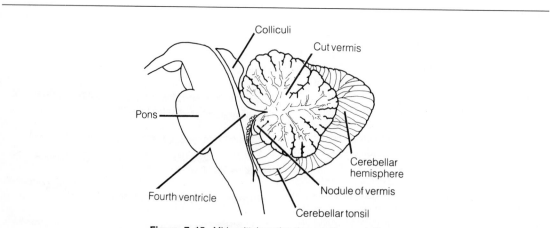

Figure 7–15. Midsagittal section through the cerebellum.

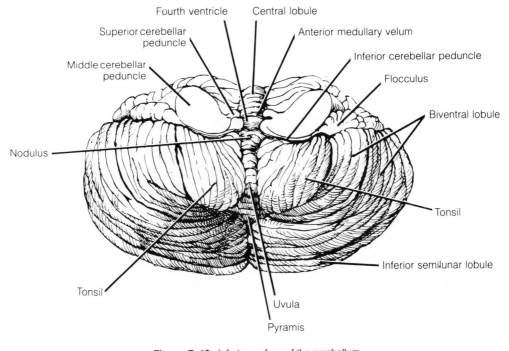

Figure 7–16. Inferior surface of the cerebellum.

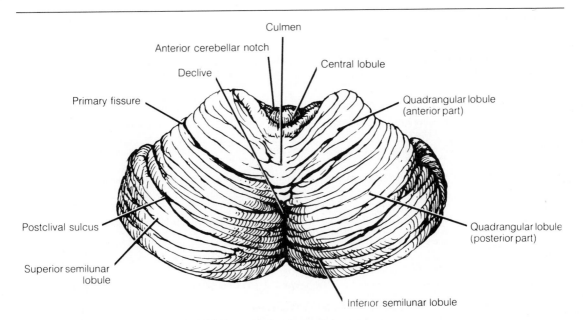

Figure 7–17. Superior surface of the cerebellum.

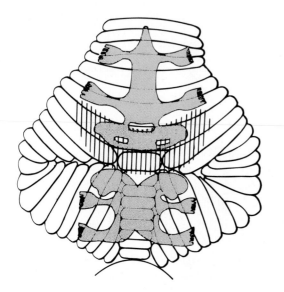

Figure 7–18. Cerebellar homunculi. Proprioceptive and tactile stimuli are projected as shown in the upper (inverted) homunculus and the lower (split) homunculus. The striped area represents the region from which evoked responses to auditory and visual stimuli are observed. (Redrawn and reproduced, with permission, from Snider R: The Cerebellum. *Sci Am* 1958;**199**:84.)

(see also Chapter 13). Afferent fibers from the ventral spinocerebellar tract also enter the cerebellum via this peduncle.

Afferents to the Cerebellum

Afferents to the cerebellum are carried primarily via the inferior and middle cerebellar peduncles, although some afferent fibers are also present in the superior cerebellar peduncles (see previous section). These afferents end in either climbing fibers or mossy fibers in the cerebellar cortex, both of which are excitatory. **Climbing fibers** originate in the inferior olivary nucleus and synapse on Purkinje cell dendrites. **Mossy fibers** are formed by afferent axons from the pontine nuclei, spinal cord, vestibular nuclei, and reticular formation: they end in specialized *glomeruli,* where they synapse with granule cell dendrites.

There are also several aminergic inputs to the cerebellum. Noradrenergic inputs, from the locus ceruleus, project widely within the cerebellar cortex. Serotonergic inputs arise in the raphe nuclei and also project to the cerebellar cortex. These inputs appear to have a modulatory effect on cerebellar activity.

Most afferent fibers (both mossy and climbing fibers) send collateral branches that provide excitatory inputs to the deep cerebellar nuclei.

Cerebellar Cortex

The cerebellar cortex consists of three layers: the subpial, outer **molecular layer**; the **Purkinje cell layer**; and the **granular layer,** an inner layer composed mainly of small granule cells (Fig 7–19 and 7–20).

The cerebellar cortex is arranged as a highly ordered array, consisting of five primary cell types (Figs 7–21 and 7–22):

- **Granule cells,** with cell bodies located in the granular layer of the cerebellar cortex, are the only excitatory neurons in the cerebellar cortex. The granule cells send their axons upward, into the molecular layer where they bifurcate in a T-like manner to become the **parallel fibers.** The nonmyelinated parallel fibers run perpendicular

Table 7–3. Functions and major terminations of the principal afferent systems to the cerebellum.*†

Afferent Tracts	Transmits	Distribution	Peduncle of Entry into Cerebellum
Dorsal spinocerebellar	Proprioceptive and exteroceptive impulses from body	Folia I–VI, pyramis and paramedian lobule	Inferior
Ventral spinocerebellar	Proprioceptives and exteroceptive impulses from body	Folia I–VI, pyramis and paramedian lobule	Superior
Cuneocerebellar	Proprioceptive impulses, especially from head and neck	Folia I–VI, pyramis and paramedian lobule	Inferior
Tectocerebellar	Auditory and visual impulses via inferior and superior colliculi	Folium, tuber, ansiform lobule	Superior
Vestibulocerebellar	Vestibular impulses from labyrinths, directly and via vestibular nuclei	Principally flocculonodular lobe	Inferior
Pontocerebellar	Impulses from motor and other parts of cerebral cortex via pontine nuclei	All cerebellar cortex except floccualonodular lobe	Middle
Olivocerebellar	Proprioceptive input from whole body via relay in inferior olive	All cerebellar cortex and deep nuclei	Inferior

* Reproduced, with permission, from Ganong WF: *Review of Medical Physiology,* 13th ed. Appleton & Lange, 1987.
† Several other pathways transmit impulses from nuclei in the brain stem to the cerebellar cortex and to the deep nuclei.

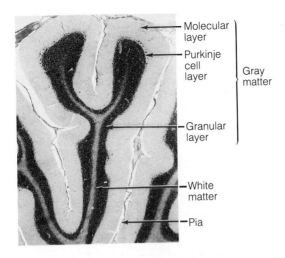

Figure 7–19. Photomicrograph of a portion of the cerebellum. Each lobule contains a core of white matter and a cortex consisting of three layers—granular, Purkinje, and molecular—of gray matter. H&E stain, × 28. (Reproduced, with permission, from Junqueira LC, Carneiro J, Kelley RO: *Basic Histology,* 7th ed. Appleton & Lange, 1992.)

through the Purkinje cell dendrites (like the wires running between telephone poles) and form excitatory synapses on these dendrites. Glutamate appears to be the neurotransmitter at these synapses.

- **Purkinje cells** provide the primary output from the cerebellar cortex. These unique neurons have their cell bodies in the Purkinje cell layer and have dendrites that fan out in a single plane like the ribs of a Japanese fan or the cross-bars on a telephone pole. The axons of Purkinje cells project ipsilaterally to

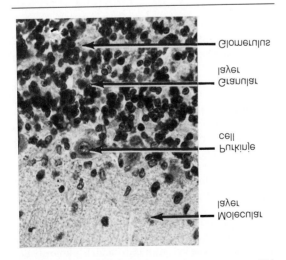

Figure 7–20. Photomicrograph of cerebellar cortex. This staining procedure does not reveal the unusually large dendritic arborization of the Purkinje cell. H&E stain, × 250. (Reproduced, with permission, from Junqueira LC, Carneiro J, Kelley RO: *Basic Histology,* 7th ed. Appleton & Lange, 1992.)

the deep cerebellar nuclei, especially the dentate nucleus, where they form inhibitory synapses.

- **Basket cells** are located in the molecular layer. These cells receive excitatory inputs from the parallel fibers and project back to Purkinje cells, which they inhibit.
- **Golgi cells** are also located in the molecular layer and receive excitatory inputs from parallel fibers and from mossy fibers. The Golgi cells send their axons back to the granule cells, which they inhibit.
- **Stellate cells** are located in the molecular layer and receive excitatory inputs, primarily from the parallel fibers. Like the basket cells, these cells give rise to inhibitory synapses on Purkinje cells.

Deep Cerebellar Nuclei

Four sets of pair deep cerebellar nuclei are embedded in the white matter of the cerebellum: fastigial, globose, emboliform, and dentate. Neurons in these nuclei project out of the cerebellum and, thus, represent the major efferent pathway from the cerebellum. Cells in the deep cerebellar nuclei receive inhibitory input (GABAergic) from Purkinje cells. They also receive excitatory inputs from sites outside the cerebellum, including pontine nuclei, inferior olivary nucleus, reticular formation, locus ceruleus, and raphe nuclei. Essentially, all inputs giving rise to climbing and mossy fibers also project excitatory collaterals to the deep cerebellar nuclei. As a result of this arrangement, cells in the deep cerebellar nuclei receive inhibitory inputs from Purkinje cells and excitatory inputs from other sources. Cells in the deep cerebellar nuclei fire tonically, at rates that reflect the balance between the opposing excitatory and inhibitory inputs that converge on them.

Efferents from the Cerebellum

Efferents from the deep cerebellar nuclei project via the superior cerebellar peduncle to the contralateral red nucleus and thalamic nuclei (especially VL, VPL). From there, projections are sent to the motor cortex. This chain of projections provides the **dento-rubro-thalamo-cortical pathway** (Fig 7–23). Via this pathway, activity in the dentate nucleus and other deep cerebellar nuclei modulates activity in the contralateral motor cortex.

In addition, neurons in the fastigial nucleus project via the inferior cerebellar peduncle to the vestibular nuclei bilaterally and to the contralateral reticular formation, pons, and spinal cord. The axons of some Purkinje cells, located in the vermis and flocculonodular lobe, also send projections to the vestibular nuclei.

As outlined in Figure 5–17, much of the input from the spinocerebellar tracts is uncrossed and enters the cerebellar hemisphere ipsilateral to its origin. Moreover, each cerebellar hemisphere projects via the dento-rubro-thalamo-cortical route to the contralateral

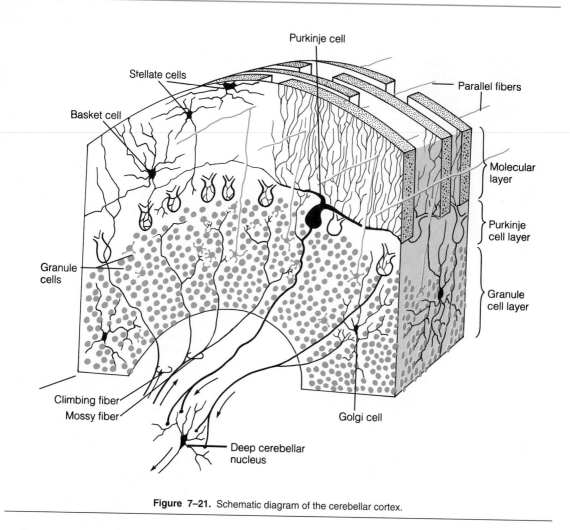

Figure 7–21. Schematic diagram of the cerebellar cortex.

motor cortex (Fig 7–23). On the basis of this anatomic arrangement, each cerebellar hemisphere participates in the coordination of motor activities for limbs on the *same side* of the body.

Cerebellum & Brain Stem in Whole-Head Sections

Magnetic resonance imaging shows the cerebellum and its relationship with the brain stem, cranial nerves, skull, and vessels (Figs 7–24 and 7–25). These images are increasingly useful in determining the location, nature (solid or cystic), and extent of cerebellar lesions (see the discussion of Chiari malformation).

Clinical Correlations

The most characteristic signs of a cerebellar disorder are **hypotonia** (diminished muscle tone) and **ataxia** (loss of the coordinated muscular contractions required for the production of smooth movements). In general, unilateral lesions of the cerebellum lead to motor disabilities *ipsilateral* to the side of the lesion. Notice that alcohol intoxication can mimic cerebellar ataxia.

Some lesions are confined to a particular subdivision of the cerebellum. For example, lesions of the **vestibulocerebellum** (involving the flocculus, nodulus, and caudal vermis) cause disturbances of equilibrium, characterized by unsteady walking and swaying when standing. **Nystagmus** (rhythmic oscillations of the eyeballs) may also be present. Because such lesions often involve midline structures, they can cause bilateral signs. Lesions of the **paleocerebellum** and **neocerebellum** usually involve portions of a cerebellar hemisphere and result in clumsy movements of the extremities (ataxia) on the same side as the cerebellar lesion. With these lesions it is difficult to clinically determine the predominant involvement of one or the other of these portions of the cerebellum.

Several types of **asynergy** (loss of coordination) can be demonstrated in patients with cerebellar lesions:

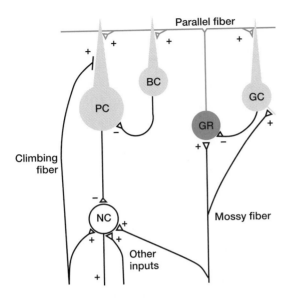

Figure 7–22. Diagram of neural connections in the cerebellum. Shaded neurons are inhibitory, and + and − signs indicate whether endings are excitatory or inhibitory. BC, basket cell; GC, Golgi cell; GR, granule cell; NC, cells within deep cerebellar nuclei; PC, Purkinje cell. The connections of the stellate cells are similar to those of the basket cells, except that they end for the most part on Purkinje cell dendrites. (Modified from Eccles JC, Ito M, Szentágothai J: *The Cerebellum as a Neuronal Machine.* Springer, 1967. Also from, Ganong WF: *Review of Medical Physiology,* 16th ed. Appleton & Lange, 1993.)

There can be the decomposition of movement into its component parts; **dysmetria,** which is characterized by the inability to place an extremity at a precise point in space (eg, touch the finger to the nose); or **intention tremor,** a tremor that arises when voluntary movements are attempted. The patient may also exhibit **adiadochokinesis (dysdiadochokinesis),** an inability to make, or difficulty in making, rapidly alternating or successive movements; ataxia of gait, with a tendency to fall toward the side of the lesion; and **rebound phenomenon,** a loss of the normal checks of agonist and antagonist muscles.

A variety of pathologic processes can affect the cerebellum. **Tumors** (especially **astrocytomas**) and **hypertensive hemorrhage** can cause cerebellar dysfunction and can compress the underlying fourth ventricle, thereby producing hydrocephalus, a neurosurgical emergency. **Cerebellar infarctions** can also cause cerebellar dysfunction, and if large, may be accompanied by edema that, again, can compress the fourth ventricle, thus producing hydrocephalus. A number of metabolic disorders (especially those involving abnormal metabolism of amino acids, ammonia, pyruvate, and lactate) and **degenerative diseases** (termed **olivo-**pontocerebellar atrophies) can also cause cerebellar degeneration.

Figure 7–26 shows a type of **Chiari malformation,** a congenital malformation characterized by displacement of the lower cerebellum into the spinal canal. This malformation is also associated with deformation of the brain stem. It can produce obstructive hydrocephalus by blocking the cerebrospinal fluid pathway from the fourth ventricle to the subarachnoid space (see Chapter 11).

CASE 6

A 60-year-old technician had a sudden onset of double vision and dizziness. Three days later (one day prior to admission), she noticed a sudden drooping of her right eyelid.

Neurologic examination showed unequal pupils (right smaller than left, both responding to light and accommodation), ptosis of the right eyelid, mild enophthalmos and decreased sweating on the right side of the face, and nystagmus on left lateral gaze. The corneal reflex was diminished on the right but normal on the left. Although pain sensation was decreased on the right side of the face, touch sensation was normal; there was minor right peripheral facial weakness. The uvula deviated to the left and mild hoarseness was noted. Muscle strength was intact, but the patient could not execute a right finger-to-nose test or make rapid alternating movements. There was an intention tremor of the right arm, and further examination revealed ataxia in the right lower extremity. Reflexes were all normal. Pain sensation was decreased on the left side of the body; senses of touch, vibration and position were intact.

What is the differential diagnosis? What is the most likely diagnosis?

CASE 7

A 27-year-old graduate student was admitted with a chief complaint of having double vision for two weeks. Earlier, he had noticed persistent tingling of all the fingers on his left hand. He also felt as though ants were crawling on the left side of his face and the left half of his tongue and thought that both legs had become weaker recently.

Neurologic examination showed a scotoma in the upper field of the left eye, weakness of the left medial rectus muscle, coarse horizontal nystagmus on left lateral gaze, and mild weakness of the left central facial muscles. All other muscles had normal strength. The deep tendon reflexes were normal on the right and livelier on the left, and there was a left extensor plantar response. The sensory system was unremarkable.

The patient was discharged a few days later, seemingly improved after corticosteroid treatment. He was

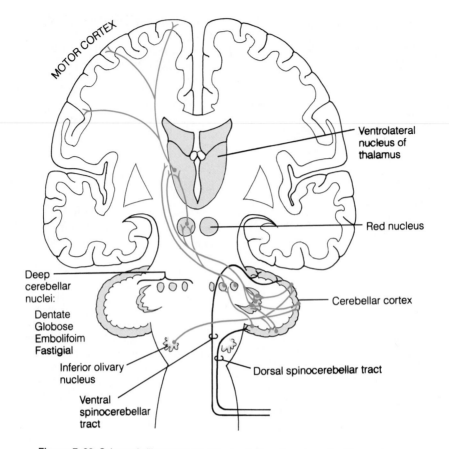

Figure 7–23. Schematic illustration of some cerebellar afferents and outflow pathways.

readmitted four months later, however, because he noticed difficulty in walking and his speech had become thickened. Neurologic examination showed the following additional findings: wide-based ataxic gait, minor slurring of speech, bilateral tremor in the finger-to-nose test, and disorganization of rapid alternating movements. A CT scan was within normal limits but

Table 7–4. Excitatory and inhibitory effects.

Excitation	Inhibition
Mossy fibers → granule cell	Basket cell → Purkinje cell body
Olive (via climbing fibers) → Purkinje cell	Stellate cell → Purkinje cell dendrite
	Golgi cell → granule cell
Granule cell → Purkinje cell	Purkinje cell → roof nuclei (including dentate)
Granule cell → Golgi cell	Purkinje cell → lat. vestib. nuclei
Granule cell → basket	Purkinje cell → Purkinje cells
Granule cell → stellate cell	Purkinje cell → Golgi cells

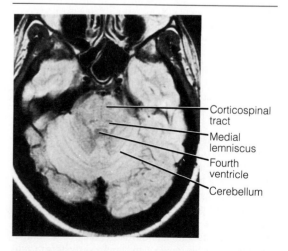

Figure 7–24. Horizontal section through the head at the level of the lower pons. Notice that the position of the pons is reversed from that of Fig 7–7D to conform with customary CT and MR procedures.

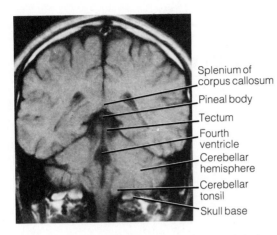

Splenium of
corpus callosum

Pineal body

Tectum

Fourth
ventricle

Cerebellar
hemisphere

Cerebellar
tonsil

Skull base

Figure 7–25. MR image of a coronal section through the head at the level of the fourth ventricle.

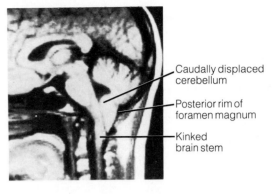

Caudally displaced
cerebellum

Posterior rim of
foramen magnum

Kinked
brain stem

Figure 7–26. MR image of a midsagittal section showing Chiari malformation (compare with Fig 1–4).

MR scans revealed numerous lesions. Lumbar puncture showed 56 mg protein with a relatively increased level of gamma globulins. All other cerebrospinal fluid findings were normal. Treatment with high doses of intravenous corticosteroids seemed to improve the neurological deficits and the patient was discharged.

What is the differential diagnosis at this point?

Two months later, the patient's symptoms recurred, and he was admitted to a nursing home. He gradually became quadriplegic, and his visual and brain stem problems increased.

What is the diagnosis?

Cases are discussed further in Chapter 25.

REFERENCES

Chan-Palay V: Cerebellar Dentate Nucleus: *Organization, Cytology and Transmitters.* Springer-Verlag, 1977.

DeArmand SJ: Structure of the Human Brain: *A Photographic Atlas,* 3rd ed. Oxford Univ Press, 1989.

Harding EA: Cerebellar and spinocerebellar disorders. In: *Neurology in Clinical Practice.* Bradley WG et al (editors). Butterworth-Heinemann, 1989.

Ito M: *The Cerebellum and Motor Control.* Raven, 1984.

Llinas RR: The cortex of the cerebellum. *Sci Am* 1975;**232**:56.

Montemurro DG, Bruni JE: *The Human Brain in Dissection.* Saunders, 1981.

Riley HA: *An Atlas of the Basal Ganglia, Brain Stem and Spinal Cord.* Williams & Wilkins, 1943.

Scheibel ME, Scheibel AB: Anatomical basis of attention: Mechanisms in vertebrate brains. In: *The Neurosciences.* Quarton GC, Melnechuck T, Schmitt FO (editors). Rockefeller Univ Press, 1967.

Wall M: Brain stem syndromes. In: *Neurology in Clinical Practice.* Bradley WG et al (editors). Butterworth-Heinemann, 1989.

8

Cranial Nerves & Pathways

ORIGIN OF CRANIAL NERVE FIBERS

The 12 pairs of cranial nerves are usually referred to by either name or roman numeral (Fig 8–1 and Table 8–1). Note that the olfactory peduncle (see Chapter 19) and the optic nerve (see Chapter 15) are not true nerves but fiber tracts of the brain, while nerve XI (the spinal accessory nerve) is derived, in part, from the upper cervical segments of the spinal cord. The remaining nine pairs relate to the brain stem.

The superficial origin of a cranial nerve is the area of the brain where the nerve emerges or enters. Cranial nerve fibers with motor (efferent) functions arise from collections of cells (motor nuclei) that lie deep within the brain stem; they are homologous to the anterior horn cells of the spinal cord. Cranial nerve fibers with sensory (afferent) functions have their cells of origin (first-order nuclei) outside the brain stem, usually in ganglia that are homologous to the dorsal root ganglia of the spinal nerves. Second-order sensory nuclei lie within the brain stem (see Chapter 7 and Fig 7–6).

Table 8–1 presents an overview of the cranial nerves. Notice that this table does not list the cranial nerves numerically, but rather groups them functionally:

- Nerves I, II, and VIII are devoted to **special sensory input.**
- Nerves III, IV, and VI control **eye movements** and **pupillary constriction.**
- Nerves XI and XII are **pure motor** (XI: sternocleidomastoid and trapezius; XII: muscles of tongue).
- Nerves V, VII, IX, and X are **mixed.**
- Note that **Nerves III, VII, IX, and X** carry **parasympathetic** fibers.

FUNCTIONAL COMPONENTS OF THE CRANIAL NERVES

A cranial nerve can have one or more functions (as shown in Table 8–1). The functional components are conveyed from or to the brain stem by six types of nerve fibers:

(1) **Somatic efferent fibers,** also called general somatic efferent fibers, innervate striated muscles that are derived from somites and are involved in eye (nerves III, IV, and VI) and tongue (nerve XII) movements.

(2) **Branchial efferent fibers,** also known as **special visceral efferent fibers,** are special somatic efferent components. They innervate muscles that are derived from the branchial (gill) arches and are involved in chewing (nerve V), making facial expressions (nerve VII), swallowing (nerves IX and X), producing vocal sounds (nerve X), and turning the head (nerve XI).

(3) **Visceral efferent fibers** are also called general visceral efferent fibers (**preganglionic parasympathetic** components of the cranial division); they course through nerves III (smooth muscles of the inner eye), VII (salivatory and lacrimal glands), IX (the parotid gland), and X (the muscles of the heart, lung, and bowel that are involved in movement and secretion; see also Chapter 20).

(4) **Visceral afferent fibers,** also called general visceral afferent fibers, convey sensation from the alimentary tract, heart, vessels, and lungs by way of nerves IX and X. A specialized visceral afferent component is involved with the sense of taste; fibers carrying gustatory impulses are present in cranial nerves VII, IX, and X.

(5) **Somatic afferent fibers,** often called general somatic afferent fibers, convey sensation from the skin and the mucous membranes of the head. They are found mainly in the trigeminal nerve (V). A small number of afferent fibers travel

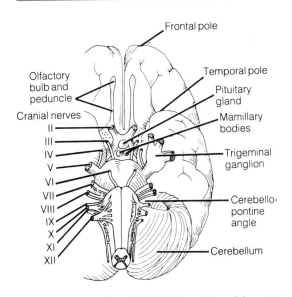

Frontal pole

Temporal pole

Olfactory
bulb and
peduncle

Pituitary
gland

Cranial nerves

II

Mamillary
bodies

III

IV

Trigeminal
ganglion

V

VI

VII

VIII

IX

Cerebello-
pontine
angle

X

XI

XII

Cerebellum

Figure 8–1. Ventral view of the brain stem with cranial nerves.

with the facial (VII), glossopharyngeal (IX), and vagus (X) nerves; these fibers terminate on trigeminal nuclei in the brain stem.

(6) **Special sensory fibers** are found in nerves I (involved in smell), II (vision), and VIII (hearing and equilibrium).

Differences Between Cranial & Spinal Nerves

Unlike the spinal nerves, cranial nerves are not found at regular intervals. They differ in other aspects as well: The spinal nerves, for example, contain neither branchial efferent nor special sensory components. Some cranial nerves contain motor components only (most motor nerves have a few proprioceptive fibers) and some contain large visceral components. Other cranial nerves are completely or mostly sensory, and still others are mixed with both types of components. The motor and sensory axons of mixed cranial nerves enter and exit at the same point on the brain stem; this point is ventral or ventrolateral except for nerve IV, which exits from the dorsal surface (Fig 8–1).

Ganglia Related to Cranial Nerves

The two types of ganglia related to cranial nerves: (1) those containing cell bodies of afferent (somatic or visceral) axons within the cranial nerves (these ganglia are somewhat analogous to the dorsal root ganglia that contain the cell bodies of sensory axons within peripheral nerves), and (2) ganglia that contain the synaptic terminals of visceral efferent axons, together with postsynaptic (parasympathetic) neurons that project peripherally (Table 8–2).

Sensory ganglia of the cranial nerves include the **semilunar (gasserian) ganglion** (nerve V), **geniculate ganglion** (nerve VII), **cochlear** and **vestibular ganglia** (nerve VIII), **inferior** and **superior glossopharyngeal ganglion** (nerve IX), **superior vagal ganglion** (nerve X), and **inferior vagal (nodose) ganglion** (nerve X).

The ganglia of the cranial **parasympathetic division** of the autonomic nervous system are the **ciliary ganglion** (nerve III), the **pterygopalatine** and **submandibular ganglia** (VIII), **otic ganglion** (IX), and **intramural ganglion** (X). The first four of these ganglia have a close association with branches of V; the trigeminal branches may course through the autonomic ganglia.

ANATOMIC RELATIONSHIPS OF THE CRANIAL NERVES

Cranial Nerve I: Olfactory Nerve

The true olfactory nerves are short connections that project from the olfactory mucosa within the nose and the olfactory bulb within the cranial cavity (Fig 8–2 and Chapter 19). There are 9–15 of these nerves on each side of the brain. The olfactory bulb lies just above the cribiform plate and below the frontal lobe (it is nestled within the **olfactory sulcus**). Axons from the olfactory bulb run within the **olfactory stalk,** synapse in the **anterior olfactory nucleus,** and terminate in the **primary olfactory cortex (pyriform cortex)** as well as the **entorhinal** cortex and amygdala.

Clinical Correlations

Anosmia (absence of the sense of smell) can result from disorders (eg, viral infections, such as the common cold) involving the nasal mucosa. The tiny olfactory nerves and bulbs can be injured as a result of head trauma. Moreover, the location of the olfactory bulb and stalk, below the frontal lobe, predisposes them to compression from frontal lobe tumors and olfactory groove meningiomas.

Cranial Nerve II: Optic Nerve

The optic nerve arises from the ganglion cells in the retina and then passes through the optic papilla to the orbit, where it is contained within meningeal sheaths. The nerve changes its name to optic tract when the fibers have passed through the optic chiasm (Figs 7–3 and 8–3). Optic tract axons project to the superior colliculus and to the lateral geniculate, which relays visual information to the cortex (see Chapter 15).

Table 8–1. Overview of cranial nerves.

		Func-tional Type*	FUNCTIONS			LOCATION OF CELL BODIES		Major Connections
			Motor Innervation	Sensory Function	Parasympathetic Function	Within Sensory Organ or Ganglia	Within Brain Stem	
Special Sensory:	I Olfactory	SS		Sense of smell		Olfactory mucosa		Mucosa projects to olfactory bulb
	II Optic	SS		Visual input from eye		Ganglion cells in retina		Projects to lateral geniculate; superior colliculus
	VIII Vestibulo-cochlear	SS		Auditory and vestibular input from inner ear		Cochlear ganglion		Projects to cochlear nuclei, then inferior colliculi, medial geniculate
						Vestibular ganglion		Projects to vestibular nuclei
Motor for Ocular System:	III Oculomotor	SE	Medial rectus, superior rectus, inferior rectus, inferior oblique				Oculomotor nucleus	Receives input from lateral gaze center (paramedial pontine reticular formation; PPRF) via median longitudinal fasciculus
		VE			Constriction of pupil		Edinger-Westphal nucl.	Projects to ciliary ganglia, then to pupil
	IV Trochlear	SE	Superior oblique				Trochlear nucl.	
	VI Abducens	SE	Lateral rectus				Abducens nucl.	Receives input from PPRF
Other Pure Motor:	XI Accessory	BE	Sternocleidomastoid, trapezius				Ventral horns at C2-C5	
	XII Hypoglossal	SE	Muscles of tongue, hyoid bone				Hypoglossal nucleus	

Mixed:

Nerve						
V Trigeminal	SA	Sensation from face, cornea, teeth, gum, palate. General sensation from anterior 2/3 of tongue		Semilunar (= gasserian or trigeminal) ganglia		Projects to sensory nucl. and spinal tract of V, then to thalamus (VPM)
	BE	Chewing muscles			Motor nucl. of V	
VII Facial	BE	Muscles of facial expression, platysma, stapedius			Facial nucl.	
	VA	Taste, anterior 2/3 of tongue (via chorda tympani)		Geniculate ganglion		Projects to solitary tract and nucleus, then to thalamus (VPM)
	VE		Submandibular, sublingual, lacrimal glands (via nervus intermedius)		Superior salivatory nucleus	
IX Glossopharyngeal	VE		Parotid gland		Inferior salivatory nucl.	
	VA	General sensation from posterior 1/3 of tongue, soft palate, auditory tube. Sensory input from carotid bodies and sinus. Taste from posterior 1/3 of tongue		Inferior (petrosal) and superior glossopharyngeal ganglia		Projects to solitary tract and nucleus
	BE	Stylopharyngeus muscle			Ambiguous nucl.	
X Vagus	BE	Soft palate and pharynx			Ambiguous nucl.	
	VE		Autonomic control of thoracic and abdominal viscera		Dorsal motor nucleus	
	SA	External auditory meatus		Superior (Jugular) ganglion		Projects to thalamus (VPM)
	VA	Sensation from abdominal and thoracic viscera		Inferior vagal (nodose) and superior ganglia		Projects to solitary tract and nucleus

*Efferent (motor)

SE-somatic; general SE
BE-branchial; special VE
VE-visceral; general VE

Afferent (sensory)

VA-visceral; general VA, special VA
SA-somatic; general SA
SS-sensory

*Most nerves with SE components have a few SA fibers for proprioception

Table 8–2. Ganglia related to cranial nerves.

Ganglion	Nerve	Functional Type	Synapse
Ciliary	III	VE (para-sympathetic)	+
Ptertgopala-tine	VII	VE (para-sympathetic)	+
Submandibu-lar	VII	VE (para-sympathetic)	+
Otic	IX	VE (para-sympathetic)	+
Intramural (in viscus)	X	VE (para-sympathetic)	+
Semilunar	V	SA	–
Geniculate	VII	VA (taste)	–
Inferior and superior	IX	SA, VA (taste)	–
Inferior and superior	X	SA, VA (taste)	–
Spiral	VIII (cochlear)	SS	–
Vestibular	VIII (vestibular)	SS	–

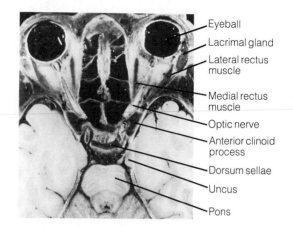

Figure 8–3. Horizontal section through the head at the level of the orbits.

Cranial Nerve III: Oculomotor Nerve

Cranial nerves III, IV, and VI control eye movements. In addition, cranial nerve III controls pupillary constriction.

The oculomotor nerve leaves the brain on the medial side of the cerebral peduncle, behind the posterior cerebral artery and in front of the superior cerebellar artery. It then passes anteriorly, parallel to the internal carotid artery in the lateral wall of the cavernous sinus, leaving the cranial cavity by way of the superior orbital fissure.

The somatic efferent portion of the nerve innervates the **levator palpebrae superioris muscle;** the **superior, medial,** and **inferior rectus muscles;** and the **inferior oblique muscle** (Fig 8–4). The visceral efferent portion innervates two smooth intraocular muscles: the **ciliary** and the **constrictor pupillae.**

Cranial Nerve IV: Trochlear Nerve

The small trochlear nerve is the only crossed cranial nerve. It originates in the lower midbrain and emerges contralaterally on the dorsal surface of the brain stem. The nerve then curves ventrally between the posterior cerebral and superior cerebellar arteries (lateral to the oculomotor nerve). It continues anteriorly in the lateral wall of the cavernous sinus and enters the orbit via the superior orbital fissure. It innervates the superior oblique muscle (Fig 8–4).

Note: Because nerves III, IV, and VI are generally grouped together for discussion, nerve V is discussed after nerve VI.

Cranial Nerve VI: Abducens Nerve

A. Anatomy: The abducens nerve emerges from the pontomedullary fissure, passes through the cavernous sinus close to the internal carotid and exits from the cranial cavity via the superior orbital fissure. Its long intracranial course makes it vulnerable to pathologic processes in the posterior and middle cranial fossae. The nerve innervates the lateral rectus muscle (Fig 8–4).

A few sensory (proprioceptive) fibers from the muscles of the eye are present in nerves III, IV, and VI and in some other nerves that innervate striated muscles.

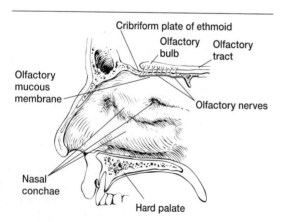

Figure 8–2. Lateral view of the olfactory bulb, tract, mucous membrane, and nerves.

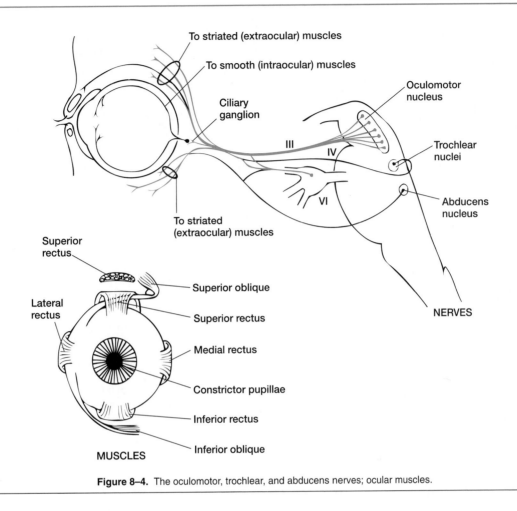

Figure 8–4. The oculomotor, trochlear, and abducens nerves; ocular muscles.

The central termination of these fibers is in the mesencephalic nucleus of V (see Chapter 7 and Fig 7–8).

B. Action of the External Eye Muscles: The actions of eye muscles operating singly and in tandem are shown in Tables 8–3 and 8–4 (Fig 8–5). The levator palpebrae superioris muscle has no action on the eyeball but lifts the upper eyelid when contracted. Closing the eyelids is performed by contraction of the orbicular muscle of the eye; this muscle is innervated by nerve VII.

C. Control of Ocular-Muscle Movements: The oculomotor system is normally precise and activates the various extraocular muscles in a highly coordinated manner (Fig 8–6). It can aid vision by accurately fixating on an object of interest without head movements or by aligning the most acute portion of each retina (the fovea) at the point of interest. When the eyes scan the environment, they do so in short, rapid movements called **saccades.** When a target moves, a different form of ocular movement—smooth pursuit—is used to keep the image in sharp focus. When the head or body moves unexpectedly, eg, when one is jolted, reflex movements of the head and eye muscles compensate and maintain fixation on the visual target. This compensatory function is achieved by the **vestibulo-ocular reflex** (see Chapter 17).

The six individual muscles that move one eye normally act together with the muscles of the other eye in controlled movement. Both eyes move in the same direction to follow an object in space, but they move by simultaneously contracting and relaxing different mus-

Table 8–3. Functions of the ocular muscles.*

Muscle	Primary Action	Secondary Action
Lateral rectus	Abduction	None
Medial rectus	Adduction	None
Superior rectus	Elevation	Adduction, intorsion
Inferior rectus	Depression	Adduction, extorsion
Superior oblique	Depression	Intorsion, abduction
Inferior oblique	Elevation	Extorsion, abduction

* Reproduced, with permission, from Vaughan D, Asbury T and Riordan-Eva P: *General Ophthalmology,* 13th ed. Appleton & Lange, 1992.

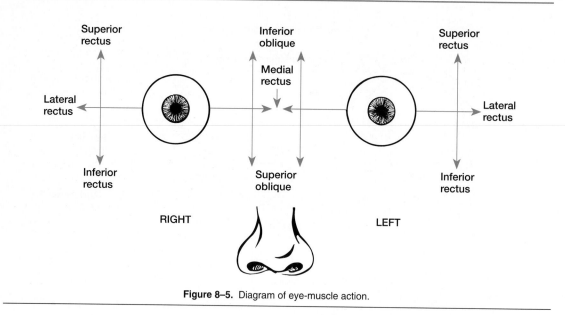

Figure 8–5. Diagram of eye-muscle action.

cles; this is called a **conjugate gaze** movement. Fixating on a single point is called **vergence,** which requires a different set of muscles, including the intraocular muscles. Each of the extraocular muscles is brought into play in conjugate gaze movements or vergence.

1. Gaze and vergence centers–Conjugate gaze and vergence are controlled from three areas in the brain stem. There are two **lateral gaze centers** in the **paramedian pontine reticular formation** near the left and right abducens nuclei and a **vergence center**

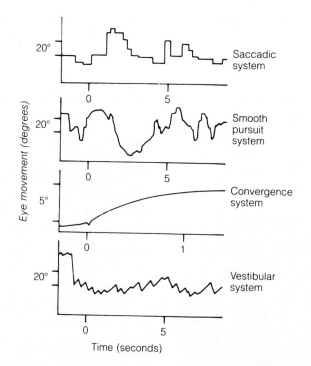

Figure 8–6. Types of eye-movement control. (Modified and reproduced, with permission, from Robinson DA: Eye movement control in primates. *Science* 1968;161:1219. Copyright 1968 by the American Association for the Advancement of Science.)

Table 8–4. Yoke muscle combinations.*

Cardinal Direc- tion of Gaze	Yoke Muscles
Eyes up, right	Right superior rectus and left inferior oblique
Eyes right	Right lateral rectus and left medial rectus
Eyes down, right	Right inferior rectus and left superior oblique
Eyes down, left	Right superior oblique and left inferior rectus
Eyes left	Right medial rectus and left lateral rectus
Eyes up, left	Right inferior oblique and left superior rectus

* Reproduced, with permission, from Vaughan D, Asbury T & Riordan-Eva P: *General Opthalmology,* 13 ed. Appleton & Lange, 1992.

in the pretectum just above the superior colliculi. Each of these three areas can be activated during head movement by the vestibular system via the medial longitudinal fasciculus (see Chapter 17). Activation of the lateral gaze center on the right produces conjugate gaze to the right and vice versa. Regions in the contralateral frontal lobe (the eye field area) influence voluntary eye movements via polysynaptic connections to the lateral gaze centers, while regions in the occipital lobe influence visual pursuit and also have connections with the vergence center (Fig 8–7).

Activity in each of the lateral gaze centers (located in the paramedian pontine reticular formation on each side, adjacent to the abducens nuclei) controls eye movements to the *ipsilateral* side. Thus, the lateral gaze center on the right is connected, via excitatory projections, to the right abducens nucleus that activates the lateral rectus muscle responsible for abduction of the right eye. The right-sided lateral gaze center also sends projections, via the medial longitudinal fasciculus, to the *contralateral* (left-sided) oculomotor nucleus, where they form excitatory synapses on oculomotor neurons innervating the medial rectus muscle (which is responsible for movement of the left eye across the midline to the right). As a result of this arrangement, activation of the right-sided lateral gaze center results in movement of both eyes to the right (Fig 8–7).

This arrangement also provides an anatomic basis for reflexes involving eye movements, such as the vestibulo-ocular reflex. Sudden rotation of the head to the left results in movement of endolymph within the semicircular canals, whose neurons project to the vestibular nuclei (Fig 8–7). These nuclei, in turn, send excitatory projections via the medial longitudinal fasciculus to the right-sided lateral gaze center (and also send inhibitory projections to the left-sided lateral gaze center). Increased activity in the right-sided lateral gaze center triggers eye movements to the right, stabilizing the image on the retina.

2. Control of pupillary size–The diameter of the pupil is affected by parasympathetic efferent fibers in the oculomotor nerve and sympathetic fibers from the superior cervical ganglion (Fig 8–8). **Constriction (miosis)** of the pupil is caused by the stimulation of parasympathetic fibers whereas, **dilation (mydriasis)** is caused by sympathetic activation. The size of both pupils is normally affected simultaneously by one or more of such causes as emotion, pain, drugs, and changes in light intensity and accommodation.

3. Reflexes–The **pupillary light reflex** is a constriction of both eyes in response to a bright light. Even if the light hits only one eye, both pupils usually constrict; this is a **consensual response.** The pathways for the reflex include optic nerve fibers (or their collaterals) to the pretectum, a nuclear area between thalamus and midbrain (Fig 8–9). Short fibers go from the pretectum to both **Edinger-Westphal** nuclei (the visceral components of the oculomotor nuclei) by way of the posterior commissure and to both ciliary ganglia by way of the oculomotor nerves. Postganglionic parasympathetic fibers to the constrictor muscles are activated, and the sympathetic nerves of the dilator muscle are inhibited. The interaction between these components of the autonomic nervous system can be used to localize a lesion in the reflex pathways.

The **accommodation reflex** involves pathways from the visual cortex in the occipital lobe to the pretectum. From here, fibers to all nuclei of nerves III, IV, and VI cause vergence of the extraocular muscles as well as parasympathetic activation of the constrictor and ciliary muscles within each eye.

D. Clinical Correlations for Nerves III, IV, and VI and Their Connections

1. Symptoms and signs–Clinical findings include strabismus, diplopia, and ptosis. **Strabismus (squint)** is the deviation of one or both eyes. In internal strabismus, the visual axes cross each other; in external strabismus, the visual axes diverge from each other. **Diplopia (double vision)** is a subjective phenomenon reported to be present when the patient is—usually—looking with both eyes; it is caused by misalignment of the visual axes. **Ptosis (lid drop)** is caused by weakness or paralysis of the levator palpebrae superioris muscle; it is seen with lesions of Nerve III and sometimes in patients with myasthenia gravis.

2. Classification of ophthalmoplegias––Lesions that cause ophthalmoplegia (paralysis) of nerves III, IV, and VI may be acute, chronic, or progressive; they may also be central or peripheral (Table 8–5).

a. Oculomotor (nerve III) paralysis. External ophthalmoplegia is characterized by divergent strabismus, diplopia, and ptosis. The eye is deviate downward and outward. Internal ophthalmoplegia is characterized by a dilated pupil and loss of light and accommodation reflexes. There may be paralysis of individual muscles of nerve III as shown in Table 8–5.

Isolated involvement of nerve III occurs as an early sign in **uncal herniation,** because of expanding hemi-

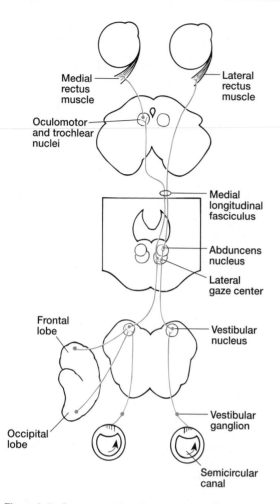

Figure 8–7. Conjugate right gaze. The impulses for voluntary conjugate movements in right lateral gaze are initiated in the left frontal lobe. Involuntary conjugate movements in right lateral gaze are initiated in the occipital lobes.

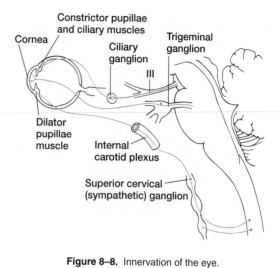

Figure 8–8. Innervation of the eye.

d. Internuclear ophthalmoplegia. Lesions of the medial longitudinal fasciculus (rostral to the abducens nuclei) interfere with conjugate movements of the eyes. A unilateral lesion of the median longitudinal fasciculus on the left, for example, produces a syndrome in which, when the patient attempts to look to the right, the left eye fails to adduct. This is because ascending influences, from the right-sided lateral gaze center, can no longer reach the left-sided oculomotor

spheric mass lesions that compress the nerve against the tentorium. Nerve III crosses the internal carotid where it joins the posterior communicating artery; **aneurisms** of the posterior communicating artery thus can compress the nerve. Isolated nerve III palsy also occurs in diabetes, presumably because of ischemic damage.

b. Trochlear (nerve IV) paralysis. This rare condition is characterized by slight convergent strabismus and diplopia on looking downward. The patient cannot look downward and inward and hence has difficulty in descending stairs. The head is tilted as a compensatory adjustment; this may be the first indication of a trochlear lesion.

c. Abducens (nerve VI) paralysis. This eye palsy is the most common, owing to the long course of nerve VI. There is weakness of eye abduction. Features of abducens paralysis include convergent strabismus and diplopia (Fig 8–10).

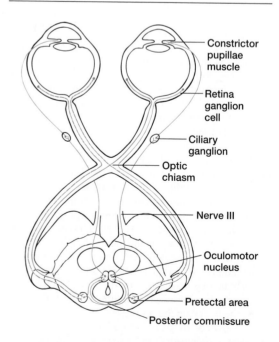

Figure 8–9. The path of the pupillary light reflex.

Table 8–5. Paralyses of individual eye muscles.*

Muscle	Nerve	Deviation of Eyeball	Diplopia Present When Looking*	Direction of Image
Medial rectus	III	Outward (external squint)	Toward nose	Vertical
Superior rectus	III	Downward and inward	Upward and outward	Oblique
Inferior rectus	III	Upward and inward	Downward and outward	Oblique
Inferior oblique	III	Downward and outward	Upward and inward	Oblique
Superior oblique	IV	Upward and outward	Downward and inward	Oblique
Lateral rectus	VI	Inward (internal squint)	Toward temple	Vertical

* Diplopia is noted only when the affected eye attempts these movements.

nucleus (see Fig 8–7). For reasons that are not clear, there is usually nystagmus (rapid, jerking movements) in the abducting eye (ie, the eye looking right). The impaired adduction of the left eye is not due to weakness of the medial rectus (because the muscle can be activated during convergence), but rather reflects disconnection of the oculomotor nucleus from the contralateral lateral gaze center. This syndrome is called **internuclear ophthalmoplegia** (it has also been termed *anterior* or *superior internuclear ophthalmoplegia*). Unilateral internuclear ophthalmoplegia is usually seen as a result of ischemic disease of the brain stem; bilateral internuclear ophthalmoplegia can be seen in patients with multiple sclerosis.

Cranial Nerve V: Trigeminal Nerve

A. Anatomy: The trigeminal nerve, shown in Figure 8–11, contains a large **sensory root,** which carries sensation from the skin and mucosa of most of the head, and a smaller **motor root,** which innervates most of the chewing muscles (masseter, temporalis, pterygoids, mylohyoid), and the tensor tympani muscle of the middle ear.

The efferent fibers of the nerve (the minor portion) originate in the **motor nucleus of V** in the pons; this cell group receives bilateral input from the corticobulbar tracts and reflex connections from the spinal

tract of nerve V and controls the muscles involved in chewing.

The sensory root (the main portion of the nerve) arises from cells in the semilunar ganglion (also known as the **gasserian** or **trigeminal ganglion**) in a pocket of dura (Meckel's cave) lateral to the cavernous sinus. It passes posteriorly between the superior petrosal sinus in the tentorium and the skull base and enters the pons.

Fibers of the **ophthalmic division** enter the cranial cavity through the superior orbital fissure. Fibers of the **maxillary division** pass through the foramen rotundum. Sensory fibers of the **mandibular division,** joined by the motor fibers involved in mastication, course through the foramen ovale.

Touch and pressure pathways pass from the nerve's main sensory nucleus via crossed fibers in the ventral trigeminothalamic-thalamic tract and via uncrossed fibers in the dorsal trigeminothalamic tract, to the ventral posteromedial (VPM) nuclei of the thalamus and higher centers. Pain and temperature pathways pass from the spinal tract and nucleus to the thalamus via the ventral trigeminothalamic tract. The reflex connections pass to the cerebellum and the motor nuclei of cranial nerves V, VII, and IX. The sensory distribution of the divisions of the face is shown in Figure 8–12 and Table 8–6.

The afferent axons for the **corneal reflex** are carried in the ophthalmic branch of nerve V and synapse in the spinal tract and nucleus of V. From there, impulses are relayed to the facial (VII) nuclei, where motor neurons that project to the orbicularis oculi muscles are activated (the efferent limb of the corneal reflex is thus carried by nerve VII). The **jaw jerk reflex** is a monosynaptic (stretch) reflex for the masseter muscle. Rapid stretch of the muscle (elicited gently with a reflex hammer) evokes afferent impulses in Ia sensory axons in the mandibular division of nerve V, which send collaterals to the mesencephalic nucleus of V, which sends excitatory projections to the motor nucleus of V. Both afferent and efferent limbs of the jaw jerk reflex thus run in nerve V.

B. Clinical Correlations: Symptoms and signs of nerve V involvement include loss of sensation of one or more sensory modalities of the nerve; impaired hearing from paralysis of the tensor tympani muscle; paral-

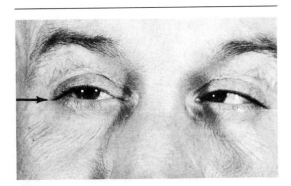

Figure 8–10. Right abducens paralysis. Right eye fails to abduct on lateral gaze.

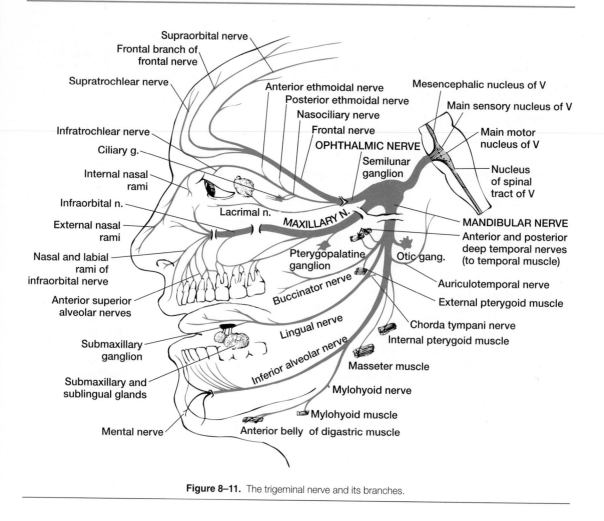

Figure 8–11. The trigeminal nerve and its branches.

ysis of the muscles of mastication, with deviation of the mandible to the affected side; loss of reflexes (cornea, jaw jerk, sneeze); trismus (lockjaw); and, in some disorders, tonic spasm of the muscles of mastication.

Because the spinal tract of V is located near the lateral spinothalamic tract in the medulla and lower pons, laterally placed lesions at these levels produce a crossed picture of pain and temperature insensibility on the *ipsi*lateral face, and on the *contra*lateral side of the body below the face. This occurs, for example, in **Wallenberg's syndrome,** in which there is damage to the lateral medulla, usually because of occlusion of the posterior inferior cerebellar artery.

Tic douloureux (trigeminal neuralgia) is characterized by severe pain in the distribution of one or more branches of the trigeminal nerve. Excruciating paroxysmal pain of short duration can be caused by pressure from a small vessel on the root entry zone of the nerve. It may follow irritation of the trigger zone, a point on the lip, face, or tongue that is sensitive to cold, pressure, or a blast of air. Involvement is usually unilateral.

Cranial Nerve VII: Facial Nerve

A. Anatomy: The facial nerve consists of the **facial nerve proper** and the **nervus intermedius** (Fig 8–13). Both parts pass through the internal auditory meatus, where the **geniculate ganglion** for the taste component lies. The facial nerve proper contains axons that arise in the facial (VII) nucleus; the nerve exits through the stylomastoid foramen; it innervates the muscles of facial expression, the platysma muscle, and the stapedius muscle in the inner ear.

The nervus intermedius sends parasympathetic preganglionic fibers to the **pterygopalatine ganglion** to innervate the lacrimal gland and via the chorda tympani nerve to the submaxillary and sublingual ganglia in the mouth to innervate the salivary glands.

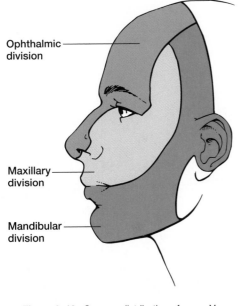

Ophthalmic
division

Maxillary
division

Mandibular
division

Figure 8–12. Sensory distribution of nerve V.

Table 8–6. Distribution of the trigeminal nerve.

Ophthalmic division
  Area of skin labeled in Fig 8–12
  Cornea, conjunctiva and intraocular structures (the sclera
    is innervated by fibers of the anterior branches of the
    ciliary plexus)
  Mucosa of paranasal sinuses (frontal, sphenoid, and eth-
    moid)
  Mucosa of upper and anterior nasal septum and lateral
    wall of nasal cavity
  Lacrimal duct

Maxillary division
  Area of skin labeled in Fig 8–12
  Mucosa of maxillary sinus
  Mucosa of posterior part of nasal septum and lower part
    of nasal cavity
  Upper teeth and gum
  Hard palate
  Soft palate and tonsil (via sphenopalatine ganglion,
    greater petrosal nerve, and nervus intermedius)

Mandibular division
  Area of skin labeled in Fig 8–12
  Mucosa of the cheek, lower jaw, floor of the mouth,
    tongue
  Proprioception from jaw muscles
  Lower teeth and gum
  Mastoid cells
  Muscles of mastication

Modified from Haymaker W: *Bing's Local Diagnosis in Neurological Disease,* 15th ed. Mosby, 1969.

The visceral afferent component of the nervus intermedius, with cell bodies in the geniculate ganglion,
carries taste sensation from the anterior two-thirds of
the tongue, via the **chorda tympani** to the solitary tract
and nucleus. The somatic afferent fibers from the skin
of the external ear are carried in the facial nerve to the
brain stem. These fibers connect there to the trigeminal nuclei and are, in fact, part of the trigeminal sensory system.

The superior salivatory nucleus receives cortical
impulses from the nucleus of the solitary tract via the
dorsal longitudinal fasciculus and reflex connections.
Visceral efferent axons run from the superior salivatory nucleus via nerve VII to the pterygopalatine and
submandibular ganglia. They synapse there with postganglionic parasympathetic neurons that innervate the
submandibular and sublingual salivary glands.

The taste fibers are run through the chorda tympani
and nervus intermedius to the solitary nucleus, which
is connected with the cerebral cortex through the medial lemnisci and the VPM nucleus of the thalamus and
with the salivatory nucleus and motor nucleus of VII
by reflex neurons. The cortical taste area is located in
the inferior central (face) region; it extends onto the opercular surface of the parietal lobe and adjacent insular cortex.

B. Clinical Correlations: The facial nucleus receives crossed and uncrossed fibers by way of the corticobulbar (corticonuclear) tract (see Fig 7–10). The facial muscles below the forehead receive contralateral
cortical innervation (crossed corticobulbar fibers
only). Therefore, a lesion rostral to the facial nucleus—
a central facial lesion—results in paralysis of the
contralateral facial muscles except the frontalis and
orbicularis oculi muscles. Because the frontalis and orbicularis oculi muscles receive bilateral cortical innervation, they are not paralyzed by lesions involving one
motor cortex or its corticobulbar pathways.

The complete destruction of the facial nucleus itself
or its branchial efferent fibers (facial nerve proper) par-
alyzes all ipsilateral face muscles; this is equivalent to
a peripheral facial lesion. **Peripheral facial paralysis
(Bell's palsy)** can occur as an idiopathic condition, but
it is seen as a complication of diabetes and can occur
as a result of tumors, sarcoidosis, AIDS, and Lyme disease. When an attempt is made to close the eyelids, the
eyeball on the affected side may turn upward (Bell's
phenomenon; Fig 8–14).

The symptoms and signs depend upon the location
of the lesion. A lesion in or outside the stylomastoid
foramen results in a flaccid paralysis (lower-motor-
neuron type) of all the muscles of facial expression in
the affected side; this can occur from a stab wound or
from swelling of the parotid gland (eg, as seen in
mumps). A lesion in the facial canal involving the
chorda tympani nerve results in reduced salivation and
loss of taste sensation from the ipsilateral anterior two-
thirds of the tongue. A lesion higher up in the canal can

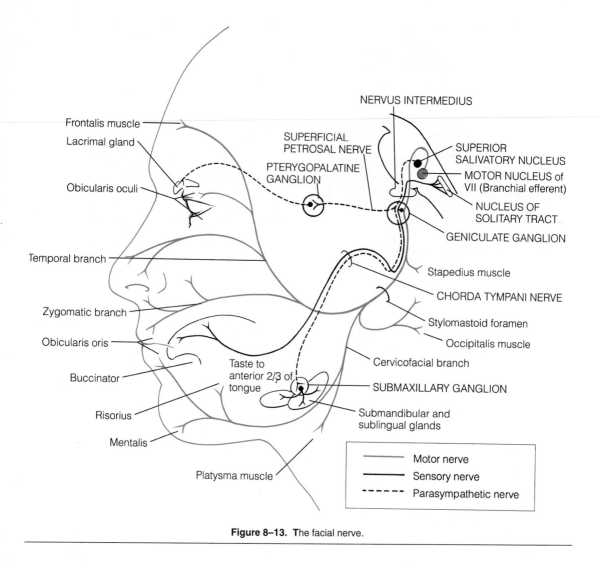

NERVUS INTERMEDIUS

SUPERFICIAL
PETROSAL NERVE

PTERYGOPALATINE
GANGLION

SUPERIOR
SALIVATORY NUCLEUS

MOTOR NUCLEUS of
VII (Branchial efferent)

NUCLEUS OF
SOLITARY TRACT

GENICULATE GANGLION

Frontalis muscle

Lacrimal gland

Obicularis oculi

Temporal branch

Stapedius muscle

CHORDA TYMPANI NERVE

Stylomastoid foramen

Occipitalis muscle

Cervicofacial branch

SUBMAXILLARY GANGLION

Submandibular and
sublingual glands

Zygomatic branch

Obicularis oris

Buccinator

Risorius

Mentalis

Platysma muscle

Taste to
anterior 2/3 of
tongue

_____ Motor nerve
——————— Sensory nerve
- - - - - - - Parasympathetic nerve

Figure 8–13. The facial nerve.

paralyze the stapedius muscle. A lesion in the middle ear involves all components of nerve VII, while a tumor in the internal auditory canal (eg, a Schwannoma) can cause dysfunction of nerves VII and VIII. (Lesions in and near the brain stem are discussed in Chapter 7.)

Cranial Nerve VIII:
Vestibulocochlear Nerve

Cranial nerve VIII is a double nerve that arises from spiral and vestibular ganglia in the labyrinth of the inner ear (Fig 8–15). It passes into the cranial cavity via the internal acoustic meatus and enters the brain stem behind the posterior edge of the middle cerebellar peduncle in the pontocerebellar angle. The cochlear nerve is concerned with hearing (audition); the vestibular nerve is part of the system of equilibrium

(position sense). The functional anatomy of the auditory system (and its clinical correlations) is discussed in Chapter 16; the vestibular system and its clinical correlations are discussed in Chapter 17.

Cranial Nerve IX:
Glossopharyngeal Nerve

A. Anatomy: Cranial nerve IX contains several types of fibers (Fig 8–16). Branchial efferent fibers from the **ambiguous nucleus** pass to the stylopharyngeus muscle.

Visceral efferent (parasympathetic preganglionic) fibers from the **inferior salivatory nucleus** pass through the tympanic plexus and lesser petrosal nerve to the **otic ganglion,** from which the postganglionic fibers pass to the **parotid gland.** The inferior saliva-

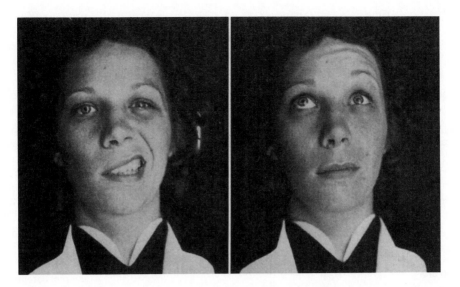

Figure 8–14. Bell's palsy. *Left:* Weakness of all the muscles on the right side of the face becomes evident when the patient tries to smile. Notice the flattened nasolabial folds and widened palpebral fissure on the right. *Right:* Weakness of the muscles of the right side of the forehead when the patient attempts to furrow the brow. (Reproduced, with permission, from Haymaker W: *Bing's Local Diagnosis in Neurological Diseases,* 15th ed. Mosby, 1969.)

tory nucleus receives cortical impulses via the dorsal longitudinal fasciculus and reflexes from the nucleus of the solitary tract.

Visceral afferent fibers arise from unipolar cells in the **inferior** (formerly **petrosal**) **ganglia.** Centrally, they terminate in the solitary tract and its nucleus, which in turn projects to the thalamus (VPM nucleus) and then to the cortex. Peripherally, the visceral afferent axons of nerve XI supply general sensation to the pharynx, soft palate, posterior third of the tongue, fauces, tonsils, auditory tube, and tympanic cavity. Through the sinus nerve, they supply special receptors in the **carotid body** and **carotid sinus** that are concerned with reflex control of respiration, blood pressure, and heart rate. Special visceral afferents supply the taste buds of the posterior third of the tongue and

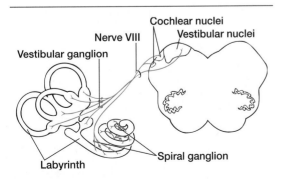

Figure 8–15. The vestibulocochlear nerve.

carry impulses via the **superior ganglia** to the gustatory nucleus of the brain stem. A few somatic afferent fibers enter by way of the glossopharyngeal nerve and end in the trigeminal nuclei.

The tongue receives its sensory innervation through multiple pathways: three cranial nerves contain taste fibers (nerve VII for anterior one-third of tongue; nerve IX for posterior one-third of tongue; nerve X for epiglottis), and the general sensory afferent fibers are mediated by nerve V (Fig 8–17); the central pathway for taste sensation is shown in Fig 8–18.

B. Clinical Correlations: The glossopharyngeal nerve is rarely involved alone (eg, by neuralgia); it is generally involved with the vagus and accessory nerves. The **pharyngeal (gag) reflex** depends on nerve IX for its sensory component, while nerve X innervates the motor component. Stroking the affected side of the pharynx does not produce gagging if the nerve is injured. The **carotid sinus reflex** depends on nerve IX for its sensory component. Pressure over the sinus normally produces slowing of the heart rate and a fall in blood pressure.

Cranial Nerve X: Vagus Nerve

A. Anatomy: Branchial efferent fibers from the ambiguous nucleus contribute rootlets to the vagus nerve and the cranial component of the accessory nerve (XI). Those of the vagus nerve pass to the muscles of the soft palate and pharynx (Fig 8–19). Those of the accessory nerve join the vagus outside the skull and pass, via the recurrent laryngeal nerve, to the intrinsic muscles of the larynx.

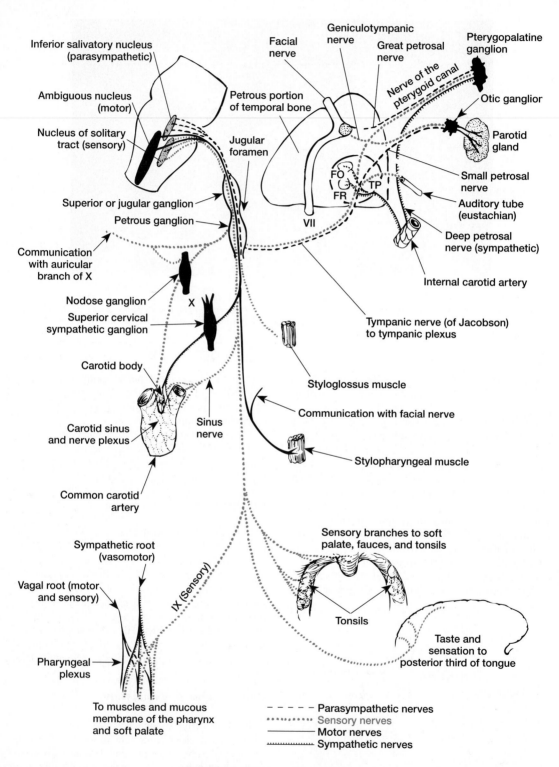

Figure 8–16. The glossopharyngeal nerve.

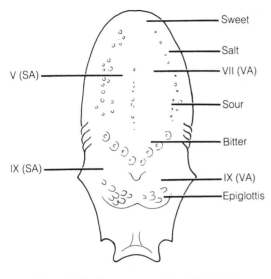

V (SA)

VII (VA)

IX (SA)

Sweet

Salt

Sour

Bitter

IX (VA)

Epiglottis

Figure 8–17. Sensory innervation of the tongue.

Visceral efferent fibers from the **dorsal motor nucleus** of the vagus course to the thoracic and abdominal viscera. Their postganglionic fibers arise in the terminal ganglia within or near the viscera. They inhibit heart rate and adrenal secretion and stimulate gastrointestinal peristalsis and gastric, hepatic, and pancreatic glandular activity (see Chapter 20).

Somatic afferent fibers of unipolar cells in the **superior** (formerly **jugular**) **ganglion** send peripheral branches via the auricular branch of nerve X to the external auditory meatus and part of the earlobe. They also send peripheral branches via the recurrent meningeal branch to the dura of the posterior fossa. Central branches pass with nerve X to the brain stem and end in the spinal tract of the trigeminal nerve and its nucleus.

Visceral afferent fibers of unipolar cells in the **inferior** (formerly **nodose**) **ganglion** send peripheral branches to the pharynx, larynx, trachea, esophagus, and the thoracic and abdominal viscera. They also send a few special afferent fibers to taste buds in the epiglottic region. Central branches run to the solitary tract and terminate in its nucleus. The visceral afferent fibers of the vagus nerve carry the sensations of abdominal distention and nausea and the impulses concerned with regulating the depth of respiration and controlling blood pressure. A few special visceral afferent fibers for taste from the epiglottis pass via the inferior ganglion to the gustatory nucleus of the brain stem.

The ambiguous nucleus receives cortical connections from the corticobulbar tract and reflex connections from the extrapyramidal and tectobulbar tracts and the nucleus of the solitary tract.

B. Clinical Correlations: Lesions of the vagus nerve may be intramedullary or peripheral. Vagus nerve lesions near the skull base often involve the glossopharyngeal and accessory nerves and sometimes the hypoglossal nerve as well (Fig 8–20).

Complete bilateral transection of the vagus nerves is fatal.

Unilateral lesions of the vagus nerve, within the cranial vault or close to the base of the skull, produce widespread dysfunction of the palate, pharynx, and larynx. The soft palate is weak and may be flaccid so the voice has a nasal twang. Weakness or paralysis of the vocal cord may result in hoarseness. There can be difficulty in swallowing and cardiac arrhythmias may be present.

Damage to the **recurrent laryngeal nerve,** which arises from the vagus, can occur as a result of invasion or compression by tumor, or as a complication of thyroid surgery. It may be accompanied by hoarseness or hypophonia but can be asymptomatic.

Cranial Nerve XI: Accessory Nerve

A. Anatomy: The accessory nerve consists of two separate components: the cranial component and the spinal component (Fig 8–21).

In the cranial component, branchial efferent fibers (from the ambiguous nucleus to the intrinsic muscles of the larynx) join the accessory nerve inside the skull, but are part of the vagus outside the skull.

In the spinal component, the branchial efferent fibers from the lateral part of the anterior horns of the first five or six cervical cord segments ascend as the spinal root of the accessory nerve through the foramen magnum and leave the cranial cavity through the jugular foramen. These fibers supply the sternocleidomastoid muscle and partly supply the trapezius muscle. The central connections of the spinal component are those of the typical lower-motor-neuron: voluntary impulses via the corticospinal tracts, postural impulses via the basal ganglia, and reflexes via the vestibulospinal and tectospinal tracts.

B. Clinical Correlations: Interruption of the spinal component leads to paralysis of the sternocleidomastoid muscle, causing the inability to rotate the head to the contralateral side, and paralysis of the upper portion of the trapezius muscle, which is characterized by a wing-like scapula and the inability to shrug the ipsilateral shoulder.

Cranial Nerve XII: Hypoglossal Nerve

A. Anatomy: Somatic efferent fibers from the **hypoglossal nucleus** in the ventromedian portion of the gray matter of the medulla emerge between the pyramid and the olive to form the hypoglossal nerve (Fig 8–22). The nerve leaves the skull through the hy-

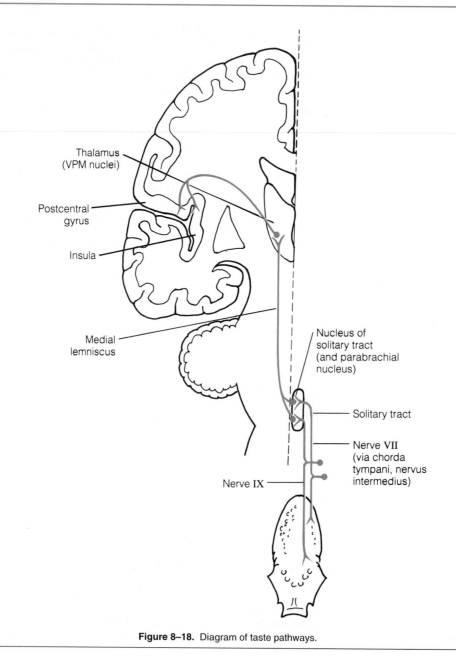

Figure 8–18. Diagram of taste pathways.

poglossal canal and passes to the muscles of the tongue. A few proprioceptive fibers from the tongue course in the hypoglossal nerve and end in the trigeminal nuclei of the brain stem. The hypoglossal nerve distributes motor branches to the geniohyoid and infrahyoid muscles with fibers derived from communicating branches of the first cervical nerve. A sensory recurrent meningeal branch of nerve XII innervates the dura of the posterior fossa of the skull.

Central connections of the hypoglossal nucleus include the corticobulbar (corticonuclear) motor system (with crossed fibers, as shown in Fig 7–10), as well as

reflex neurons from the sensory nuclei of the trigeminal nerve and the nucleus of the solitary tract (not shown).

B. Clinical Correlations: Peripheral lesions that affect the hypoglossal nerve usually come from mechanical causes (Fig 8–23). Nuclear and supranuclear lesions can have many causes (eg, tumors, bleeding, demyelination).

Lesions of the medulla produce characteristic symptoms that are related to the involvement of the nuclei of the last four cranial nerves that lie within the medulla and the motor and sensory pathways through it. Ex-

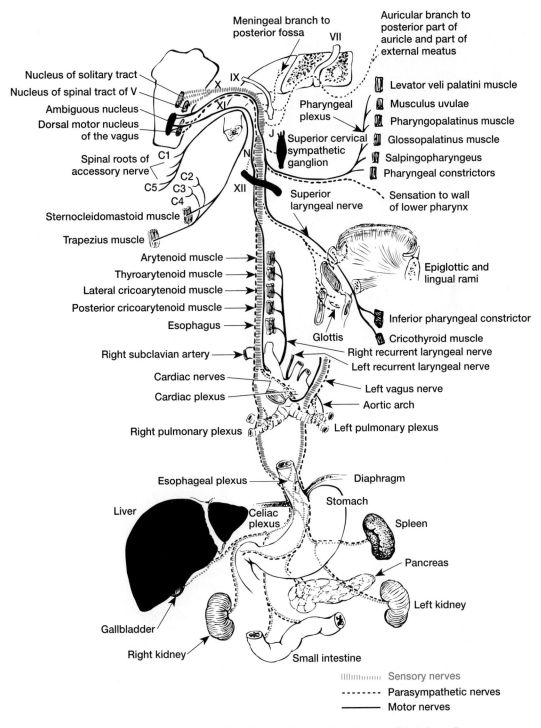

Meningeal branch to posterior fossa

Auricular branch to posterior part of auricle and part of external meatus

VII

IX

X

XI

Nucleus of solitary tract

Nucleus of spinal tract of V

Ambiguous nucleus

Dorsal motor nucleus of the vagus

Spinal roots of accessory nerve

C1

C2

C5 C3

C4

XII

J

N

Pharyngeal plexus

Superior cervical sympathetic ganglion

Levator veli palatini muscle

Musculus uvulae

Pharyngopalatinus muscle

Glossopalatinus muscle

Salpingopharyngeus

Pharyngeal constrictors

Sensation to wall of lower pharynx

Superior laryngeal nerve

Sternocleidomastoid muscle

Trapezius muscle

Arytenoid muscle

Thyroarytenoid muscle

Lateral cricoarytenoid muscle

Posterior cricoarytenoid muscle

Esophagus

Right subclavian artery

Cardiac nerves

Cardiac plexus

Right pulmonary plexus

Epiglottic and lingual rami

Glottis

Inferior pharyngeal constrictor

Cricothyroid muscle

Right recurrent laryngeal nerve

Left recurrent laryngeal nerve

Left vagus nerve

Aortic arch

Left pulmonary plexus

Esophageal plexus

Liver

Celiac plexus

Diaphragm

Stomach

Spleen

Pancreas

Left kidney

Gallbladder

Right kidney

Small intestine

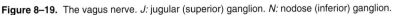

Sensory nerves

Parasympathetic nerves

Motor nerves

Figure 8–19. The vagus nerve. *J:* jugular (superior) ganglion. *N:* nodose (inferior) ganglion.

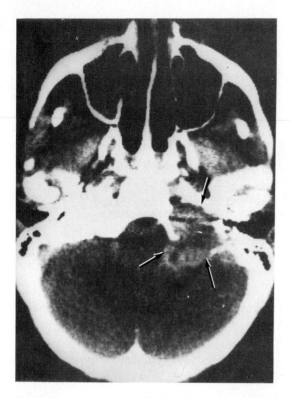

Figure 8–20. CT image through horizontal section through the head at the level of the posterior fossa. A large mass (arrows) has eroded the left jugular foramen.

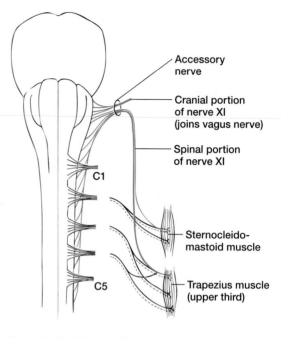

Figure 8–21. Schematic illustration of the accessory nerve, viewed from below.

tramedullary lesions of the posterior fossa may involve the roots of the last four cranial nerves between their emergence from the medulla and their exit from the skull.

CASE 8

A 24-year-old medical student noticed while shaving one morning that he was unable to move the left side of his face. He worried that a serious problem, possibly a stroke, might have occurred. He had suffered from influenza-like symptoms the week before this sudden attack.

Neurologic examination showed that the patient could not wrinkle his forehead on the left side, neither could he show his teeth or purse his lips on that side. Taste sensation was abnormal in the left anterior two-thirds of the tongue, and he had trouble closing his left eye. A test to determine tear secretion showed that secretion on the right side was normal, but the left lacrimal gland produced little fluid. Loud noises

caused discomfort in the patient, who was in good health otherwise, and there were no additional signs or symptoms.

What is the differential diagnosis? What is the most likely diagnosis?

CASE 9

A 56-year-old mailman complained of attacks of severe stabbing pains in the right side of the face. These pain attacks had started to appear about six months earlier and had lately seemed to come more often. The pain would occur several times a day, lasting only a few seconds. He was unable to shave, because touching his right cheek would trigger an excruciating pain (he now had a full beard). On windy days the attacks seemed to occur more frequently. Sometimes drinking or eating would trigger the pain, and he had lost weight recently. He had seen a dentist who had not found any tooth-related problems.

The neurologic examination was almost entirely normal; however, when testing his face for touch and pain sensibility, a pain attack was set off each time his right cheek was touched.

What is the most likely diagnosis? Would a radiologic examination be useful?

Cases are discussed further in Chapter 25. Tests designed to determine the function of cranial nerves are described in Appendix A.

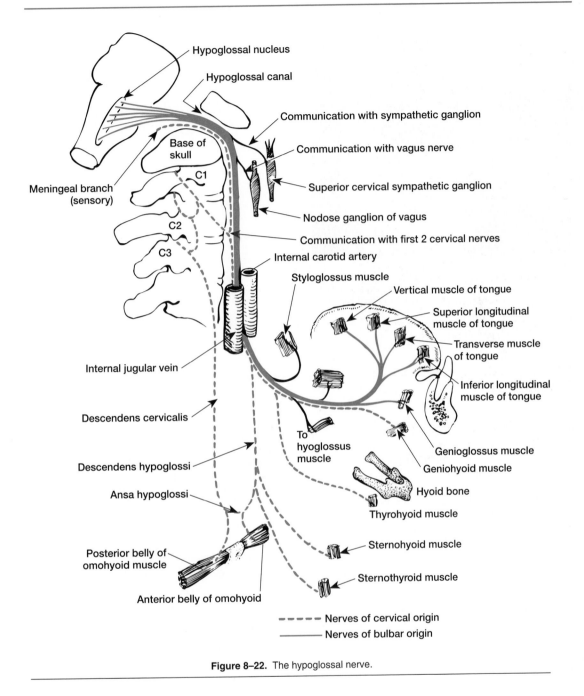

Figure 8–22. The hypoglossal nerve.

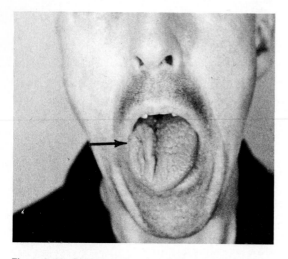

Figure 8–23. Right hypoglossal paralysis. Atrophy of the right side of the tongue and deviation of the tongue to the right occurred two months after surgical section of the right hypoglossal nerve.

REFERENCES

Bannister R: *Brain's Clinical Neurology,* 6th ed. Oxford Univ Press, 1984.

Bender MB: Brain control of conjugate horizontal and vertical eye movements. *Brain* 1980;**103:**23.

Foley JM: The cranial mononeuropathis. *New Engl J Med* 1969;**281:**905.

Hanson MR, Sweeney PJ: Lower cranial neuropathies. In: *Neurology in Clinical Practice.* Bradley WG et al (editors), Butterworth-Heinnemann, 1989.

Leigh RJ, Zee DS: *The Neurology of Eye Movements.* FA Davis Publ, 1983.

Samii M, Jannetta PJ (editors): *The Cranial Nerves.* Springer-Verlag, 1981.

Sears ES, Patton JG, Fernstermacher MJ: Diseases of the cranial nerves and brain stem. In: *Comprehensive Neurology.* Raven, 1991.

Diencephalon

9

The diencephalon, which is part of the cerebrum, includes the thalamus and its geniculate bodies, the hypothalamus, the subthalamus, and the epithalamus (Fig 9–1). The third ventricle lies between the halves of the diencephalon. A small groove on the lateral wall of the slim third ventricle—the hypothalamic sulcus—separates the thalamus and epithalamus dorsally and the hypothalamus and subthalamus inferiorly. The development of the diencephalon is reviewed briefly in Chapter 10 (see Figs 10–1, 10–3, and 10–4).

THALAMUS

Landmarks

Each half of the brain contains a thalamus (**dorsal thalamus),** a large, ovoid, gray mass of nuclei. Its broad posterior end, the **pulvinar,** extends over the medial and lateral **geniculate bodies** (Fig 9–2). The narrower rostral end of the thalamus contains the **anterior thalamic tubercle.** In many individuals there is a short **interthalamic adhesion (massa intermedia)** between the thalami, across the narrow third ventricle (see Fig 9–1); this adhesion has no functional significance.

White Matter

The **thalamic radiations** are the fiber bundles that emerge from the lateral surface of the thalamus and terminate in the cerebral cortex. The **external medullary lamina** is a layer of myelinated fibers on the lateral surface of the thalamus close to the internal capsule. The **internal medullary lamina** is a vertical sheet of white matter that bifurcates in its anterior portion and thus divides the gray matter of the thalamus into lateral, medial, and anterior portions (Fig 9–3).

Thalamic Nuclei

There are five groups of thalamic nuclei, each with specific fiber connections (Fig 9–3; Table 9–1).

A. Anterior Nuclear Group: This group forms the anterior tubercle of the thalamus and is bordered by the limbs of the internal lamina. It receives fibers from the mamillary bodies via the mamillothalamic tract and projects to the cingulate cortex of the cerebrum.

B. Nuclei of the Midline: These groups of cells are located just beneath the lining of the third ventricle and in the interthalamic adhesion. They connect with the hypothalamus and central periaqueductal gray matter. The **centromedian nucleus** connects with the cerebellum and corpus striatum.

C. Medial Nuclei: These include most of the gray substance medial to the internal medullary lamina: the **intralaminar nuclei** as well as the dorsomedial nucleus, which projects to the frontal cortex.

D. Lateral Nuclear Mass: This constitutes a large part of the thalamus anterior to the pulvinar between the internal and external medullary laminas. The mass includes a **reticular nucleus** between the external medullary lamina and the internal capsule; a **ventral anterior nucleus** (VA), which connects with the corpus striatum; a **ventral lateral** (VL), which projects to the cerebral motor cortex; a **dorsolateral nucleus,** which projects to the parietal lobe cortex; and a **ventral posterior** (also known as ventral basal) group, which ends in the postcentral gyrus and receives fibers from the medial lemniscus and the spinothalamic and trigeminal tracts. The ventral posterior group is divided into the **ventral posterolateral (VPL) nucleus,** which relays sensory input from the body, and the **ventral posteromedial (VPM) nucleus,** which relays sensory input from the face. The ventral posterior nuclei project information via the internal capsule to the sensory cortex of the cerebral hemisphere (see Chapter 10).

E. Posterior Nuclei: These include the pulvinar nucleus, the medial geniculate nucleus, and the lateral geniculate nucleus. The **pulvinar nucleus** is a large posterior nuclear group that connects with the parietal and temporal lobe cortices. The **medial geniculate nucleus,** which lies lateral to the midbrain under the pulvinar, receives acoustic fibers from the lateral lemniscus

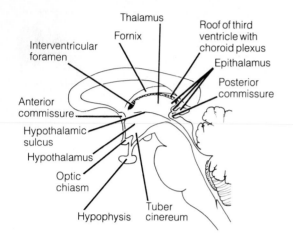

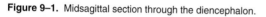

Figure 9–1. Midsagittal section through the diencephalon.

and inferior colliculus. It projects fibers via the acoustic radiation to the temporal lobe cortex. The **lateral geniculate nucleus** receives most of the fibers of the optic tract and projects via the geniculocalcarine radiation to the visual cortex around the calcarine fissure. The geniculate nuclei or bodies appear as oval elevations below the posterior end of the thalamus (see Fig 9–2).

Functional Divisions

Depending on the anatomic connections, the thalamus can be divided into five functional nuclear groups: sensory, motor, limbic, multimodal, and intralaminar (Table 9–1).

The **sensory nuclei** (ventral posterior group and geniculate bodies) are involved in relaying and modifying sensory signals from the body, face, retina, cochlea, and taste receptors (see also Chapter 14). The thalamus (rather than the sensory cortex) is thought to be the crucial structure for the perception of some types

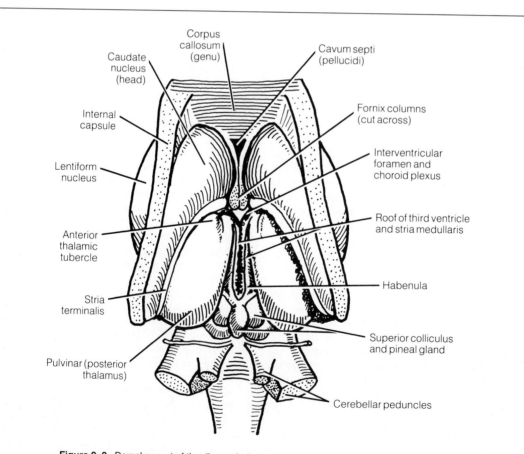

Figure 9–2. Dorsal aspect of the diencephalon after partial removal of the corpus callosum.

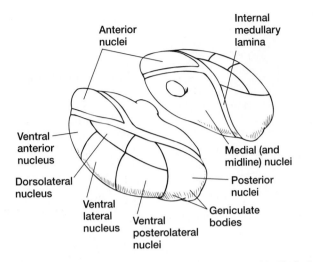

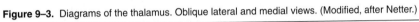

Figure 9–3. Diagrams of the thalamus. Oblique lateral and medial views. (Modified, after Netter.)

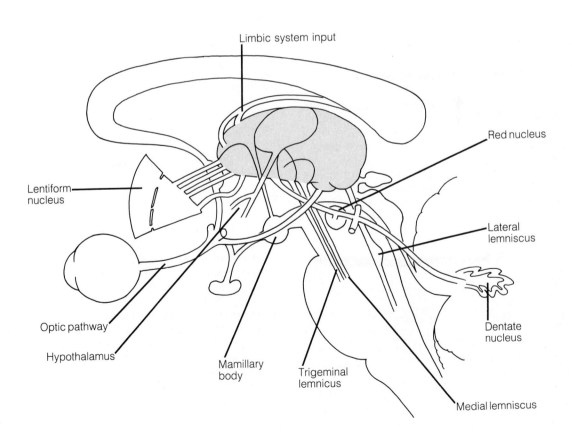

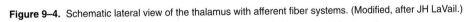

Figure 9–4. Schematic lateral view of the thalamus with afferent fiber systems. (Modified, after JH LaVail.)

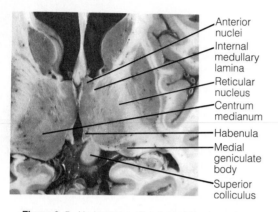

Anterior nuclei
Internal medullary lamina
Reticular nucleus
Centrum medianum
Habenula
Medial geniculate body
Superior colliculus

Figure 9–5. Horizontal section through the thalamus.

of sensation, especially pain, and the sensory cortex may function to give finer detail to the sensation.

The thalamic **motor nuclei** (ventral anterior and lateral) convey motor information from the cerebellum and globus pallidus to the precentral motor cortex. The nuclei have also been called motor relay nuclei on the basis of these connections (see also Chapter 13).

There are three anterior **limbic nuclei** interposed between the mamillary nuclei of the hypothalamus and the cingulate gyrus of the cerebral cortex. The dorsomedial nucleus receives input from the olfactory cortex and amygdala regions and projects reciprocally to the prefrontal cortex and the hypothalamus (see also Chapter 19).

The **multimodal nuclei** (pulvinar, posterolateral, and dorsolateral) have connections with the association areas in the parietal lobe (see Chapter 10). Other diencephalic regions may contribute to these connections.

Other, nonspecific thalamic nuclei include the **intralaminar** and reticular **nuclei** and the centrum medianum; the projections of these nuclei are not known

Table 9–1. Functional divisions of thalamic nuclei.

Type	Nucleus
Sensory	Lateral geniculate Medial geniculate Ventral posterolateral Ventral posteromedial
Motor	Ventral anterior Ventral lateral
Limbic	Anterior Dorsomedial
Multimodal	Pulvinar Lateral posterior (posterolateral) Lateral dorsal (dorsolateral)
Intralaminar	Reticular Centrum medianum Intralaminar

in detail. Interaction with cortical motor areas, the caudate nucleus, the putamen, and the cerebellum has been demonstrated.

Clinical Correlations

The *thalamic syndrome* is characterized by immediate hemianesthesia, with the threshold of sensitivity to pinprick, heat, and cold rising later. When a sensation is felt, sometimes referred to as thalamic hyperpathia, it is disagreeable and unpleasant. The syndrome usually appears during recovery from a thalamic infarct; rarely, persistent burning or boring pain can occur (*thalamic pain syndrome*).

HYPOTHALAMUS

Landmarks

The hypothalamus lies below and in front of the thalamus; it forms the floor and lower walls of the third ventricle (see Fig 9–1). External landmarks of the hypothalamus are the **optic chiasm;** the **tuber cinereum,** with its infundibulum extending to the posterior lobe of the hypophysis; and the **mamillary bodies** lying between the cerebral peduncles (Fig 9–6).

The hypothalamus can be divided into an anterior portion, the chiasmatic region, including the lamina terminalis; the central hypothalamus, including the tuber cinereum and the infundibulum; and the posterior portion, the mamillary area (Fig 9–7).

The right and left sides of the hypothalamus can each be further divided into a medial hypothalamic area that contains many nuclei and a lateral hypothalamic area that contains fiber systems (eg, the medial forebrain bundle) and diffuse lateral nuclei.

Hypothalamic Nuclei

Each half of the medial hypothalamus can be divided into three parts (Fig 9–8): the **supraoptic portion,** which is farthest anterior and contains the **supraoptic, suprachiasmatic,** and **paraventricular nuclei;** the **tuberal** portion, which lies immediately behind the supraoptic portion and contains the **ventromedial, dorsomedial,** and **arcuate nuclei** in addition to the median eminence; and the **mamillary** portion. This last part is farthest posterior and contains the **posterior nucleus** and several **mamillary nuclei.** There is also the **preoptic area,** a region that lies anterior to the hypothalamus, between the optic chiasm and the anterior commissure.

Fiber Connections

Afferent connections to the hypothalamus include part of the medial forebrain bundle, which sends fibers

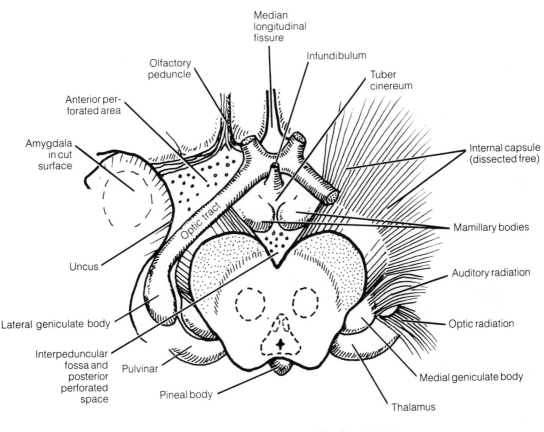

Figure 9–6. Diencephalon from below, with adjacent structures.

to the hypothalamus from nuclei in the **parolfactory area** and **corpus striatum;** thalamohypothalamic fibers from the medial and midline thalamic nuclei; and the fornix, which brings fibers from the hippocampus to the mamillary bodies. These connections also include the **stria terminalis,** which brings fibers from the **amygdala; pallidohypothalamic fibers,** which lead from the **lentiform nucleus** to the **ventromedial hypothalamic nucleus;** and the inferior mamillary peduncle, which sends fibers from the tegmentum of the midbrain. These and other connections are shown in Table 9–2.

Efferent tracts from the hypothalamus include the **hypothalamohypophyseal tract,** which runs from the supraoptic and paraventricular nuclei to the **neurohypophysis;** the **mamillotegmental tract** (part of the medial forebrain bundle) going to the tegmentum; and the **mamillothalamic tract (tract of Vicq d'Azyr),** from the mamillary nuclei to the anterior thalamic nuclei. There are also the **periventricular system,** including the dorsal fasciculus to the lower brain levels; the **tuberohypophyseal tract,** which goes from the tuberal portion of the hypothalamus to the posterior pituitary; and fibers from the septal region, by way of the fornix, to the hippocampus (see Chapter 19).

Functions

Although the hypothalamus is small (it weighs 4 gm—about 0.3 of the total brain weight), the hypothalamic region has important regulatory functions as outlined in Table 9–3.

A. Eating: A tonically active feeding center in the lateral hypothalamus evokes eating behavior. A satiety center in the ventromedial nucleus stops hunger and inhibits the feeding center when a high blood glucose level is reached after food intake. Damage to the feeding center leads to anorexia (loss of appetite) and severe loss of body weight; lesions of the satiety center lead to hyperphagia (overeating) and obesity.

B. Autonomic Function: Although anatomically discrete centers have not been identified, the posterolateral and dorsomedial areas of the hypothalamus function as a sympathetic (catecholamine) activating region, while an anterior area functions as a parasympathetic activating region. The evidence for this is derived from studying the effects of lesions in humans and animals (see also Chapter 20).

C. Body Temperature: When some regions of the hypothalamus are appropriately stimulated, they evoke autonomic responses that result in loss, conser-

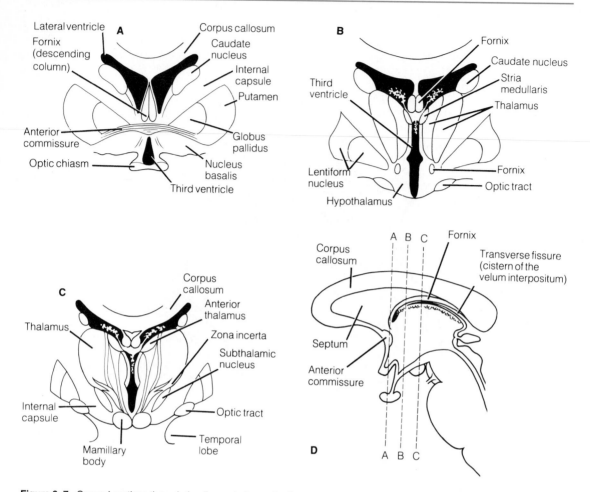

Figure 9–7. Coronal sections through the diencephalon and adjacent structures. *A:* Section through the optic chiasm and the anterior commissure. *B:* Section through the tuber cinereum and the anterior portion of the thalamus. *C:* Section through the mamillary bodies and middle thalamus. *D:* Key to the section levels.

vation, or production of body heat (Table 9–4). A fall in body temperature, for example, causes vasoconstriction, which conserves heat, and shivering, which produces heat. A rise in body temperature results in sweating and cutaneous vasodilation. Normally, the hypothalamic set-point, or thermostat, lies just below 37°C of body temperature. A higher temperature, or fever, is the result of a change in the set-point, eg, by pyrogens in the blood.

D. Water Balance: Hypothalamic influence on vasopressin secretion by the posterior pituitary is activated by osmoreceptors that are stimulated by any increase in blood osmolarity. Pain, stress, and emotional states also stimulate vasopressin secretion. Lack of secretion caused by hypothalamic or pituitary lesions, for example, can result in polyuria (increased urine excretion) and polydipsia (increased thirst).

E. Anterior Pituitary Function: The hypothalamus exerts a direct influence on secretions of the anterior pituitary and an indirect influence on secretions

of other endocrine glands by releasing or inhibiting hormones carried by the pituitary portal vessels (Fig 9–9). It thus regulates many endocrine functions, including reproduction, sexual behavior, thyroid and adrenal cortex secretions, and growth.

F. Circadian Rhythm: Many body functions (eg, temperature, corticosteroid levels, oxygen consumption) are cyclically influenced by light-intensity changes that have a circadian (day-to-day) rhythm. A retinosuprachiasmatic pathway reacts to changes in light intensity. The suprachiasmatic nucleus itself functions as an independent clock with a period of about 25 hours per cycle; lesions in this nucleus cause the loss of all circadian cycles.

G. Expression of Emotion: The hypothalamus is involved in the expression of rage, fear, aversion, sexual behavior, and pleasure. Patterns of expression and behavior are subject to limbic system influence and, in part, to changes in visceral system function (see Chapters 19 and 20).

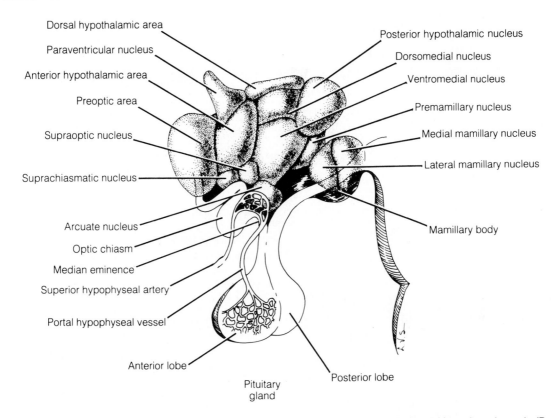

Figure 9–8. The human hypothalamus, with a superimposed diagrammatic representation of the portal-hypophyseal vessels. (Reproduced, with permission, from Ganong WF: Review of Medical Physiology, 16th ed. Appleton & Lange, 1993.)

Clinical Correlations

Several clinical problems related to dysfunction of the hypothalamus have been discussed in the previous paragraphs (Table 9–5). Lesions in the hypothalamus are most often caused by tumors that arise from either the hypothalamus itself (eg, glioma, hamartoma, germinoma) or adjacent structures (eg, pituitary adenoma, craniopharyngioma, thalamic glioma). Somnolence or even coma may be the result of bilateral lesions of the lateral hypothalamus and its reticular formation components (see Chapter 18). Even relatively minor destruction in the hypothalamus can cause a considerable loss of function.

SUBTHALAMUS

Landmarks

The subthalamus is the zone of brain tissue that lies between the dorsal thalamus and the tegmentum of the midbrain. The hypothalamus lies medial and rostral to the subthalamus; the internal capsule lies lateral to it (see Fig 9–7C). The **subthalamic nucleus,** or **body of Luys,** is a cylindrical mass of gray substance dorsolateral to the upper end of the substantia nigra; it extends posteriorly as far as the lateral aspect of the red nucleus.

Fiber Connections

The subthalamus receives fibers from the globus pallidus and projects back to it (Chapter 13); the projections from the globus pallidus to the subthalamic nucleus form part of the efferent descending path from the corpus striatum. Fibers from the globus pallidus also occupy the **fields of Forel,** which lie anterior to the red nucleus and contain cells that may be a rostral extension of reticular nuclei. The ventromedial portion is usually designated as field H, the dorsomedial portion as field H_1, and the ventrolateral portion as field H_2. The **fasciculus lenticularis** (field H_2) runs medially from the globus pallidus and is joined by the **ansa lenticularis,** which bends acutely in field H. The **thalamic fasciculus** extends through field H_1 to the anterior ventral nucleus of the thalamus. The **zona incerta** is a thin zone of gray substance above the fasciculus lenticularis. The tracts and nuclear areas of the subthalamus are involved in several functional pathways for sensory, motor, and reticular function (see Chapters 13, 14, and 18).

Table 9–2. Principal pathways to and from the hypothalamus.*

Tract	Type†	Description
Medial forebrain bundle	A, E	Connects limbic lobe and midbrain via lateral hypothalamus, where fibers enter and leave it; includes direct amygdalohypothalamic fibers, which are sometimes referred to as a separate pathway.
Fornix	A, E	Connects hippocampus to hypothalamus; mostly mamillary bodies.
Stria terminalis	A	Connects amygdala to hypothalamus, especially ventromedial region.
Mamillary peduncle	A	Diverges from sensory pathways in midbrain to enter hypothalamus; may be the pathway by which sensory stimuli enter.
Ventral noradrenergic bundle	A	Axons of noradrenergic neurons projecting from nucleus of solitary tract and other hindbrain nuclei to paraventricular nuclei and other parts of hypothalamus.
Dorsal noradrenergic bundle	A	Axons of noradrenergic neurons projecting from locus ceruleus to dorsal hypothalamus.
Serotoinergic neurons	A	Axons of serotonin-secreting neurons projecting from raphe nuclei to hypothalamus.
Adrenergic neurons	A	Axons of epinephrine-secreting neurons from medulla to ventral hypothalamus.
Retinohypothalamic fibers	A	Optic nerve fibers to suprachiasmatic nuclei from optic chiasm.
Periventricular system (including dorsal longitudinal fasciculus of Schütz)	A, E	Interconnects hypothalamus and midbrain; efferent projections to spinal cord, afferent from sensory pathways.
Mamillothalmic tract of Vicq d'Azyr	E	Connects mamillary nuclei to anterior thalamic nuclei.
Mamillotegmental tract	E	Connects hypothalamus with reticular portions of midbrain.
Hypothalamohypophyseal tract (supraopticohypophyseal and paraventriculohypophyseal tracts)	E	Axons of neurons in supraoptic and paraventricular nuclei; end in pituitary stalk and posterior pituitary.

* Modified, with permission, from Ganong WF: *Review of Medical Physiology,* 16th ed. Appleton & Lange, 1993.
† A = principally afferent; E = principally efferent.

Clinical Correlations

Lesions in the subthalamic nucleus usually result in hemiballismus, a motor disorder that affects one side of the body. (In rare cases, the lesions cause ballismus, affecting both sides.) Intermittent flailing of the affected extremities may lead to severe trauma or fractures; muscle-relaxant drugs may give temporary relief.

EPITHALAMUS

The epithalamus consists of the habenular trigones on each side of the third ventricle, the pineal body (pineal gland, or epiphysis cerebri), and the habenular commissure (see Fig 9–1).

Habenular Trigone

The habenular trigone is a small triangular area in front of the superior colliculus. It contains the **habenular nuclei,** which receive fibers from the stria medullaris thalami and are joined via the habenular commissure. The **habenulopeduncular tract** extends from the habenular nucleus to the interpeduncular nucleus in the midbrain. The function of these structures in humans is not known.

Pineal Body

The pineal body is a small mass that normally lies in the depression between the superior colliculi (see Figs 9–1 and 9–10). Its base is attached by the pineal stalk. The ventral lamina of the stalk is continuous with the posterior commissure and the dorsal lamina with the habenular commissure. At their proximal ends, the laminas of the stalk are separated, forming the pineal recess of the third ventricle. The pineal body is said to secrete hormones that are absorbed into its blood vessels.

Clinical Correlations

A tumor in the pineal region may obstruct the cerebral aqueduct or cause inability to move the eyes in the vertical plane (Parinaud's syndrome). One type of tumor (germinoma) produces precocious sexual development, and interruption of the posterior commissure abolishes the consensual light reflex.

CIRCUMVENTRICULAR ORGANS

Several small areas in or near the wall of the third ventricle, the aqueduct, and the fourth ventricle may be

Table 9–3. Principal hypothalamic regulatory mechanisms.*

Function	Afferents From	Integrating Areas
Temperature regulation	Cutaneous cold receptors; temperature-sensitive cells in hypothalamus	Anterior hypothalamus (response to heat), posterior hypothalamus (response to cold)
Neuroendrocrine contol of Catecholamines	Emotional stimuli, probably via limbic system	Dorsomedial and posterior hypothalamus
Vasopressin	Osmoreceptors, volume receptors, others	Supraoptic and paraventricular nuclei
Oxytocin	Touch receptors in breast, uterus, genitalia	Supraoptic and paraventricular nuclei
Thyroid-stimulating hormone (thyrotropin, TSH) via thyrotropin-stimulating hormone (TRH)	Temperature receptors, perhaps others	Dorsomedial nuclei and neighboring areas
Adrenocorticotropic hormone (ACTH) and β-lipotropin (β-LPH) via corticotropin-releasing hormone (CRH)	Limbic system (emotional stimuli); reticular formation ("systemic" stimuli); hypothalamic or anterior pituitary cells sensitive to circulating blood cortisol level; suprachiasmatic nuclei (diurnal rhythm)	Paraventricular nuclei
Follicle-stimulating hormone (FSH) and luteinizing hormone (LH) via luteinizing-hormone-releasing hormone (LHRH)	Hypothalamic cells sensitive to estrogens; eyes, touch receptors in skin and genitalia of reflex ovulating species	Preoptic area, other areas
Prolactin via prolactin-inhibiting hormone (PIH) and prolactin-releasing hormone (PRH)	Touch receptors in breasts, other unknown receptors	Arcuate nucleus, other areas (hypothalamus inhibits secretion)
Growth hormone via somatostatin and growth-hormone-releasing hormone (GRH)	Unknown receptors	Periventricular nucleus, arcuate nucleus
"Appetitive" behavior Thirst	Osmoreceptors, subfornical organ	Lateral superior hypothalamus
Hunger	"Glucostat" cells sensitive to rate of glucose utilization	Ventromedial satiety center, lateral hunger center; also limbic components
Sexual behavior	Cells sensitive to circulating estrogen and androgen, others	Anterior ventral hypothalamus plus (in the male) piriform cortex
Defensive reactions Fear, rage	Sense organs and neocortex, paths unknown	In limbic system and hypothalamus
Control of various endocrine and activity rhythms	Retina via retinohypothalamic fibers	Suprachiasmatic nuclei

* Reproduced and modified, with permission, from Ganong WF: *Review of Medical Physiology,* 16th ed. Appleton & Lange, 1993.

of functional importance with regard to cerebrospinal fluid composition, hormone secretion into the ventricles, and the maintenance of normal cerebrospinal fluid pressure (Fig 9–10). Most of the research has been performed on experimental animals. The functions of the habenula, the pineal body, and the pituitary gland in humans have been discussed previously.

CASE 10

A 21-year-old mailman was referred to the neurology service for an evaluation of severe headaches, from which he said he had been suffering for six months. He reported that the pain was not constant but had become more pronounced during the past month, and he felt that his eyesight had deteriorated in the past few weeks. He also stated that he now often felt cold, even in warm weather.

Neurologic examination showed partial (incomplete) bitemporal hemianopia. There was no clear papilledema, but the disks had become flattened and slightly pale. The patient had indicated that he was sexually inactive; further examination showed underdeveloped testes and the absence of pubic and axillary hair.

What is the differential diagnosis? Which neuroradiologic procedures are needed? What is the most likely diagnosis?

Cases are discussed further in Chapter 25.

Table 9–4. Temperature-regulating mechanisms.*

Activated by cold:	Result
Shivering	
Hunger	Increased
Increased voluntary activity	heat
Increased secretion of norepinephrine and epinephrine	production
Cutaneous vasoconstriction	Decreased
Curling up	heat
Horripilation	loss
Activated by heat:	
Cutaneous vasodilation	Increased
Sweating	heat
Increased respiration	loss
Anorexia	Decreased
Apathy and inertia	heat
	production

* Reproduced, with permission, from Ganong WF: *Review of Medical Physiology,* 16th ed. Appleton & Lange, 1993.

Table 9–5. Symptoms and signs in 60 cases of hypothalamic disease.*

	Percentage of Cases
Endocrine and metabolic findings	
Precocious puberty	40
Hypogonadism	32
Diabetes insipidus	35
Obesity	25
Abnormalities of temperature regulation	22
Emaciation	18
Bulimia	8
Anorexia	7
Neurologic findings	
Eye signs	78
Pyramidal and sensory deficits	75
Headache	65
Extrapyramidal signs	62
Vomiting	40
Psychic disturbances, rage attacks, etc	35
Somnolence	30
Convulsions	15

* Data from Bauer HG: Endocrine and other clinical manifestations of hypothalamic disease. *J Clin Endocrinol* 1954;**14**:13. See also Kahana L et al: Endocrine manifestations of intracranial extrasellar lesions. *J Clin Endocrinol* 1962;**22**:304. Table reproduced, with permission, from Ganong WF: *Review of Medical Physiology,* 16th ed. Appleton & Lange, 1993.

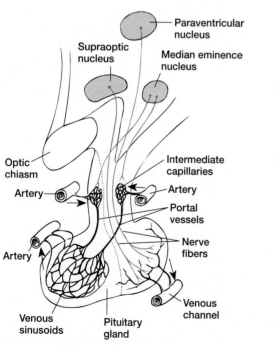

Figure 9–9. Schematic view of the pituitary portal system of vessels and neurohypophyseal pathways.

Figure 9–10. Location of the circumventricular organs. There is no blood-brain barrier in these organs (see Chapter 11).

REFERENCES

Ganong WF: Brain mechanisms regulating the secretions of the pituitary gland. Pages 549–564 in: *The Neurosciences.* Schmitt FO, Worden FG (editors). MIT Press, 1974.

Ganten D, Pfaff D (editors): *Morphology of Hypothalamus and its Connections.* Springer Verlag, 1980.

Hensel H: *Thermoreception and Temperature Regulation.* Monographs of the Physiological Society. No 38. Academic Press, 1981.

Jones EG: Functional subdivisions and synaptic organization of the mammalian thalamus. *Int Rev Physiol* 1981;**25:**173.

Meijer JH, Rietveld WJ: Neurophysiology of the suprachiasmatic circadian pacemaker in rodents. *Physiol Rev* 1989, Vol 89.

Morgan PJ, Panksepp J (editors): *Handbook of the Hypothalamus.* Marcel Dekker, 1979.

Purpura DP, Yahr MD (editors): *The Thalamus.* Columbia Univ Press, 1986.

Steriade M, Llinas RR: The functional states of the thalamus. *Physiol Rev* 1988, Vol 68.

Wurtman RJ, Axelrod J, Kelly DE: *The Pineal.* Academic Press, 1968.

Cerebral Hemispheres/ Telencephalon

The paired cerebral hemispheres include the **cerebral cortex** (which consists of six lobes on each side: frontal, parietal, temporal, occipital, insular, and limbic), the underlying **cerebral white matter,** and a complex of deep gray matter masses, the **basal ganglia.** From a phylogenetic point of view the cerebral hemispheres, particularly the cortex, are relatively new. The cortex is particularly well-developed in humans and is responsible for many aspects of higher nervous activity including language, reasoning, and many aspects of learning and memory.

DEVELOPMENT

The **telencephalon (endbrain)** gives rise to the left and right cerebral hemispheres (Fig 10–1). The hemispheres undergo a pattern of extensive differential growth; in the later stages, they resemble an arch over the lateral fissure (Fig 10–2).

The derivatives of the neural tube, or **neuraxis,** include the spinal cord, the brain stem, and the diencephalon. The upper end of the neural tube just below the anterior commissure (see section, "White Matter") is the lamina terminalis. The cerebral hemispheres and the cerebellum, however, are not considered part of the neuraxis.

The basal ganglia arise from the base of the primitive telencephalic vesicles (Fig 10–3). The growing hemispheres gradually cover most of the diencephalon and the upper part of the brain stem. Fiber connections (commissures) between the hemispheres are formed first at the rostral portions as the anterior commissure, later extending posteriorly as the **corpus callosum** (Fig 10–4).

ANATOMY OF THE CEREBRAL HEMISPHERES

The two cerebral hemispheres make up the largest portion of the brain. As seen from their external sur-

face, the cerebral hemispheres appear as highly convoluted masses of gray matter that are organized into a folded structure. The crests of the cortical folds **(gyri)** are separated by furoughs **(sulci)** or deeper **fissures.** The folding of the cortex into gyri and sulci permits the cranial vault to contain a large area of cortex (nearly 2½ square feet)—more than 50% of which is hidden within the sulci and fissures.

Main Sulci & Fissures

The surfaces of the cerebral hemispheres contain many fissures and sulci that separate the frontal, parietal, occipital, and temporal lobes from each other and the insula (Figs 10–5 and 10–6). Fissures are visible earlier during development and separate important and often large functional areas. Some gyri are relatively constant in location and contour, while others show considerable variation.

The **lateral cerebral fissure (Sylvian fissure)** separates the temporal lobe from the frontal and parietal lobes. This fissure resulted from the differential growth pattern of the adjacent cerebral hemisphere (see Fig 10–2). The insula, a portion of cortex that did not grow much during development, lies deep within the fissure (Fig 10–7). The **circular sulcus (circuminsular fissure)** surrounds the insula and separates it from the adjacent frontal, parietal, and temporal lobes.

The hemispheres are separated by a deep median fissure, the **longitudinal cerebral fissure.** The **central sulcus** (the **sulcus of Rolando**) arises about the middle of the hemisphere, beginning near the longitudinal cerebral fissure and extending downward and forward to about 2.5 cm above the lateral cerebral fissure (see Fig 10–5). The central sulcus separates the frontal lobe from the parietal lobe. The **parieto-occipital fissure** passes along the medial surface of the posterior portion of the cerebral hemisphere and then runs downward and forward as a deep cleft (see Fig 10–6). The fissure separates the parietal lobe from the occipital lobe. The **calcarine fissure** begins on the medial surface of the hemisphere near the occipital pole and ex-

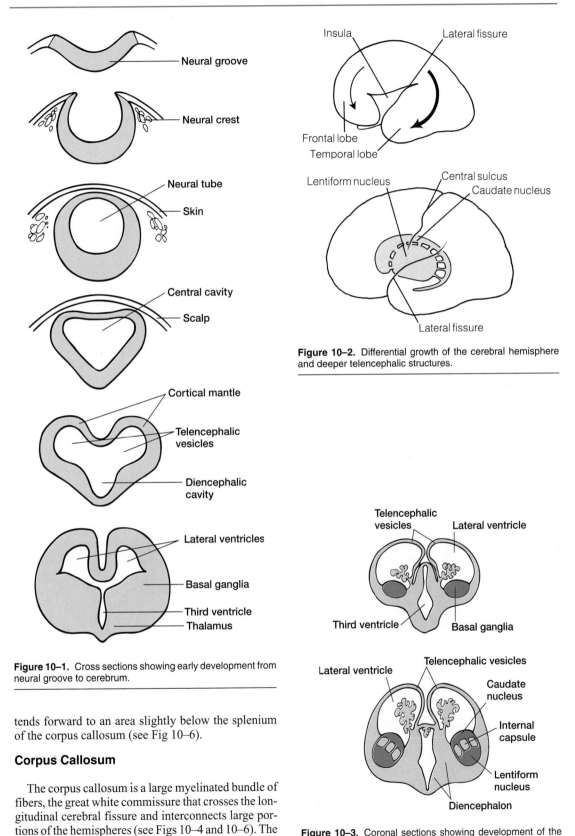

Figure 10–1. Cross sections showing early development from neural groove to cerebrum.

Figure 10–2. Differential growth of the cerebral hemisphere and deeper telencephalic structures.

Figure 10–3. Coronal sections showing development of the basal ganglia in the floor of the lateral ventricle.

tends forward to an area slightly below the splenium of the corpus callosum (see Fig 10–6).

Corpus Callosum

The corpus callosum is a large myelinated bundle of fibers, the great white commissure that crosses the longitudinal cerebral fissure and interconnects large portions of the hemispheres (see Figs 10–4 and 10–6). The body of the corpus callosum is arched; its anterior

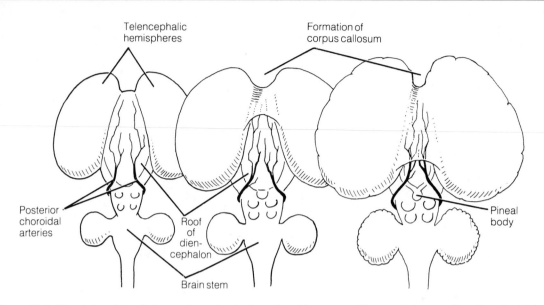

Figure 10–4. Dorsal view of developing cerebrum showing formation of the corpus callosum, which covers the subarachnoid cistern and vessels over the diencephalon.

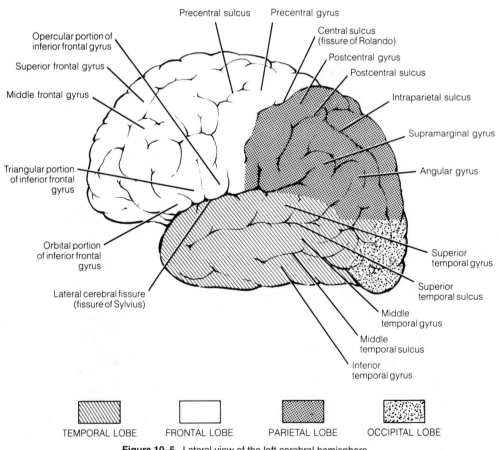

Figure 10–5. Lateral view of the left cerebral hemisphere.

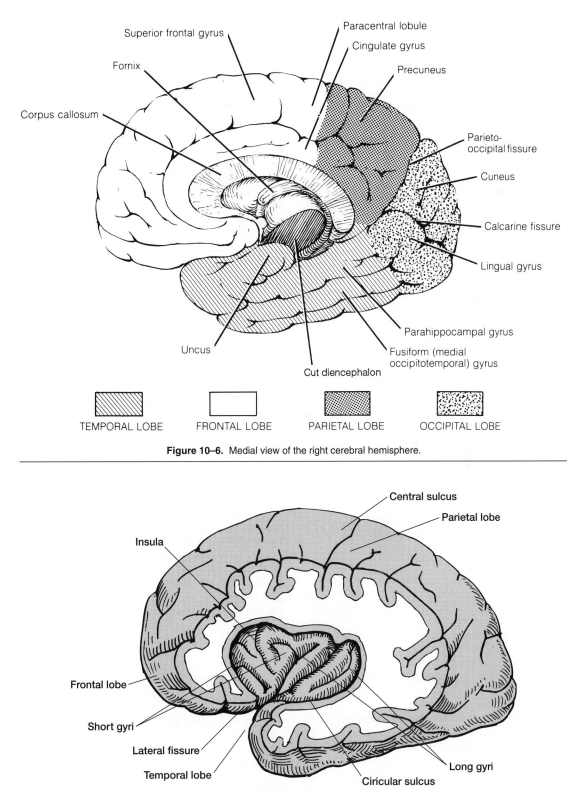

Figure 10–6. Medial view of the right cerebral hemisphere.

Figure 10–7. Dissection of the left hemisphere to show the insula.

curved portion, the **genu,** continues anteroventrally as the rostrum. The thick posterior portion terminates in the curved **splenium,** which lies over the midbrain.

Most parts of the cerebral cortex are connected with their counterparts in the opposite hemisphere by axons that run in the corpus callosum. The corpus callosum is the largest of the interhemispheric commissures, and is largely responsible for coordinating the activities of the two cerebral hemispheres.

Frontal Lobe

The frontal lobe extends from the frontal pole to the central sulcus and the lateral fissure (Figs 10–5 and 10–6). The **precentral sulcus** lies anterior to the **precentral gyrus** and parallel to the central sulcus. The **superior** and **inferior frontal sulci** extend forward and downward from the precentral sulcus, dividing the lateral surface of the frontal lobe into three parallel gyri: the **superior, middle,** and **inferior frontal gyri.** The inferior frontal gyrus is divided into three parts by the anterior horizontal and ascending rami of the lateral cerebral fissure. The orbital part lies rostral to the anterior horizontal ramus; the triangular, wedge-shaped portion lies between the anterior horizontal and anterior ascending rami; and the opercular part is between the ascending ramus and the precentral sulcus.

The **orbital sulci** and **gyri** are irregular in contour and location. The **olfactory sulcus** lies beneath the olfactory tract on the orbital surface; lying medial to it is the **straight gyrus (gyrus rectus).** The **cingulate gyrus** is the crescent-shaped, or arched, convolution on the medial surface between the cingulate sulcus and the corpus callosum. The **paracentral lobule** is the **quadrilateral gyrus** around the end of the central sulcus on the medial surface of the hemisphere and is the continuation of the precentral and postcentral gyri.

Parietal Lobe

The parietal lobe extends from the central sulcus to the parieto-occipital fissure; laterally, it extends to the level of the lateral cerebral fissure (Figs 10–5 and 10–6). The **postcentral sulcus** lies behind the postcentral gyrus. The **intraparietal sulcus** is a horizontal groove that sometimes unites with the postcentral sulcus. The **superior parietal lobule** lies above the horizontal portion of the intraparietal sulcus and the **inferior parietal lobule** lies below it.

The **supramarginal gyrus** is the portion of the inferior parietal lobule that arches above the ascending end of the posterior ramus of the lateral cerebral fissure. The **angular gyrus** arches above the end of the superior temporal sulcus and becomes continuous with the middle temporal gyrus. The **precuneus** is the posterior portion of the medial surface between the parieto-occipital fissure and the ascending end of the cingulate sulcus.

Occipital Lobe

The pyramid-shaped occipital lobe is situated behind the parieto-occipital fissure (Figs 10–5 and 10–6). The **lateral occipital sulcus** extends transversely along its lateral surface, dividing the occipital lobe into a superior and an inferior gyrus. The calcarine fissure divides the medial surface of the occipital lobe into the cuneus and the lingual gyrus. The cortex on the banks of the calcarine fissure (termed the **striate cortex** because it contains a light band of myelinated fibers in layer IV) is the site of termination of visual afferents from the lateral geniculate body; this region of cortex thus functions as the **primary visual cortex.** The wedge-shaped **cuneus** lies between the calcarine and parieto-occipital fissures, and the **lingual (lateral occipitotemporal) gyrus** is between the calcarine fissure and the posterior part of the collateral fissure. The posterior part of the **fusiform (medial occipitotemporal) gyrus** is on the basal surface of the occipital lobe.

Temporal Lobe

The temporal lobe lies below the lateral cerebral fissure and extends back to the level of the parieto-occipital fissure on the medial surface of the hemisphere (Figs 10–5 and 10–6). The lateral surface of the temporal lobe is divided into the parallel **superior, middle,** and **inferior temporal gyri,** which are separated by the **superior** and **middle temporal sulci.** The **inferior temporal sulcus** extends along the lower surface of the temporal lobe from the temporal pole to the occipital lobe. The **transverse temporal gyrus** occupies the posterior part of the superior temporal surface. The **fusiform gyrus** is medial, and the inferior temporal gyrus is lateral to the inferior temporal sulcus on the basal aspect of the temporal lobe. The **hippocampal fissure** extends along the inferomedian aspect of the lobe from the area of the splenium of the corpus callosum to the uncus. The **parahippocampal gyrus** lies between the hippocampal fissure and the anterior part of the collateral fissure. Its anterior part, the most medial portion of the temporal lobe, curves in the form of a hook; it is known as the **uncus.**

Insula

The insula is a sunken portion of the cerebral cortex (Fig 10–7). It lies deep within the lateral cerebral fissure and can be exposed by separating the upper and lower lips **(opercula)** of the lateral fissure. The deep circular sulcus bounds the insula. Several short gyri, formed by shallow sulci, occupy the anterior portion of the insula; a long gyrus occupies the posterior part.

Limbic System Components

The cortical components of the limbic system include the cingulate, parahippocampal, and subcallosal gyri as well as the hippocampal formation. These form a ring of cortex—much of which is phylogenetically old, with a relatively primitive microscopic structure—that forms a border (limbus) between the diencephalon and more lateral neocortex of the cerebral hemispheres. The anatomy and function of these components are discussed in Chapter 19.

Basal Forebrain Nuclei and Septal Area

Several poorly-defined cell islands, located beneath the basal ganglia deep in the hemisphere, project widely to the cortex. These include the **basal forebrain nuclei** (also known as the **nuclei of Meynert** or **substantia innominata**), which send widespread cholinergic projections throughout the cerebral cortex. Located just laterally are the **septal nuclei,** which receive afferent fibers from the hippocampal formation and reticular system and send axons to the hippocampus, hypothalamus, and midbrain.

White Matter

The white matter of the adult cerebral hemisphere contains myelinated nerve fibers of many sizes as well as neuroglia (mostly oligodendrocytes) (Fig 10–8 and Table 10–1). The white center of the cerebral hemisphere, sometimes called the **centrum semiovale,** contains myelinated transverse fibers, projection fibers, and association fibers.

A. Transverse (Commissural) Fibers: Transverse fibers interconnect the two cerebral hemispheres. The **corpus callosum** comprises the largest bundle of fibers; most of these arise from parts of the neocortex of one cerebral hemisphere and terminate in the corresponding parts of the opposite cerebral hemisphere. The **anterior commissure** connects the two olfactory

Table 10–1. Myelinated nerve fibers in the cerebral hemisphere.

Type of Fiber	Name	Function
Transverse (commisural)	Corpus callosum Anterior commissure Hippocampal commissure	Connect homologous areas of the 2 cerebral hemispheres
Projection	Corticopetal (afferent) fibers	Connect the thalamus to the cerebral cortex
	Corticofugal (efferent) fibers	Connect the cerebral cortex's lower portions of the brain or the spinal cord
Association	Short association (U) fibers Long association fibers Uncinate fasciculus Arcuate fasciculus Longitudinal fasciculi (inferior and superior) Occipitofrontal fasciculus Cingululm	Connect gyri, lobes, or widely separated areas within each cerebral hemisphere

bulbs and temporal lobe structures. The **hippocampal commissure,** or **commissure of the fornix,** joins the two hippocampi; it is variable in size (see also Chapter 19).

B. Projection Fibers: These fibers connect the cerebral cortex with lower portions of the brain or the spinal cord. The **corticopetal (afferent) fibers** include the geniculocalcarine radiation from the lateral geniculate body to the calcarine cortex, the auditory radiation from the medial geniculate body to the auditory cortex, and thalamic radiations from the thalamic nuclei to specific cerebrocortical areas. Afferent fibers tend to terminate in the more superficial cortical layers (layers I to IV; see next section), with thalamocortical afferents (especially the specific thalamocortical afferents that arise in the ventral tier of the thalamus, lateral geniculate, and medial geniculate) terminating in layer IV.

Corticofugal (efferent) fibers proceed from the cerebral cortex to the thalamus, brain stem, or spinal cord. Projection efferents to the spinal cord and brain stem tend to arise from large pyramidal neurons in deeper cortical layers (layer V).

C. Association Fibers: These fibers connect the various portions of a cerebral hemisphere and permit the cortex to function as a coordinated whole. The association fibers tend to arise from small pyramidal cells in cortical layers II and III (Fig 10–9).

Short association fibers, or **U fibers,** connect adjacent gyri; those located in the deeper portions of the

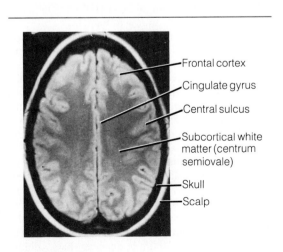

Frontal cortex

Cingulate gyrus

Central sulcus

Subcortical white matter (centrum semiovale)

Skull

Scalp

Figure 10–8. MRI of a horizontal section through the upper head.

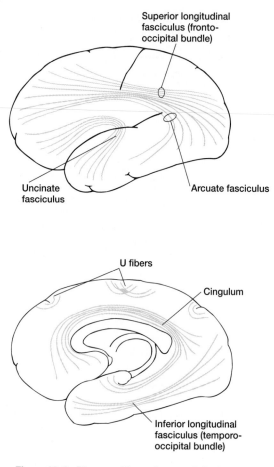

Figure 10–9. Diagram of the major association systems.

white matter are the intracortical fibers and those just beneath the cortex are called subcortical fibers.

Long association fibers connect more widely separated areas. The **uncinate fasciculus** crosses the bottom of the lateral cerebral fissure and connects the inferior frontal lobe gyri with the anterior temporal lobe. The **cingulum,** a white band within the cingulate gyrus, connects the anterior perforated substance and the parahippocampal gyrus. The **arcuate fasciculus** sweeps around the insula and connects the superior and middle frontal convolutions (which contain the speech motor area) with the temporal lobe (which contains the speech comprehension area). The **superior longitudinal fasciculus** connects portions of the frontal lobe with occipital and temporal areas. The **inferior longitudinal fasciculus,** which extends parallel to the lateral border of the inferior and posterior horns of the lateral ventricle, connects the temporal and occipital lobes. The **occipitofrontal fasciculus** extends backward from the frontal lobe, radiating into the temporal and occipital lobes.

MICROSCOPIC STRUCTURE OF THE CORTEX

The cerebral cortex contains three types of neurons: **pyramidal cells** (shaped like a teepee with an apical dendrite reaching from the upper end toward the cortical surface, and basilar dendrites extending horizontally from the cell body); **stellate neurons** (star-shaped, with dendrites extending in all directions); and **fusiform neurons** (found in deeper layers with a large dendrite that ascends toward the surface of the cortex). The axons of pyramidal and fusiform neurons form the projection and association fibers, with large layer V pyramidal neurons projecting their axons to the spinal cord and brain stem, smaller layer II and III pyramidal cells sending association axons to other cortical areas, and fusiform neurons giving rise to corticothalamic projections. Stellate neurons are interneurons whose axons remain within the cortex.

A. Types of Cortices: The cortex of the cerebrum is considered to comprise two types: allocortex and isocortex. The **allocortex (archicortex)** is found predominantly in the limbic system cortex and contains fewer layers than the isocortex (three in most regions) (see Chapter 19). The **isocortex (neocortex)** is more commonly found in most of the cerebral hemisphere and contains six layers. The **juxtallocortex (mesocortex)** forms the transition between the allocortex and isocortex. It contains 3–6 layers and is found in regions such as the cingulate gyrus and the insula.

B. Layers: The isocortex consists of up to six layers of cells (the organization of these layers is referred to as **cytoarchitecture**) (Fig 10–10).

The outermost **molecular layer (I)** contains nonspecific afferent fibers that come from within the cortex or from the thalamus.

The **external granular layer (II)** is a rather dense layer composed of small cells.

The **external pyramidal layer (III)** contains pyramidal cells, frequently in row formation.

The **internal granular layer (IV)** is usually a thin layer with cells similar to those in the external granular layer.

These cells receive specific afferent fibers from the thalamus. The **internal pyramidal layer (V)** contains, in most areas, pyramidal cells that are fewer in number but larger in size than those in the external pyramidal layer. These cells project to distal structures (eg, brain stem and spinal cord).

The **fusiform (multiform) layer (VI)** consists of irregular fusiform cells whose axons enter the adjacent white matter.

C. Columns: Although the cortex is arranged in layers, its constituent groups of neurons with similar functions are interconnected in vertically oriented columns about 30–100 μm in diameter. Each column appears to be a functional unit, consisting of cells with related properties. For example, in the somatosensory

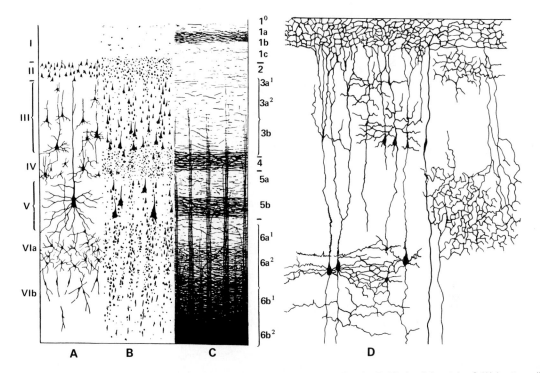

Figure 10–10. Diagram of the structure of the cerebral cortex. **A:** Golgi neuronal stain. **B:** Nissl cellular stain. **C:** Weigert myelin stain. **D:** Neuronal connections. Roman and Arabic numerals indicate the layers of the isocortex (neocortex); 4: external line of Baillarger (line of Gennari in the occipital lobe); 5b: internal line of Baillarger. (A, B, and C reproduced, with permission, from Ranson SW, Clark SL: *The Anatomy of the Nervous System,* 10th ed. Saunders, 1959. **D** reproduced, with permission, from Ganong WF: *Review of Medical Physiology,* 16th ed. Appleton & Lange, 1993.)

cortex all of the neurons in a column are activated by a single type of sensory receptor and all receive inputs from a similar part of the body. Similarly, within the visual cortex all of the cells within a column receive input from the same part of the retina (hence, from the same part of the visual world) and are tuned to respond to stimuli with similar orientations. It is the vast number of such local circuits that gives the brain its complex functions.

D. Myeloarchitecture: Myelinated fiber layers between the cortical layers give the appearance of white lines. The **line of Gennari** in the striated area of the occipital lobe is prominent and visible to the naked eye (Fig 10–10); it forms the outer portion of the internal granular layer (IV). Elsewhere in the cortex, this line is thinner and is known as the **external line of Baillarger.** The **internal line of Baillarger** is formed at the inner aspect of the ganglionic layer (V).

E. Classification of Principal Areas: Division and classification of the cerebral cortex have been attempted by many investigators on the basis of cytoarchitecture. Inferences concerning its structure and function have been drawn largely from observations on animals, especially primates.

The most commonly employed system is **Brodmann's** classification system, which uses numbers to label individual areas of the cortex that Brodmann be-

lieved differed from others (Figs 10–11 and 10–12). The areas have been used as a reference base for the localization of physiologic and pathologic processes. Ablation and stimulation, electrically and with various chemicals, have led to functional localizations. The principal areas and their functional correlations are shown in Figures 10–11 to 10–13 (some of the major cortical areas are listed in Table 10–2).

1. Frontal lobe–Area 4 is the **primary motor area** in the precentral gyrus. Large pyramidal neurons (Betz cells) and smaller neurons in this area give rise to many (but not all) axons that descend as the corticospinal tract. The motor cortex is organized somatotopically: The lips, tongue, face, and hands are represented in order within a map-like homunculus on the lower part of the convexity of the hemisphere (notice that these body parts have a magnified size as projected onto the cortex, reflecting the large amount of cortex devoted to fine finger control and buccolingual movements); the arm, trunk, and hip are then represented in order higher on the convexity; and the foot, lower leg, and genitals are draped into the interhemispheric fissure (Fig 10–14).

Area 6 (the premotor area) contains a second motor map and several other motor zones, including the **supplementary motor area** (located on the medial aspect of the hemisphere), are clustered nearby.

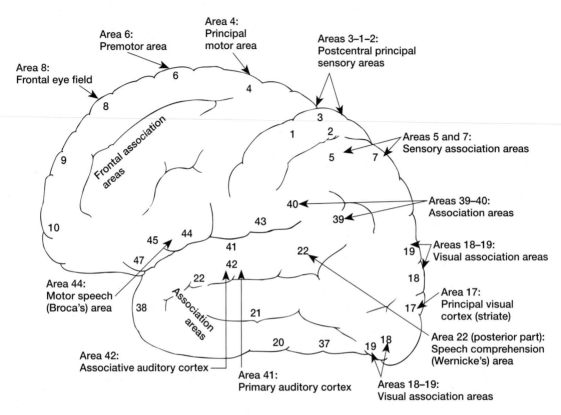

Figure 10–11. Lateral aspect of the cerebrum. The cortical areas are shown according to Brodmann with functional localizations.

Area 8 (the frontal eye field) is concerned with eye movements.

Within the inferior frontal gyrus, **areas 44 and 45 (Broca's area)** are located anterior to the motor cortex controlling the lips and tongue. Broca's area is an important area for speech.

Anterior to these areas, the **prefrontal cortex** has extensive reciprocal connections with the dorsomedial and ventral anterior thalamus and with the limbic system. This **association area** receives inputs from multiple sensory modalities and integrates them. When prefrontal areas are injured, patients become either apathetic (in some cases motionless and mute) or uninhibited and distractible, with loss of social graces and impaired judgment.

2. Parietal lobe–Areas 3, 1, and 2 are the **primary sensory areas,** which are somatotypically represented (again in the form of a homunculus) in the postcentral gyrus (Fig 10–15). This area receives somatosensory input from the VPL and VPM nuclei in the thalamus. The remaining areas are sensory or multimodal association areas.

3. Occipital lobe–Area 17 is the **striate**—the **primary visual**—**cortex.** The geniculocalcarine radiation relays visual input from the lateral geniculate to the striate cortex. Upper parts of the retina (lower parts

of the visual field) are represented in upper parts of area 17, while lower parts of the retina (upper parts of the visual field) are represented in the lower part of area 17. **Areas 18 and 19** are **visual association areas.**

4. Temporal lobe–Area 41 is the **primary auditory cortex; area 42** is the **associative (secondary) auditory cortex.** Together, these areas are referred to as **Heschl's gyrus.** They receive input (via the auditory radiations) from the medial geniculate. The surrounding temporal cortex **(area 22)** is auditory association cortex. In the posterior part of area 22 (in the posterior 1/3 of the superior temporal gyrus) is **Wernicke's area,** which plays an important role in the comprehension of language. The remaining temporal areas are multimodal association areas.

PHYSIOLOGY OF THE CORTEX

The functions of the olfactory receptive cortex and related areas are discussed in Chapter 19.

Primary Motor Projection Cortex

A. Location and Function: The primary motor projection cortex (area 4; see Chapter 13) is located on

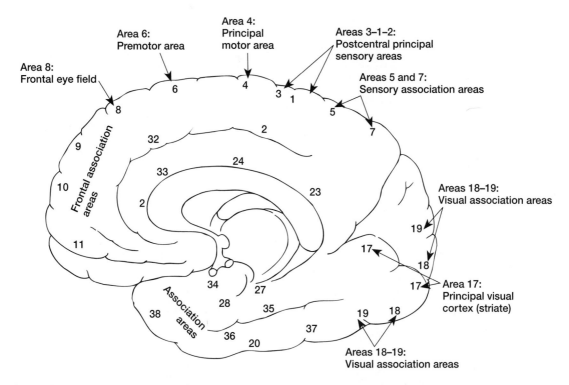

Figure 10–12. Medial aspect of the cerebrum. The cortical areas are shown according to Brodmann with functional localizations.

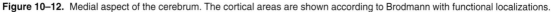

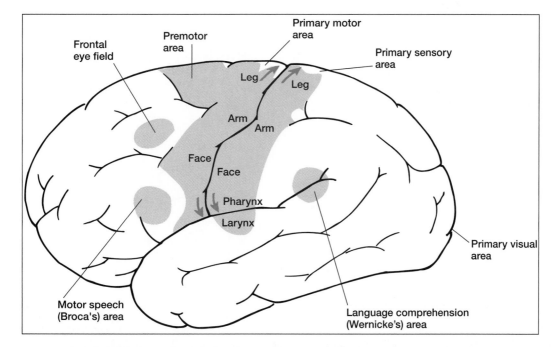

Figure 10–13. Lateral view of the left hemisphere showing the functions of the cortical areas.

Table 10–2. Specialized cortical areas.

	Brodmann's Area	Name		Function	Connections
Frontal Lobe:	4	Primary motor cortex		Voluntary muscle activation	Contributes to corticospinal tract
	6	Premotor cortex			
	8	Frontal eye field		Eye movements	Sends projections to lateral gaze center (paramedium pontine reticular formation)
	44, 45	Broca's area		Motor aspects of speech	Projects to Wernicke's area via arcuate fasciculus
Parietal Lobe:	3, 1, 2	Primary sensory cortex		Somatosensory	Input from VPL, VPM
Occipital Lobe:	17	Striate cortex = primary visual cortex		Processing of visual stimuli	Input from lateral geniculate only Projects to areas 18, 19
	18, 19	Extrastriate = visual association cortex		Processing of visual stimuli	Input from area 17
Temporal Lobe:	41	Primary auditory cortex		Processing of auditory stimuli	Input from medial geniculate
	42	Associative auditory cortex			
	22	Wernicke's area		Language comprehension	Inputs from auditory association cortex, visual association cortex, Broca's area (via arcuate fasciculus)

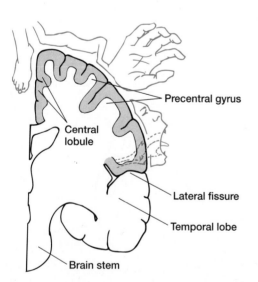

Figure 10–14. Motor homunculus drawn on a coronal section through the precentral gyrus. The figure shows the location of cortical control of various body parts.

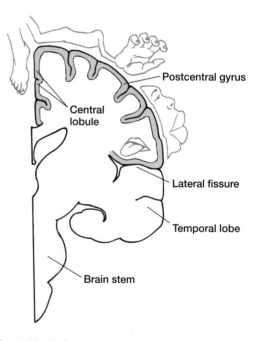

Figure 10–15. Sensory homunculus drawn overlying a coronal section through the postcentral gyrus. The figure shows the location of the cortical representation of various body parts.

the anterior wall of the central sulcus and the adjacent portion of the precentral gyrus, corresponding generally to the distribution of the giant pyramidal (Betz) cells. These cells control voluntary movements of skeletal muscle on the opposite side of the body, with the impulses traveling over their axons in the corticobulbar and corticospinal tracts to the branchial and somatic efferent nuclei in the brain stem and to the ventral horn in the spinal cord.

A somatotopic representation within the motor areas, mapped by electrical stimulation during brain surgery, appears in Figure 10–14. Secondary and tertiary areas of motor function can be mapped roughly around the primary motor cortex where stimulation produces gross movements. Contralateral conjugate deviation of the head and eyes occurs upon stimulation of the posterior part of the middle frontal gyrus (area 8), termed the frontal eye fields.

B. Clinical Correlations: Irritative lesions of the motor centers may cause seizures that begin as focal twitching and spread (in a somatotopic manner, reflecting the organization of the homunculus) to involve large muscle groups (jacksonian epilepsy). As abnormal electrical discharge spreads across the motor cortex, the seizure "marches" along the body. There may also be modification of consciousness and postconvulsive weakness or paralysis. Destructive lesions of the motor cortex (area 4) produce contralateral flaccid paresis, or paralysis, of affected muscle groups. Spasticity is more apt to occur if area 6 is also ablated.

Primary Sensory Projection Cortex

A. Location and Function: The primary sensory projection cortex for sensory information received from the skin and mucosa of the body and face is located in the postcentral gyrus and is called the **somatesthetic area** (areas 3, 1, and 2; see Fig 10–15). From the thalamic radiations, this area receives fibers that convey touch and proprioceptive (muscle, joint, and tendon) sensations from the opposite side of the body (see also Chapter 14).

Experimental studies indicate that a relatively wide portion of the adjacent frontal and parietal lobes can be considered a secondary sensory cortex since this area also receives sensory stimuli. The primary **sensorimotor area** is therefore considered capable of functioning as both a motor and a sensory cortex, with the portion of the cortex anterior to the central sulcus predominantly motor and that behind it predominantly sensory.

The **cortical taste area** is located close to the facial sensory area and extends onto the opercular surface of the lateral cerebral fissure (see Fig 8–18). This cortical area receives gustatory information, which is relayed from the solitary nucleus in the medulla via the ventral

posteromedial (VPM) nucleus of the thalamus (see Figs 7–6 and 8–18).

B. Clinical Correlations: Irritative lesions of this area produce **paresthesias** (eg, numbness, abnormal sensations of tingling, electric shock, or pins and needles) on the opposite side of the body. Destructive lesions produce objective impairments in sensibility, such as an impaired ability to localize or measure the intensity of painful stimuli and impaired perception of various forms of cutaneous sensation. Complete anesthesia on a cortical basis is rare.

Primary Visual Receptive Cortex and Visual Association Cortex

A. Location and Function: The primary visual receptive (striate) cortex (area 17) is located in the occipital lobe. It lies in the cortex of the calcarine fissure and adjacent portions of the cuneus and the lingual gyrus.

In primates, an extensive posterior portion of the occipital pole is concerned primarily with macular vision; the more anterior parts of the calcarine cortex are concerned with peripheral vision. The visual cortex in the right occipital lobe receives impulses from the right half of each retina, while the left visual cortex (area 17) receives impulses from the left half of each retina. The upper portion of area 17 represents the upper half of each retina, while the lower portion represents the lower half. Visual association is a function of areas 18 and 19. Area 19 can receive stimuli from the entire cerebral cortex; area 18 receives stimuli mainly from area 17 (see also Chapter 15).

B. Clinical Correlations: Irritative lesions of area 17 can produce such visual hallucinations as flashes of light, rainbows, brilliant stars, or bright lines. Destructive lesions can cause contralateral homonymous defects of the visual fields without destruction of macular vision. Injury to areas 18 and 19 can produce visual disorganization with defective spatial orientation in the homonymous halves of the visual field.

Primary Auditory Receptive Cortex

A. Location and Function: The primary auditory receptive area (41; see also Chapter 16) is located in the transverse temporal gyrus, which lies in the superior temporal gyrus toward the lateral cerebral fissure. The auditory cortex on each side receives the auditory radiation from the cochlea of both ears, and there is point-to-point projection of the cochlea upon the acoustic area (tonotopia). In humans, low tones are projected or represented in the frontolateral portion and high tones in the occipitomedial portion of area 41. Low tones are detected near the apex of the cochlea and high tones near the base. Area 22, which includes Wernicke's area (in the posterior 1/3 of the superior temporal gyrus in the dominant usually left hemisphere), is involved in high-order auditory discrimination and speech comprehension.

B. Clinical Correlations: Irritation of the region in or near the primary auditory receptive area in humans causes buzzing and roaring sensations. A unilateral lesion in this area may cause only mild hearing loss, but bilateral lesions can result in deafness. Damage to area 22 in the dominant hemisphere produces a syndrome of pure word deafness (in which words cannot be understood although hearing is not impaired) or Wernicke's aphasia.

BASAL GANGLIA

The term *basal ganglia* refers to masses of gray matter deep within the cerebral hemispheres. The term is debatable, however, because these masses are nuclei rather than ganglia—and some of them are not basal. Anatomically, the basal ganglia include the **caudate nucleus,** the **putamen,** the **globus pallidus,** and other gray areas at the base of the forebrain.

Terminology used to describe the basal ganglia is summarized in Table 10–3. Sheets of myelinated fibers, including the **internal capsule,** run between the nuclei comprising the basal ganglia imparting a striped appearance (Figs 10–16 and 10–17); thus, classical neuroanatomists termed the caudate nucleus, putamen, and globus pallidus collectively the **corpus striatum.** The caudate nucleus and putamen develop together and contain similar cells and, together, are termed the **striatum.** Lateral to the internal capsule, the putamen and globus pallidus abut each other to form a lens-shaped mass termed the **lenticular nuclei.** Functionally, the basal ganglia and their interconnections and neurotransmitters form an associated motor system (the **extrapyramidal system**) that includes nuclei in the subthalamus and midbrain (see Chapter 13).

Caudate Nucleus

The caudate nucleus, an elongated gray mass whose pear-shaped head is continuous with the putamen, lies adjacent to the inferior border of the anterior horn of the lateral ventricle. The slender end curves backward and downward as the tail; it enters the roof of the temporal horn of the lateral ventricle and tapers off at the level of the amygdala. The caudate nucleus and putamen (striatum) constitute the major site of input to the basal ganglia; the circuitry is described in Chapter 13.

Lenticular Nucleus

The lenticular nucleus is situated between the insula and the internal capsule. The external medullary lamina divides the nucleus into two parts, the putamen and the globus pallidus. The putamen is the larger, convex gray mass lying lateral to and just beneath the insular cortex. The striped appearance of the corpus striatum is caused by the white fasciculi of the internal capsule that are situated between the putamen and the caudate nucleus. The globus pallidus is the smaller, triangular median zone whose numerous myelinated fibers make it appear lighter in color. A medullary lamina divides the globus pallidus into two portions. The globus pallidus is the major outflow nucleus of the basal ganglia.

Claustrum & External Capsule

The claustrum is a thin layer of gray substance situated just beneath the insular cortex and separated from the more median putamen by the thin lamina of white matter known as the external capsule.

Fiber Connections

Most portions of the basal ganglia are interconnected by two-way fiber systems (Fig 10–18). The caudate nucleus sends many fibers to the putamen, which in turn sends short fibers to the globus pallidus. The putamen and globus pallidus receive some fibers from the substantia nigra, and the thalamus sends fibers to the caudate nucleus. Efferent fibers from the corpus striatum leave via the globus pallidus. Some fibers pass through the internal capsule and form a bundle, the **fasciculus lenticularis,** on the medial side. Other fibers sweep the medial border of the internal capsule to form a loop, the **ansa lenticularis.** Both these sets of fibers have some terminals in the subthalamic and red nuclei; others continue upward to the thalamus via the **thalamic fasciculus** (Fig 10–18). As described further in Chapter 13, this rich system of interconnections forms a basis for the control of movement and posture.

Internal Capsule

The internal capsule is a broad band of myelinated fibers that separates the lentiform nucleus from the medial caudate nucleus and thalamus. It consists of an anterior limb and a posterior limb. The capsule is not one of the basal ganglia, but a related fiber bundle. In horizontal section, it presents a *V* appearance, with the

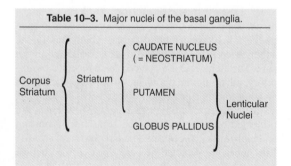

Table 10–3. Major nuclei of the basal ganglia.

Corpus Striatum	Striatum	CAUDATE NUCLEUS (= NEOSTRIATUM)	
		PUTAMEN	Lenticular Nuclei
		GLOBUS PALLIDUS	

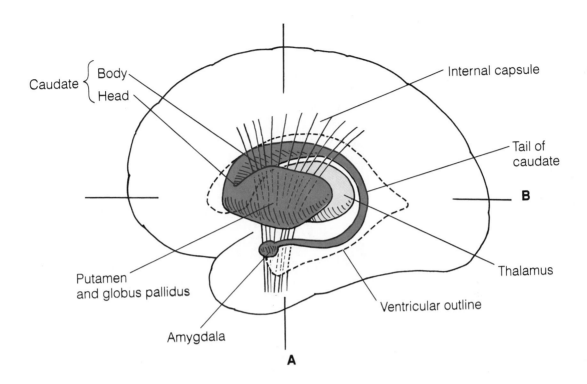

Figure 10–16. Spatial relationships between basal ganglia, thalamus, and internal capsule as viewed from the left side. Sections through planes A and B are shown in Figures 10–17A and 10–17B.

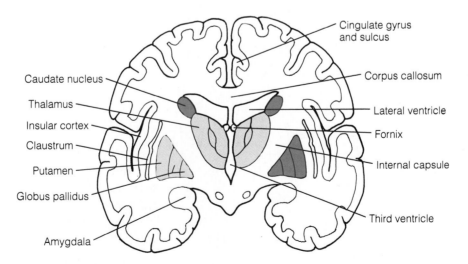

Figure 10–17. **A:** Frontal section through cerebral hemispheres showing basal ganglia and thalamus.

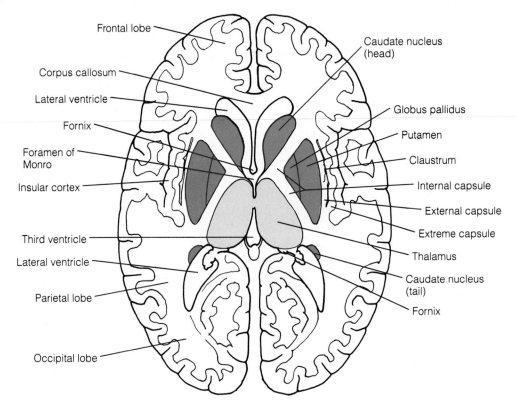

Figure 10-17B: Horizontal section through cerebral hemispheres.

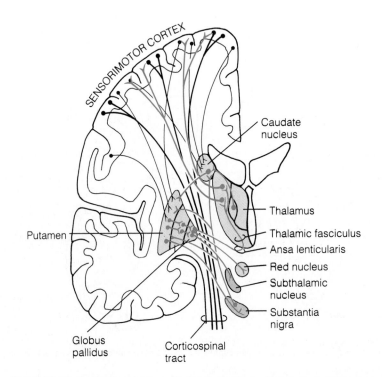

Figure 10–18. Connections between the basal ganglia, the thalamus, and the cortex.

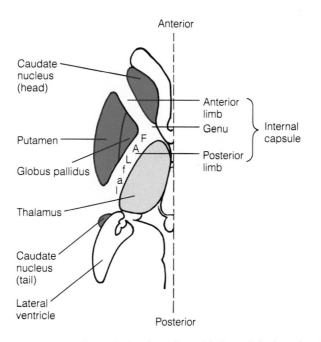

Figure 10–19. Relationships between internal capsule, basal ganglia, and thalamus in horizontal section. Notice that descending motor fibers for the face, arm, and leg (F, A, L) run in front of ascending sensory fibers (f, a, l) in the posterior limb of the internal capsule. (Modified after Greenberg DA, Aminoff MJ, Simon RP: *Clinical Neurology*, 2nd ed. Appleton & Lange, 1993.)

genu (apex) pointing medially (Figs 10–19 and 10–20).

The **anterior limb** of the internal capsule separates the lentiform nucleus from the caudate nucleus. It contains thalamocortical and corticothalamic fibers that join the lateral thalamic nucleus and the frontal lobe cortex, frontopontine tracts from the frontal lobe to the pontine nuclei, and fibers that run transversely from the caudate nucleus to the putamen.

The **posterior limb** of the internal capsule, located between the thalamus and the lentiform nucleus, contains major ascending and descending pathways. The corticobulbar and corticospinal tracts run in the anterior one-half of the posterior limb, with the fibers to the face and arm (Fig 10–19F, A) in front of the fibers to the leg (Fig 10–19L). Corticorubral fibers from the frontal lobe cortex to the red nucleus accompany the corticospinal tract.

The posterior one-third of the posterior limb contains third-order sensory fibers from the posterolateral nucleus of the thalamus to the postcentral gyrus. As with the more anteriorly located corticospinal and corticobulbar fibers, there is a somatotopic organization of the sensory fibers in the posterior limb, with the face and arm (f,a) ascending in front of the fibers for the leg (l) (Figure 10–18). As a result of its orderly organization, small lesions of the internal capsule can compromise motor and sensory function in a selective manner. For example, small infarcts (termed "lacunar" infarcts), owing to occlusion of small penetrating arter-

ial branches, can selectively involve the anterior part of the posterior limb of the internal capsule, producing "pure motor" strokes (an example is shown in Fig 4–1).

Lower horizontal sections through the head show the descending fibers of the internal capsule contained in the crus cerebri, the ventral part of the cerebral peduncle of the midbrain (Fig 10–21).

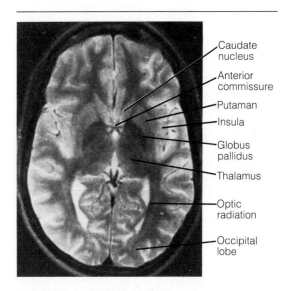

Figure 10–20. MRI of a horizontal section through the head.

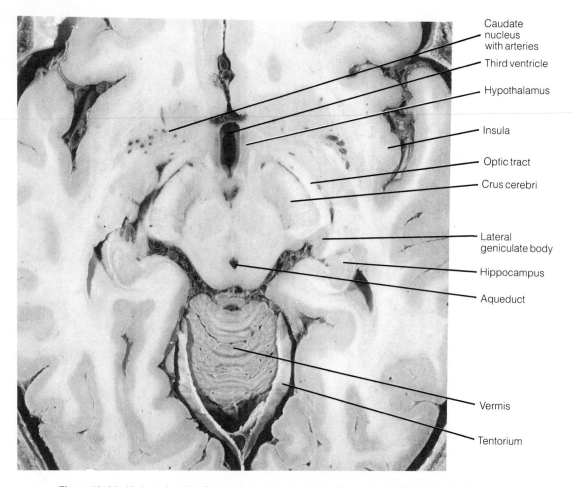

Caudate nucleus with arteries

Third ventricle

Hypothalamus

Insula

Optic tract

Crus cerebri

Lateral geniculate body

Hippocampus

Aqueduct

Vermis

Tentorium

Figure 10–21. Horizontal section through the head at the level of the midbrain. (Compare with Figure 7–9.)

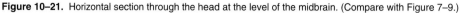

CASE 11

A 44-year-old woman was brought to a clinic by her husband, who gave a history of disorientation, confusion, and of distractibility and forgetfulness. These symptoms had become more severe in the last several months. The patient had recently begun to complain of headaches and after she had what she described as "a fit," her husband insisted she see a doctor.

Neurologic examination showed apathy and difficulty focusing attention, impairment of memory, left papilledema, facial asymmetry, lack of movement on the right side of the face, and general weakness but symmetric reflexes in the remainder of the body. An electroencephalogram showed an abnormal slow-wave focus in the left hemisphere. Imaging studies showed a calcified multifocal mass in the left frontoparietal region.

What is the differential diagnosis based on the above findings?

A brain biopsy was performed and a diagnosis made. By the next day, the patient had become comatose with dilated fixed pupils and she died soon afterward. At autopsy, findings included small hemorrhages in the brain stem and extensive pathologic changes in the forebrain.

What happened after the brain biopsy? What is the most likely diagnosis?

CASE 12

A 12-year-old girl began to have increasingly severe ear pain and fever. A few days later, her mother noticed a discharge from the left ear and took her to her family physician. The doctor prescribed antibiotics. One week later, the girl developed a severe, constant, left-frontal headache with swelling around the left eye. The following week, she developed left-sided facial weakness.

What is the differential diagnosis at this point?

The girl was then referred to a neurologist. At the time of admission, she was lethargic and confused, spoke unintelligibly, displayed silly behavior, and had a temperature of 100°F (37.8°C). Neurologic examination showed confusion of past and recent events, severe difficulty in naming objects, bilateral papilledema, normal extraocular movements, minor left peripheral facial paralysis, and decreased hearing ability on the left. The patient resisted neck flexion. An electroencephalogram showed slow-wave activity in the left hemisphere, especially in the frontotemporal region. CT scanning revealed a lesion in the left frontotemporal area.

What is the most likely diagnosis?
Cases are discussed further in Chapter 25.

REFERENCES

Alexander GE, Crutcher MD: Functional architecture of basal ganglia circuits. *Trends Neurosci* 1990;**13**:266.

Freund H: Abnormalities of motor behavior after cortical lesions in humans. In: *The Nervous System, vol V, part 2. Higher Functions of the Brain.* Plum F (editor). American Physiology Society 1987;763–810.

Gilbert C, Hirsch JA, Wiesel TN: Lateral interactions in the visual cortex. *Cold Spring Harb Symp Quant Biol* 1990;**55**:663.

Hubel DH: *Eye, Brain, and Vision.* Scientific American Library, 1988.

Mountcastle VB: Central nervous mechanisms in mechanoreceptive sensibility. In: *The Nervous System, vol. III. Sensory Processes.* Darian-Smith I (editor). American Physiology Society 1984;789.

Schmitt FO et al: *The Organization of the Cerebral Cortex.* MIT Press, 1981.

Strick PL: Anatomical organization of motor areas in the frontal lobe. In: *Functional Recovery in Neurological Disease.* Waxman SG (editor). Raven, 1988;293–312.

Yahr MD (editor): *The Basal Ganglia.* Raven, 1976.

11

Ventricles & Coverings of the Brain

VENTRICULAR SYSTEM

Within the brain substance is a communicating system of five cavities that are lined with ependyma and filled with cerebrospinal fluid (CSF). These cavities are designated as the two lateral ventricles, the third ventricle (between the halves of the diencephalon), the cerebral aqueduct, and the fourth ventricle within the brain stem (Fig 11–1).

Lateral Ventricles

The irregularly shaped lateral ventricles are the largest of the ventricles; they include two central portions (body and atrium) and three extensions (horns).

The **choroid plexus** of the lateral ventricle is a fringe-like vascular process of pia mater containing capillaries of the choroid arteries. It projects into the ventricular cavity and is covered by an epithelial layer of ependymal origin (Figs 11–2 and 11–3). The attachment of the plexus to the adjacent brain structures is known as the **tela choroidea.** The choroid plexus extends from the interventricular foramen, where it joins with the plexuses of the third ventricle and opposite lateral ventricle, to the end of the inferior horn (there is no choroid plexus in the anterior and posterior horns). The arteries to the plexus consist of the **anterior choroidal artery,** a branch of the internal carotid artery that enters the plexus at the inferior horn, and the lateral **posterior choroidal arteries,** which are branches of the posterior cerebral artery.

The **anterior (frontal) horn** is in front of the interventricular foramen. Its roof and anterior border are formed by the corpus callosum; its vertical medial wall by the septum pellucidum; and the floor and lateral wall by the bulging head of the caudate nucleus. During development and early life, the septum contains the **cavum septi pellucidi** (erroneously called the fifth ventricle). This fluid-filled cavity (its posterior portion is called the **cavum vergae**) may persist; it sometimes extends to the splenium.

The central part, or body, of the lateral ventricle is the long, narrow portion that extends from the interventricular foramen to a point opposite the splenium of the corpus callosum. Its roof is formed by the corpus callosum and its medial wall by the posterior portion of the septum pellucidum. The floor contains (from medial to lateral side) the fornix, the choroid plexus, the lateral part of the dorsal surface of the thalamus, the stria terminalis, the vena terminalis, and the caudate nucleus. The **atrium,** or **trigone,** is a wide area of the body that connects with the posterior and inferior horns (Fig 11–4).

The **posterior (occipital) horn** extends into the occipital lobe. Its roof is formed by fibers of the corpus callosum. On its medial wall is the **calcar avis,** an elevation of the ventricular wall produced by the calcarine fissure.

The **inferior (temporal) horn** traverses the temporal lobe, whose white substance forms its roof. Along the medial border are the stria terminalis and the tail of the caudate nucleus. The amygdaloid nuclear complex bulges into the upper terminal part of the inferior horn, whose floor and medial wall are formed by the fimbria, hippocampus, and collateral eminence.

The two **interventricular foramens** are oval apertures between the column of the fornix and the anterior end of the thalamus. The two lateral ventricles communicate with the third ventricle through these foramens, which are sometimes referred to as the foramens of Monro (see Fig 11–1).

Third Ventricle

The third ventricle is a narrow vertical cleft between the two halves of the diencephalon (see Figs 11–1 to 11–4). The roof of the third ventricle is formed by a thin tela choroidea (a layer of ependyma) and pia mater from which a small choroid plexus extends into the lumen of the ventricle (see Fig 9–1). This plexus is supplied by the medial posterior choroidal artery from the posterior cerebral artery. The lateral walls are formed

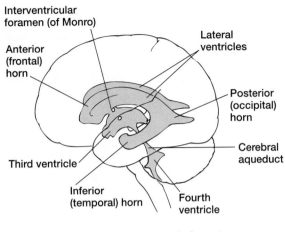

Figure 11–1. The ventricular system.

mainly by the medial surfaces of the two thalami. The lower lateral wall and the floor of the ventricle are formed by the hypothalamus; the anterior commissure and the lamina terminalis form the rostral limit.

The **optic recess** is an extension of the third ventricle between the lamina terminalis and the optic chiasm. The hypophysis is attached to the apex of its downward extension, the funnel-shaped **infundibular recess.** A small **pineal recess** projects into the stalk of the pineal body. A variable, often large, extension of the third ventricle above the epithalamus is known as the **suprapineal recess.** The **interthalamic adhesion,** a band of gray matter, crosses the cavity of the ventricle and joins the external walls. This band, which is present in about 60% of all brains, has no functional significance.

Cerebral Aqueduct

The cerebral aqueduct is a narrow, curved channel running from the posterior third ventricle into the fourth; it contains no choroid plexus (see Figs 11–1 and 11–4).

Fourth Ventricle

The fourth ventricle is a pyramid-shaped cavity bounded ventrally by the pons and medulla oblongata (see Figs 7–16, 11–1, and 11–3); its floor is also known as the **rhomboid fossa.** The **lateral recess** extends as a narrow, curved extension of the ventricle on the dorsal surface of the inferior cerebellar peduncle. The fourth ventricle extends under the **obex** into the central canal of the medulla.

The incomplete roof of the fourth ventricle is formed by the anterior and posterior medullary vela. The **anterior medullary velum** extends between the dorsomedial borders of the superior cerebellar peduncles, and its dorsal surface is covered by the adherent lin-

gula of the cerebellum. The **posterior medullary velum** extends caudally from the cerebellum. The point at which the fourth ventricle passes up into the cerebellum is called the **apex,** or **fastigium.**

The **lateral aperture (foramen of Luschka)** is the opening of the lateral recess into the subarachnoid space near the flocculus of the cerebellum. A tuft of choroid plexus is commonly present in the aperture and partly obstructs the flow of cerebrospinal fluid from the fourth ventricle to subarachnoid space. The **medial aperture (foramen of Magendie)** is an opening in the caudal portion of the roof of the ventricle. Most of the outflow of cerebrospinal fluid from the fourth ventricle passes through this aperture, which varies in size.

The **tela choroidea** of the fourth ventricle is a layer of pia and ependyma that contains small vessels and lies in the posterior medullary velum; it forms the choroid plexus of the fourth ventricle and is supplied by branches of the posterior inferior cerebellar arteries.

MENINGES & SPACES

Three membranes, or meninges, envelop the brain: the dura, the arachnoid, and the pia. The dura, the outer membrane, is separated from the thin arachnoid by a potential compartment, the **subdural space,** which normally contains only a few drops of cerebrospinal fluid. An extensive **subarachnoid space** containing cerebrospinal fluid and the major arteries separates the arachnoid from the *pia,* which completely invests the brain. The arachnoid and the pia, known collectively as *leptomeninges,* are connected by thin strands of tissue, the arachnoid trabeculae. The pia, together with a narrow extension of the subarachnoid space, accompanies the vessels deep into the brain tissue; this space is called the **perivascular space** or Virchow-Robin space.

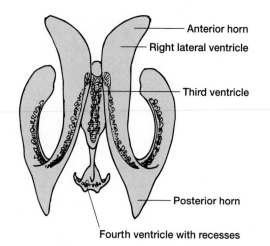

Anterior horn

Right lateral ventricle

Third ventricle

Posterior horn

Fourth ventricle with recesses

Figure 11–3. Dorsal view of the choroid plexus in the ventricular system. Notice the absence of choroid in the aqueduct and the anterior and posterior horns.

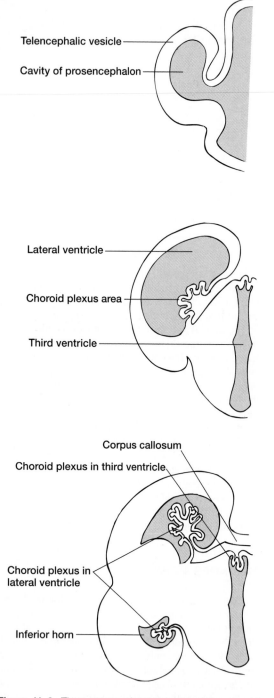

Telencephalic vesicle

Cavity of prosencephalon

Lateral ventricle

Choroid plexus area

Third ventricle

Corpus callosum

Choroid plexus in third ventricle

Choroid plexus in lateral ventricle

Inferior horn

Figure 11–2. Three stages of development of the choroid plexus in the lateral ventricle (coronal sections).

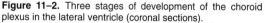

Dura

The cranial dura, or **pachymeninx,** is a tough, fibrous structure with an inner **(meningeal)** layer and an outer **(periosteal)** layer (Figs 11–4 and 11–5). The dural layers over the brain are generally fused, except where they separate to provide space for the venous sinuses (most of the dura's venous sinuses lie between the dural layers) and where the inner layer forms septa between brain portions. The outer layer is firmly attached to the inner surface of the cranial bones and sends vascular and fibrous extensions into the bone itself; the inner layer is continuous with the spinal dura.

One of the dural septa, the curved **falx cerebri,** extends down into the longitudinal fissure between the cerebral hemispheres (Figs 11–5 and 11–6). The anterior falx cerebri is narrower than the posterior end. It attaches to the inner surface of the skull in midplane, from the crista galli to the internal occipital protuberance, where it becomes continuous with the tentorium cerebelli.

The **tentorium cerebelli** separates the occipital lobes from the cerebellum. It is a roughly transverse membrane that attaches at the rear and side to the skull at the transverse sinuses; at the front, it attaches to the petrous portion of the temporal bone and to the clinoid processes of the sphenoid bone. Toward the midline, it slopes up and fuses with the falx cerebri. The free, curved, anterior border leaves a large opening, the **incisura tentorii** (tentorial notch), for passage of the upper brain stem, aqueduct, and vessels.

The **falx cerebelli** projects between the cerebellar hemispheres from the inner surface of the occipital bone to form a small triangular dural septum.

The **diaphragma sellae** forms an incomplete lid over the hypophysis in the sella turcica by connecting

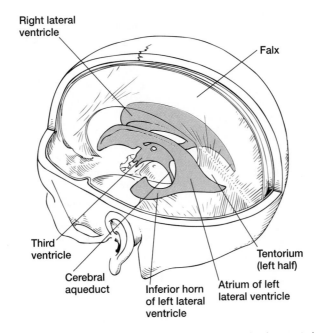

Right lateral
ventricle

Falx

Third
ventricle

Cerebral
aqueduct

Inferior horn
of left lateral
ventricle

Atrium of left
lateral ventricle

Tentorium
(left half)

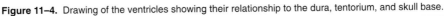

Figure 11–4. Drawing of the ventricles showing their relationship to the dura, tentorium, and skull base.

the clinoid attachments of the two sides of the tentorium cerebelli. The pituitary stalk passes through the opening in the diaphragma.

Arachnoid

The arachnoid, a delicate avascular membrane, covers the subarachnoid space, which is filled with cerebrospinal fluid. The inner surface of the arachnoid is connected to the pia by fine (but inconstantly present) **arachnoid trabeculae** (Fig 11–5). The cranial arachnoid closely covers the inner surface of the dura mater but is separated from it by the subdural space, which contains a thin film of fluid. The arachnoid does not dip into the sulci or fissures except to follow the falx and the tentorium.

Arachnoid granulations consist of many microscopic villi (Fig 11–5B). They have the appearance of berry-like clumps protruding into the superior sagittal sinus or its associated venous lacunae and into other sinuses and large veins. With advancing age, the granulations increase in size and number, sometimes pushing against or through the periosteal dura and causing bone resorption and depressions in the skull cap. The granulations are sites of absorption of cerebrospinal fluid.

The **subarachnoid space** between the arachnoid and the pia is relatively narrow over the surface of the cerebral hemisphere, but it becomes much wider in areas at the base of the brain. These widened spaces, the

subarachnoid **cisterns,** are often named after neighboring brain structures (Fig 11–7). They communicate freely with adjacent cisterns and the general subarachnoid space.

The **cisterna magna** results from the bridging of the arachnoid over the space between the medulla and the cerebellar hemispheres; it is continuous with the spinal subarachnoid space. The **pontine cistern** on the ventral aspect of the pons contains the basilar artery and some veins. Below the cerebrum lies a wide space between the two temporal lobes. This space is divided into the **chiasmatic cisterna** above the optic chiasm, the **suprasellar cistern** above the diaphragma sellae, and the **interpeduncular cistern** between the cerebral peduncles. The space between frontal, parietal, and temporal lobes is called the **cistern of the lateral fissure (cistern of Sylvius).**

Pia

The pia is a thin connective-tissue membrane that covers the brain surface and extends into sulci and fissures and around blood vessels throughout the brain (see Fig 11–5). It also extends into the transverse cerebral fissure under the corpus callosum. There it forms the tela choroidea of the third and lateral ventricles and combines with the ependyma and choroid vessels to form the choroid plexus of these ventricles. The pia and ependyma pass over the roof of the fourth ventricle and form its tela choroidea for the choroid plexus there.

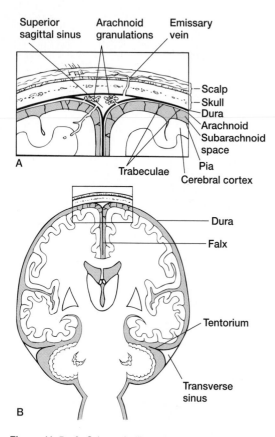

Figure 11–5. ***A:*** Schematic illustration of a coronal section through the brain and coverings. ***B:*** Enlargement of the area at the top of A.

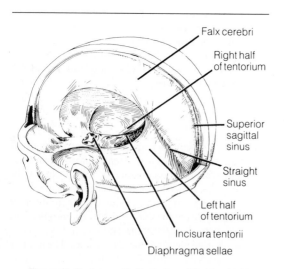

Figure 11–6. Schematic illustration of the dural folds.

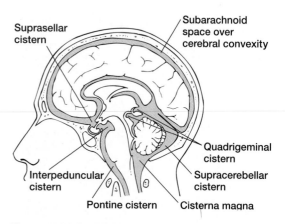

Figure 11–7. Schematic illustration of the brain showing spaces that contain cerebrospinal fluid.

Clinical Correlations

The dura may become partly calcified or even ossified with age. In some cases, often in association with longstanding hydrocephalus, the falx is fenestrated.

Several types of herniation of the brain can occur. The tentorium separates the supratentorial and the infratentorial compartments, and the two spaces communicate by way of the incisura that contains the midbrain. Both the falx and the tentorium form incomplete separations, and a mass or expanding lesion may displace a portion of the brain around these septa, resulting in either **subfalcial** or **transtentorial herniation.** The latter type may be downward (uncal, or caudal transtentorial, herniation) or upward (rostral transtentorial herniation). The herniation of the cerebellar tonsils into the foramen magnum by a lesion is often called **coning.** Transtentorial herniations, especially the caudal type, are potentially life-threatening because they can distort or compress the brain stem and damage its vital regulatory centers for respiration, consciousness, blood pressure, and other functions (see Chapter 20).

Various types of lesions can occur in one or more intracranial compartments: the brain itself (tumor, bleeding, abscess); the extracellular space (edema); the vascular compartment (venous obstruction, arteriovenous malformation, bleeding); and the spaces containing cerebrospinal fluid (obstructions).

CEREBROSPINAL FLUID

Function

The cerebrospinal fluid provides mechanical support of the brain and acts like a protective water jacket. It controls brain excitability by regulating the ionic composition, carries away metabolites (the brain has no lymphatic vessels), and provides some protection from pressure changes (venous volume versus cerebrospinal fluid volume).

Composition & Volume

Normal cerebrospinal fluid is clear, colorless, and odorless. Its more important average normal values are shown in Table 11–1.

The cerebrospinal fluid is present, for the most part, in a system that comprises two communicating parts. The internal portion of the system consists of two lateral ventricles, the interventricular foramens, the third ventricle, the cerebral aqueduct, and the fourth ventricle. The external part consists of the subarachnoid spaces and cisterns. Communication between the internal and external portions occurs through the two lateral apertures of the fourth ventricle (foramens of Luschka) and the median aperture of the fourth ventricle (foramen of Magendie). In adults, the total volume of cerebrospinal fluid in all the spaces combined is normally about 150 mL; the internal (ventricular) portion of the system contains about half this amount. Between 400 and 500 mL of cerebrospinal fluid is produced and reabsorbed daily.

Pressure

The normal mean cerebrospinal fluid pressure is 70–180 mm of water; periodic changes occur with heartbeat and respiration. The pressure rises if there is an increase in intracranial volume (eg, with tumors), blood volume (with hemorrhages), or cerebrospinal fluid volume (with hydrocephalus), because the adult skull is a rigid box of bone that cannot accommodate the increased volume without a rise in pressure.

Circulation

Much of the cerebrospinal fluid originates from the choroid plexuses within the lateral ventricles of the brain. The fluid passes through the interventricular foramens into the midline third ventricle; more cerebrospinal fluid is produced here by the choroid plexus in the ventricle's roof (Fig 11–8). The fluid then moves through the cerebral aqueduct within the midbrain and passes into the rhombus-shaped fourth ventricle, where the choroid plexus adds more fluid. The fluid leaves the ventricular system through the midline and lateral apertures of the fourth ventricle and enters the subarachnoid space. From here it may flow over the

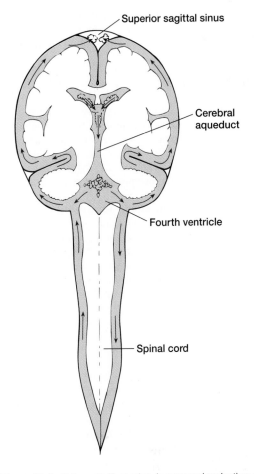

Figure 11–8. Schematic illustration, in a coronal projection, of the circulation (arrows) of cerebrospinal fluid.

cerebral convexities or into the spinal subarachnoid spaces. Some of it is reabsorbed (by diffusion) into the small vessels in the pia or ventricular walls and the remainder passes via the arachnoid villi into the venous blood (of sinuses or veins) in various areas—mostly over the superior convexity. A minimum pressure of cerebrospinal fluid must be present to maintain reabsorption. There exists, therefore, a continuous circulation of cerebrospinal fluid in and around the brain, in which production and reabsorption are in balance.

A clear concept of the route of the circulation through the ventricles into and through the subarachnoid spaces is of great practical and clinical impor-

Table 11–1. Normal cerebrospinal fluid findings.

Area	Appearance	Pressure (in mm of water)	Cells (per μL)	Protein	Miscellaneous
Lumbar	Clear and colorless	70–180	0–5	15–45 mg/dL	Glucose 50–75 mg/dL
Ventricular	Clear and colorless	70–190	0–5 (lymphocytes)	5–15 mg/dL	

tance. Magnetic resonance imaging can show that the flow of cerebrospinal fluid is faster through (and just downstream from) narrow stretches in the pathway (Fig 11–9).

Clinical Correlations

Blocking the circulatory pathway of cerebrospinal fluid usually leads to dilatation of the ventricles upstream (hydrocephalus), because the production of fluid usually continues despite the obstruction (Figs 11–10 to 11–14 and Table 11–2). There are two types of hydrocephalus: noncommunicating and communicating.

In **noncommunicating (obstructive) hydrocephalus,** which occurs more frequently than the other type, the cerebrospinal fluid of the ventricles cannot reach the subarachnoid space because there is obstruction of one or both interventricular foramens, the cerebral aqueduct (the most common site of obstruction, Figs 11–9 and 11–10), or the outflow foramens of the fourth ventricle (median and lateral apertures). A block at any of these sites leads rapidly to dilatation of one or more ventricles. The production of cerebrospinal fluid continues, and in the acute obstruction phase, there may be a transependymal flow of cerebrospinal fluid. The gyri are flattened against the inside of the skull. If the skull is still pliable, as it is in most children under two years of age, the head may enlarge (Fig 11–11).

In **communicating hydrocephalus,** the obstruction is in the subarachnoid space and can be the result of prior bleeding or meningitis, which caused thickening of the arachnoid with a resultant block of the return-flow channels (Fig 11–14). If the intracranial pressure is raised because of excess cerebrospinal fluid (more production than reabsorption), the central canal of the spinal cord may dilate. In some patients, the spaces filled by cerebrospinal fluid are uniformly enlarged

without an increase in intracranial pressure. This **normal-pressure hydrocephalus** may be accompanied by atrophy of the brain in the elderly (see Chapter 23) or have an uncertain origin (a lesion or trauma causing blood to be present in the subarachnoid space has been suggested).

Various procedures have been developed to bypass the obstruction in noncommunicating hydrocephalus or to improve absorption in general. Examples of these shunts are shown in Figure 11–15.

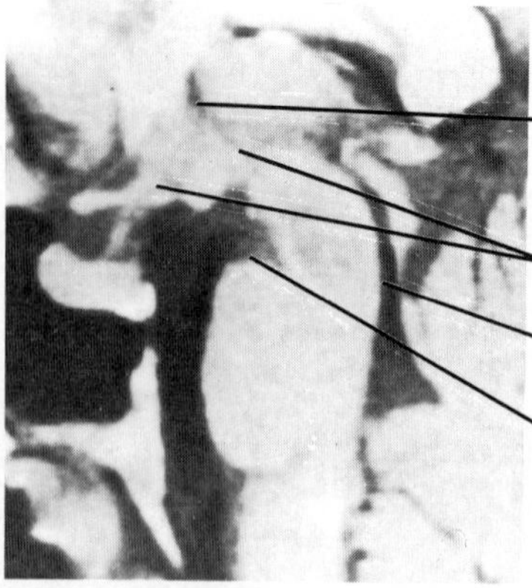

BARRIERS IN THE NERVOUS SYSTEM

Several functionally important types of barriers exist in the nervous system and all play a role in maintaining a constant environment within and around the brain so that normal function continues and foreign or harmful substances are kept out. Some are readily visible, such as the three investing membranes (meninges), the dura, arachnoid and pia (see Chapter 6); others are distinct only when examined with an ultramicroscope or electron microscope.

Blood-Brain Barrier

The blood-cerebrospinal-fluid barrier, the vascular endothelial barrier, and the arachnoid barrier together form the blood-brain barrier. This barrier is absent in several specialized regions of the brain: the basal hypothalamus, the pineal gland, the area postrema of the fourth ventricle, and several small areas near the third ventricle. Highly permeable fenestrated capillaries are present in these regions.

A. Blood-Cerebrospinal-Fluid Barrier: About 60% of the cerebrospinal fluid is formed by active transport (through the membranes) from the blood vessels in the choroid plexus. Epithelial cells of the plexus, joined by tight junctions, form a continuous layer that selectively permits the passage of some substances but not others (see Chapter 12).

B. Vascular-Endothelial Barrier: Collectively, the blood vessels within the brain have a very large surface area that promotes the exchange of oxygen, CO_2, amino acids, and sugars between blood and brain. Because other substances are kept out, the chemical composition of the extracellular fluid of the nervous system differs markedly from that of cell plasma. The blocking function is achieved by tight junctions between endothelial cells. There is evidence that neither the processes of astrocytes nor the basal laminas of endothelial cells prevent diffusion, even for molecules as large as proteins.

C. Arachnoid Barrier: Blood vessels of the dura are far more permeable than those of the brain, but because the outermost layer of cells of the arachnoid forms a barrier, substances diffusing out of dural vessels do not enter the cerebrospinal fluid of the subarachnoidal space. The cells are joined by tight junc-

Figure 11–9. Magnetic resonance image of a midsagittal section through a normal head, demonstrating the fast flow of cerebrospinal fluid.

Fast flow through interventricular foramen

Slow flow in third ventricle

Fast flow in aqueduct

Slow flow in interpeduncular cistern

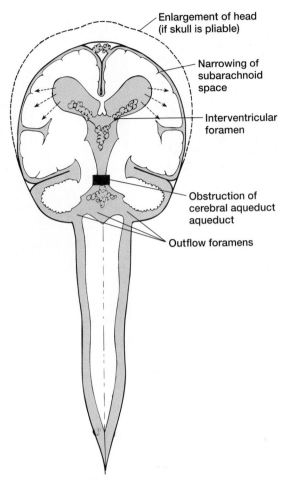

Figure 11–10. Schematic illustration of the effects of obstruction of the cerebral aqueduct causing noncommunicating hydrocephalus. Arrows indicate transependymal flow (compare with Fig 11–8). Other possible sites of obstruction are the interventricular foramen and the outflow foramens of the fourth ventricle.

tions, and their permeability characteristics are similar to those of the blood vessels of the brain itself.

Ependyma

The ependyma lining the cerebral ventricles is continuous with the epithelium of the choroid plexus (Fig 11–16). Except for the ependyma of the lower third ventricle, most ependymal cells do not have tight junctions and cannot prevent the movement of macromolecules between ventricles and brain tissue.

Blood-Nerve Barrier

Large nerves consist of bundles of axons embedded in an **epineurium.** Each bundle is surrounded by a

Table 11–2. Hydrocephalus.

Type	Cause	Effect
Noncommunicating (obstructive)	Obstruction of interventricular foramen	Enlargement of lateral ventricle
	Obstruction of cerebral aqueduct	Enlargement of lateral and third ventricles
	Obstruction of outflow foramens of fourth ventricle	Enlargement of all ventricles
Communicating	Obstruction of perimesencephalic cistern (occlusion of incisura tentorii)	Enlargement of all ventricles; widening of posterior fossa cisterns
	Obstruction of subarachnoid CSF flow over the cerebral convexities	Enlargement of all ventricles; widening of all basal cisterns

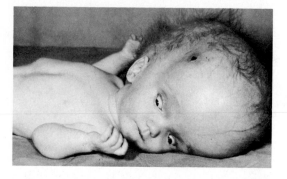

Figure 11–11. Hydrocephalus in a 14-month-old infant.

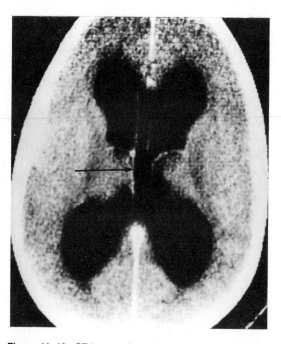

Figure 11–13. CT image of a horizontal section through the head of a 7-year-old child with noncommunicating hydrocephalus owing to the obstruction of the outflow foramens by a medulloblastoma.

layer of cells called the **perineurium;** connective tissue within each bundle is the **endoneurium.** Blood vessels of the epineurium, which are similar to those of the dura, are permeable to macromolecules but the endoneurial vessels, similar to those of the arachnoid, are not.

SKULL

The skull (cranium), which is rigid in adults but pliable in newborn infants, surrounds the brain and meninges completely and forms a strong mechanical protection. In adults, skull contents that increase beyond the capacity of the intact cranium can cause herniation. Increased cranial pressure in infants may cause the fontanelles to bulge or the head to begin to enlarge abnormally (see Fig 11–11).

The skull consists of two major portions: the **neurocranium,** which contains the brain and consists of the skull base and cap **(calvaria),** and the skeleton of the face, the **viscerocranium** (Fig 11–17). The anatomy of the neurocranium and orbit will be discussed in this chapter.

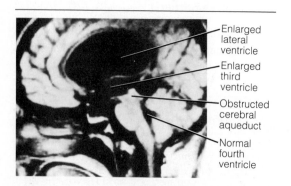

Enlarged lateral ventricle

Enlarged third ventricle

Obstructed cerebral aqueduct

Normal fourth ventricle

Figure 11–12. MRI of a midsagittal section through the head of a 3-year-old child with aqueductal stenosis (compare with Fig 1–4). The lateral ventricles are greatly dilated and the third ventricle is moderately enlarged.

Basal View of the Skull

The anterior portion of the base of the skull, the hard palate, projects below the level of the remainder of the inferior skull surface. The **choanae,** or posterior nasal apertures, are behind and above the hard palate. The pterygoid plates lie lateral to the choanae (Figs 11–18 and 11–19).

At the base of the lateral pterygoid plate is the **foramen ovale,** which transmits the third branch of the trigeminal nerve, the accessory meningeal artery, and (occasionally) the superficial petrosal nerve. Posterior to the foramen ovale is the **foramen spinosum,** which transmits the middle meningeal vessels. At the base of the styloid process is the **stylomastoid foramen,** through which the facial nerve exits.

The **foramen lacerum** is a large irregular aperture at the base of the medial pterygoid plate. Its inferior portion is closed by a fibrocartilaginous plate above the auditory tube. Within its superior aspect is the **carotid canal.** The internal carotid artery, which emerges from this aperture, crosses only the superior part of the foramen lacerum.

Lateral to the foramen lacerum is a groove, the **sulcus tubae auditivae,** that contains the cartilaginous part of the **auditory (eustachian) tube.** It is continuous posteriorly with the canal in the temporal bone that forms the bony part of the auditory tube. Lateral to the groove is the lower orifice of the carotid canal, which

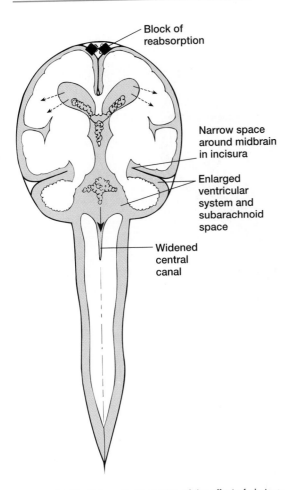

- Block of reabsorption
- Narrow space around midbrain in incisura
- Enlarged ventricular system and subarachnoid space
- Widened central canal

Figure 11–14. Schematic illustration of the effect of obstruction of reabsorption of cerebrospinal fluid causing communicating hydrocephalus. Arrows indicate transependymal flow (compare with Figs 11–8 and 11–10). Another possible site of obstruction is at the narrow space around the midbrain in the incisura.

transmits the internal carotid artery and the carotid plexus of the sympathetic nerves.

Behind the carotid canal is the large **jugular foramen,** which is formed by the petrous portion of the temporal and occipital bones and can be divided into three compartments. The anterior compartment contains the inferior petrosal sinus; the intermediate compartment contains the glossopharyngeal, vagus, and spinal accessory nerves; and the posterior compartment contains the sigmoid sinus and meningeal branches from the occipital and ascending pharyngeal arteries.

Posterior to the basilar portion of the occipital bone is the **foramen magnum,** which transmits the medulla and its membranes, the spinal accessory nerves, the vertebral arteries, the anterior and posterior spinal arteries, and ligaments connecting the occipital bone with the axis. The foramen magnum is bounded laterally by the **occipital condyles.**

Behind each condyle is the condyloid fossa, perforated on one or both sides by the **posterior condyloid canal** (which may transmit an emissary vein from the transverse sinus). Farther forward is the **anterior condylar canal,** or **hypoglossal canal,** which transmits the hypoglossal nerve and a meningeal artery.

Interior of the Skull

A. Calvaria: The inner surface of the calvaria (skull cap) is concave, with depressions for the convolutions of the cerebrum and numerous furrows for the branches of the meningeal vessels. Along the midline is a longitudinal groove, narrow anteriorly and posteriorly wide, that contains the superior sagittal sinus. The margins of the groove provide attachment for the falx cerebri. There are several depressions on either side of the groove for the arachnoid granulations of the lateral lacunae. At the rear are the openings of the parietal emissary foramens (when these are present). The **sutures** of the calvaria (**sagittal, coronal, lambdoid,** and others) are meshed lines of union between adjacent skull bones.

B. Floor of the Cranial Cavity: The internal or superior surface of the skull base forms the floor of the cranial cavity (Figs 11–19 and 11–20; Table 11–3). It is divided into three fossae: anterior, middle, and posterior. The floor of the anterior fossa lies higher than the floor of the middle fossa, which in turn lies higher than the floor of the posterior fossa.

1. Anterior cranial fossa—The floor of this is formed by the orbital plates of the frontal bone, the cribriform plates of the ethmoid, and the lesser wings and anterior part of the sphenoid. It is limited at the rear by the posterior borders of the lesser wings of the sphenoid and by the anterior margins of the chiasmatic groove.

The lateral segments of the anterior cranial fossa are the roofs of the orbital cavities, which support the frontal lobes of the cerebrum. The medial segments form the roof of the nasal cavity. The medial segments lie alongside the **crista galli,** which together with the frontal crest afford attachment to the falx cerebri. A **foramen caecum** is usually present in front of the crista galli; it transmits an emissary vein that connects to the superior sagittal sinus.

The **cribriform plate** of the ethmoid bone lies on either side of the crista galli and supports the olfactory bulb. This plate is perforated by foramens for the olfactory nerves. Internal openings of the anterior and posterior ethmoidal foramens are in the lateral wall of the olfactory groove. The cranial openings of the **optic canals** lie just behind the flat portion of the sphenoid bone (**planum sphenoidal).**

2. Middle cranial fossa—This is deeper than the anterior cranial fossa and is narrow centrally and wide peripherally. It is bounded at the front by the posterior margins of the lesser wings of the sphenoid and the anterior clinoid processes. It is bounded posteriorly

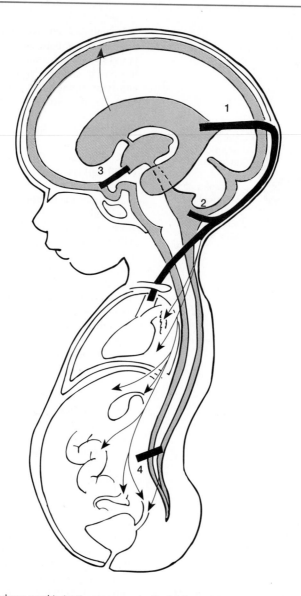

Figure 11–15. Shunting procedures used to treat noncommunicating hydrocephalus. *1:* Ventriculocaval shunt. *2:* Ventriculocisternal shunt. *3:* Anterior ventriculostomy. *4:* Spinoperitoneal shunt. Lighter lines and arrows indicate other shunts.

by the superior angles of the petrous portion of the temporal bones and by the dorsum sellae. It is bounded laterally by the temporal squamae and the greater wings of the sphenoid (Figs 11–20 and 11–21).

The narrow medial portion of the fossa presents the **chiasmatic groove** and the **tuberculum sellae** anteriorly; the chiasmatic groove ends on either side at the **optic canal,** which transmits the optic nerve and ophthalmic artery. Behind the optic canal, the **anterior clinoid process** is directed posteriorly and medially and provides attachment for the tentorium cerebelli. In back of the tuberculum sellae is a deep depression, the **sella turcica;** this structure, whose name means "Turkish saddle" (which it resembles), is especially important because it contains the hypophyseal fossa in which

the hypophysis (pituitary) lies. The sella turcica is bounded posteriorly by a quadrilateral plate of bone, the **dorsum sellae,** whose sides project anteriorly as the **posterior clinoid processes.** These attach to slips of the tentorium cerebelli. Below each posterior clinoid process is a notch for the abducens nerve.

On either side of the sella turcica is the broad and shallow **carotid groove,** curving upward from the foramen lacerum to the medial side of the anterior clinoid process. This groove contains the internal carotid artery, surrounded by a plexus of sympathetic nerves.

The lateral segments of the middle fossa are deeper than its middle portion; they support the temporal lobes of the brain and show depressions that mark the convolutions of the brain. These segments are traversed by

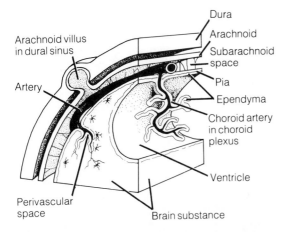

Figure 11–16. Schematic illustration of the relationships and the barriers between the brain, the meninges, and the vessels.

furrows for the anterior and posterior branches of the **middle meningeal vessels,** which pass through the **foramen spinosum.**

The **superior orbital fissure** is situated in the anterior portion of the middle cranial fossa. It is bounded above by the lesser wing, below by the greater wing, and in the middle by the body of the sphenoid. The superior orbital fissure transmits into the orbital cavity the oculomotor nerve, the trochlear nerve, the ophthalmic division of the trigeminal nerve, the abducens nerve, some filaments from the cavernous plexus of the sympathetic nerves, the ophthalmic veins, and the orbital branch of the middle meningeal artery.

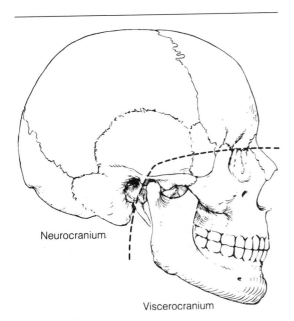

Figure 11–17. Lateral view of the skull.

The maxillary division of the trigeminal nerve passes through the **foramen rotundum,** which is located behind the medial wall of the superior orbital fissure. Behind the foramen rotundum is the **foramen of Vesalius,** which transmits an emissary vein or a cluster of small venules; it can be large, small, multiple, or absent in different skulls. The **foramen ovale,** which transmits the mandibular division of the trigeminal nerve, the accessory meningeal artery, and the lesser superficial petrosal nerve, is posterior and lateral to the foramen rotundum.

The **foramen lacerum** is medial to the foramen ovale. Its inferior segment is filled by fibrocartilage. Its superior segment transmits the internal carotid artery, which is surrounded by a plexus of sympathetic nerves. The anterior wall of the foramen lacerum is pierced by the pterygoid canal.

The **arcuate eminence,** which marks the position of the superior semicircular canal, lies on the upper surface of the petrous portion of the temporal bone. Medially, there is a groove leading to the hiatus of the facial canal for transmission of the greater petrosal nerve and the petrosal branch of the middle meningeal artery. There is, below, a smaller groove for passage of the lesser petrosal nerve, and near the apex of the petrous bone is the depression for the semicircular ganglion of V and for the irregular orifice of the carotid canal.

3. Posterior cranial fossa—This fossa is larger and deeper than the middle and anterior cranial fossae. It is formed by the occipital bone, the dorsum sellae and clivus of the sphenoid bone, and portions of the temporal and parietal bones (Figs 11–19 and 11–20).

The posterior fossa, or **infratentorial compartment,** contains the cerebellum, pons, medulla, and part of the midbrain. It is separated from the middle cranial fossa in and near the midline by the dorsum sellae of the sphenoid bone and on either side by the superior angle of the petrous portion of the temporal bone **(petrous pyramid).** This angle provides attachment for the tentorium cerebelli and is grooved for the superior petrosal sinus.

The **foramen magnum** lies in the center of the fossa. Just above the tubercle is the **anterior condylar canal,** or **hypoglossal canal,** which transmits the hypoglossal nerve and a meningeal branch for the ascending pharyngeal artery. In front of the foramen magnum, the basilar part of the occipital bone and the posterior part of the body of the sphenoid bone support the pons and the medulla. These bones are joined by a synchondrosis in young people. On either side, the petro-occipital fissure is continuous posteriorly with the jugular foramen. The margins of the petro-occipital fissure are grooved for the **inferior petrosal sinus.**

The **jugular foramen** lies between the lateral part of the occipital bone and the petrous portion of the temporal bone. The anterior portion of the foramen transmits the inferior petrosal sinus, the posterior portion transmits the transverse sinus and some meningeal branches from the occipital and ascending

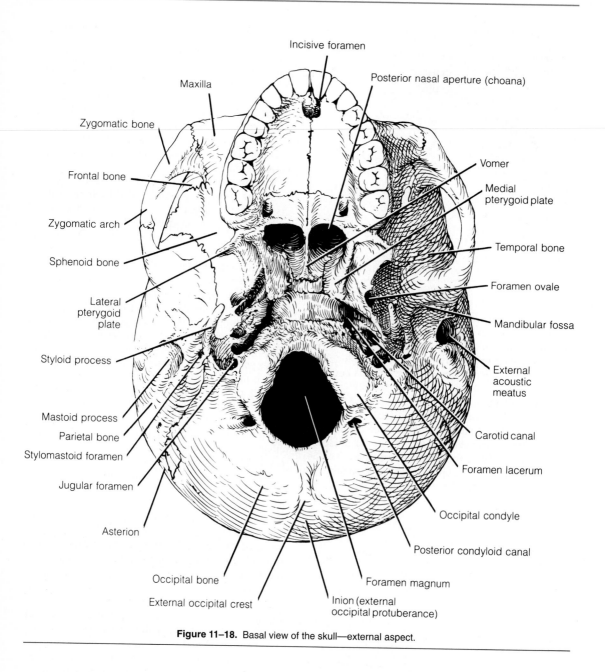

Figure 11–18. Basal view of the skull—external aspect.

pharyngeal arteries, and the intermediate portion transmits the glossopharyngeal, vagus, and spinal accessory nerves.

Above the jugular foramen lies the **internal acoustic meatus** for the facial and acoustic nerves and the internal auditory artery. The inferior occipital fossae, which support the hemispheres of the cerebellum, are separated by the internal occipital crest, which serves for attachment of the falx cerebelli and contains the **occipital sinus.** The posterior fossae are surrounded by deep grooves for the **transverse sinuses.**

Clinical Correlations

Trauma to the skull can result in fractures. By itself, a fracture of the calvaria or the base is not a very serious problem; however, there are often complications. Fractures with meningeal tears can lead to leaks of cerebrospinal fluid and possibly intracranial infection; fractures with vascular tears can lead to extradural (epidural) hemorrhages, especially if branches of large meningeal arteries are torn; and depressed fractures can cause brain contusions with bleeding and tissue destruction. Contusion may also be present on the side

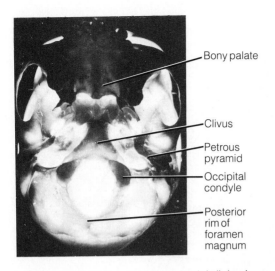

Figure 11–19. Basal view of transilluminated skull showing areas of thick and thin bone.

Labels:
- Bony palate
- Clivus
- Petrous pyramid
- Occipital condyle
- Posterior rim of foramen magnum

Table 11–3. Structures passing through openings in the cranial floor.

Foramens	Structures
Cribriform plate of ethmoid	Of-factory nerves
Optic foramen	Optic nerve, ophthalmic artery, meninges
Superior orbital fissure	Oculomotor, trochlear, and abducens nerves; ophthalmic division of trigeminal nerve; superior ophthalmic vein
Foramen rotundum	Maxillary division of trigeminal nerve, small artery and vein
Foramen ovale	Mandibular division of trigeminal nerve, vein
Foramen lacerum	Internal carotid artery, sympathetic plexus
Foramen spinosum	Middle meningeal artery and vein
Internal acoustic meatus	Facial and vestibulocochlear nerves, internal auditory artery
Jugular foramen	Glossopharyngeal, vagus, and spinal accessory nerves; sigmoid sinus
Hypoglossal canal	Hypoglossal nerve
Foramen magnum	Medulla and meninges, spinal accessory nerve, vertebral arteries, anterior and posterior spinal arteries

opposite to the impact (contrecoup contusion), at a site where the brain has rubbed against bony edges such as the tip of the temporal lobe, the occipital pole, or the orbital surface of the frontal lobe, or where the corpus callosum and pericallosal artery have rubbed against the edge of the falx.

Infection **(osteomyelitis), Paget's disease (osteitis deformans),** or skull tumors can affect the skull. Chronic hypertrophic anterior osteitis, in which the squama of the frontal bone is abnormally thickened, is seen in about 5% of human skulls.

CASE 13

A 63-year-old unemployed man was brought to the hospital because he had a fever and had a depressed level of consciousness. His landlady stated that he had lost weight for several months and had lately complained of fever, poor appetite, and cough. On the day of admission, he had been found in a stuporous state and had felt hot to the touch.

During the general physical examination, the patient was uncooperative and thrashed about in bed. Findings included a rigid neck, a harsh systolic murmur heard along the left sternal margin, a body temperature of 40° C (104° F), and a pulse rate of 140.

The red blood count showed 3.8 million/μL and the white blood count was 18,000/μ-L with 80% polymorphonuclear leukocytes. The blood glucose level was 120 mg/dL. Lumbar puncture results showed pressure, 300 mm of water; white blood count, 20,000/μL (with mostly polymorphonuclear leukocytes); glucose, 18 mg/dL; and protein, unknown (test results were lost). Gram's stain of the cerebrospinal fluid sediment revealed gram-positive rod-shaped diplococci (pneumococci).

What is the most likely diagnosis?

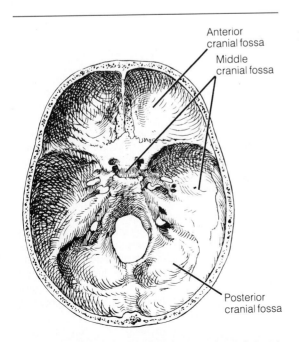

Figure 11–20. Floor of the cranial cavity—internal aspect.

Labels:
- Anterior cranial fossa
- Middle cranial fossa
- Posterior cranial fossa

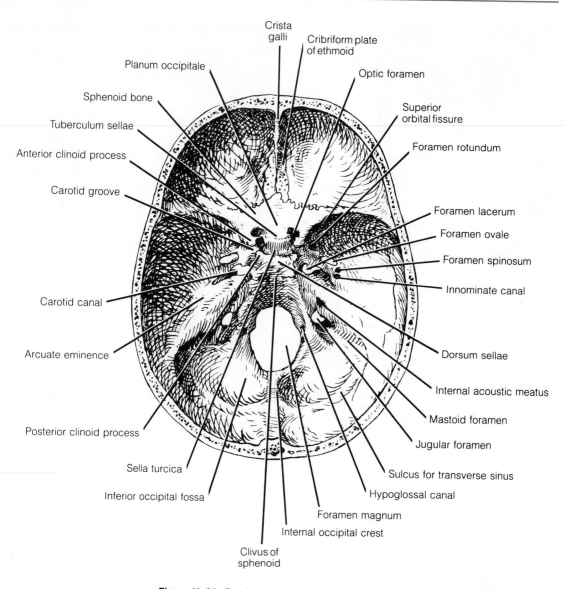

Figure 11–21. Basal view of the skull—internal aspect.

CASE 14

A 21-year-old right-handed motorcyclist was brought into the emergency room. He had been found lying unconscious without a helmet in the street, having apparently slipped going around a curve. From the position at the scene it appeared that his head had probably hit the curb. He had several facial abrasions and a swelling above his right ear. While in the emergency room he regained consciousness. He appeared dazed and complained of headache, but did not speak clearly.

Neurologic examination showed no papilledema. His pupils were equal, round, and reactive to light (PERRL), extraocular movements were normal, and there was questionable left facial weakness. There were no other neurologic deficits. Other findings included a blood pressure of 120/80 mg Hg, a pulse rate of 75/min, and a respiratory rate of 17/min.

What is the differential diagnosis at this time? What neuroradiologic or other diagnostic procedures are indicated?

The patient was kept under observation in the emergency room. Because of a sudden influx of emergency patients, however, repeat neurologic examination was not performed until several hours later. By that time, the patient had become stuporous, his right pupil was dilated, the blood pressure was 150/90 mg Hg, pulse rate 55/min, and respiratory rate 12/min. Emergency surgery was undertaken.

What is the most likely diagnosis?

Cases are discussed further in Chapter 25.

REFERENCES

Fishman RA: *Cerebrospinal Fluid in Diseases of the Nervous System.* Saunders, 1980.

Heimer L: *The Human Brain and Spinal Cord.* Springer-Verlag, 1983.

Rapoport SI: *Blood-Brain Barrier in Physiology and Medicine.* Raven, 1976.

Romanes GJ: *Cunningham's Textbook of Anatomy,* 12th ed. Oxford Univ Press, 1983.

Waddington MM: *Atlas of the Human Skull.* Academic Books, 1983.

12

Vascularization

About 18% of the total blood volume in the body circulates in the brain, which accounts for about 2% of the body weight. The blood transports oxygen, nutrients, and other substances necessary for proper functioning of the brain tissues and carries away metabolites. The brain uses about 20% of the oxygen absorbed in the lungs; the remainder goes to the rest of the body. A constant flow of oxygen must be maintained. Loss of consciousness occurs in less than 15 seconds after blood flow to the brain has stopped, and irreparable damage to the brain tissue occurs within five minutes. **Cerebrovascular disease, or stroke,** occurs as a result of vascular compromise or hemorrhage in the CNS and is one of the most frequent sources of neurologic disability in our society. Nearly one-half of the admissions to many busy neurologic services are because of strokes. Cerebrovascular disease is discussed later in this chapter.

Cerebral angiography is a commonly used neuroradiologic procedure that results in the visualization of cerebral arteries, precapillaries, veins, and sinuses. Normal and abnormal angiograms are discussed in Chapter 23. **Ultrasonography** permits the noninvasive visualization of the cerebral vasculature. **PET** and **SPECT scanning** are also emerging as very useful methods for the measurement of cerebral blood flow in humans, and **functional MRI scanning** can visualize regions of the brain with a high metabolic rate.

ARTERIAL SUPPLY OF THE BRAIN

Characteristics of the Cerebral Arteries

The **circle of Willis** (named after the English neuroanatomist, Sir Thomas Willis) shows many variations between individuals. The posterior communicating arteries may be large on one or both sides (embryonic type); the posterior cerebral artery may be thin in its first stretch (embryonic type); and the anterior communicating artery may be absent, double, or thin. Although occlusion of most of the major cerebral arteries usually produces a characteristic clinical picture, these variants of the circle (actually an irregular hexagon) make it difficult to predict whether functionally adequate anastomosis will readily occur in any given individual if a major supply vessel on one side suddenly becomes blocked.

The course of the large arteries (at least in their initial stretches) is largely ventral to the brain in a relatively small region. The arteries course in the subarachnoid space, often for a considerable distance, before entering the brain itself; rupture of a vessel thus may cause a subarachnoid hemorrhage.

Each major artery supplies a certain territory, separated by **border zones (watershed areas)** from other territories; sudden occlusion in a vessel affects its territory immediately, sometimes irreversibly. Often, a superficial layer of cortex receives blood from the meningeal arteries and thus survives, but in isolation.

Principal Arteries

The arterial blood for the brain enters the cranial cavity by way of two pairs of large vessels (Figs 12–1 and 12–2): the **internal carotid arteries,** which branch off the common carotids, and the **vertebral arteries,** which come from the subclavian arteries. The vertebral arterial system supplies the brain stem, cerebellum, occipital lobe, and parts of the thalamus, while the carotids normally supply the remainder of the forebrain. The carotids are interconnected via the **anterior cerebral arteries** and the **anterior communicating artery;** the carotids are also connected to the **posterior cerebral arteries** of the vertebral system by way of two **posterior communicating arteries,** part of the circle of Willis.

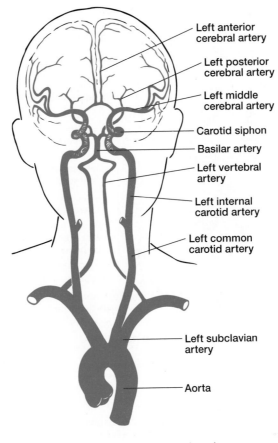

Figure 12–1. Major cerebral arteries.

Vertebrobasilar Territory

After passing through the foramen magnum in the base of the skull, the two vertebral arteries form a single midline vessel, the **basilar artery** (Figs 12–2, 12–3 and see 7–11); this vessel terminates in the interpeduncular cistern in a bifurcation as the left and right posterior cerebral arteries. These may be thin, large, or asymmetric, depending on retention of the embryonic pattern (in which the carotid supplies the posterior cerebral arteries).

Several pairs of small circumferential arteries arise from the vertebral arteries and their fused continuation, the basilar artery. These are the **posterior** and **anterior inferior cerebellar arteries,** the **superior cerebellar arteries,** and several smaller branches, such as the **pontine and internal auditory arteries.** All these vessels can show considerable asymmetry and variability. The small **penetrating arteries,** which branch off the basilar artery, supply vital centers in the brain stem (Fig 12–4).

Carotid Territory

The **internal carotid artery** passes through the **carotid canal** of the skull, then curves forward within the cavernous sinus and up and backward through the dura, forming the **carotid siphon** before reaching the brain (see Fig 12–3). The first branch is usually the **ophthalmic artery.** In addition to their links with the vertebral system, the carotids branch into a large middle and a smaller anterior cerebral artery on each side (Fig 12–5). The two anterior cerebral arteries usually meet over a short distance in midplane to form a short but functionally important **anterior communicating artery.** This vessel forms a link in the anastomoses between the left and right hemispheres, which is especially important when one internal carotid becomes occluded. The **anterior choroidal artery,** directly off the internal carotid, carries blood to the choroid plexus of the lateral ventricles as well as to several adjacent brain structures.

Cortical Supply

The **middle cerebral artery** supplies many deep structures and much of the lateral aspect of the cerebrum; it breaks up into several large branches that course in the depth of the lateral fissure, over the insula, before reaching the convexity of the hemisphere.

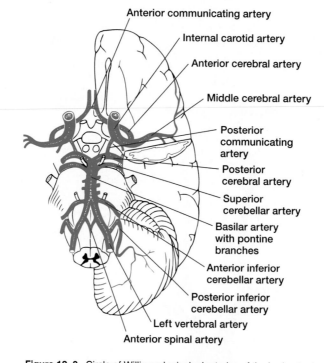

Anterior communicating artery

Internal carotid artery

Anterior cerebral artery

Middle cerebral artery

Posterior communicating artery

Posterior cerebral artery

Superior cerebellar artery

Basilar artery with pontine branches

Anterior inferior cerebellar artery

Posterior inferior cerebellar artery

Left vertebral artery

Anterior spinal artery

Figure 12–2. Circle of Willis and principal arteries of the brain stem.

The **anterior cerebral artery** and its branches course around the genu of the corpus callosum to supply the anterior frontal lobe and the medial aspect of the hemisphere; they extend quite far to the rear. The **posterior cerebral artery** curves around the brain stem, supplying mainly the occipital lobe and the choroid plexuses of the third and lateral ventricles and the lower surface of the temporal lobe (Figs 12–6 and 12–7). By comparing the territories irrigated by the anterior, middle, and posterior cerebral arteries on the one hand, and the homunculus on the other, the student can predict the deficits caused by a stroke affecting the territories irrigated by each of these arteries (Fig 12–6). For example, in a stroke affecting the territory of the middle cerebral artery, weakness and sensory loss are most severe in the contralateral face and arm, while the leg may be only mildly affected or unaffected. In contrast, in a stroke affecting the territory irrigated by the anterior cerebral artery, weakness is most pronounced in the contralateral leg.

Cerebral Blood Flow & Autoregulation

Many physiologic and pathologic factors can affect the blood flow in the arteries and veins of the brain (Table 12–1). Under normal conditions of autonomic regulation, the pressure in the small cerebral arteries is maintained at 450 mm of water. This ensures adequate perfusion of the cerebral capillary beds despite changes in systemic blood pressure. Increased activity in one cortical area is usually accompanied by a shift in blood volume to that area.

VENOUS DRAINAGE

Types of Channels

The venous drainage of the brain and coverings includes the veins of the brain itself, the dural **venous sinuses,** the dura's **meningeal veins,** and the **diploic veins** between the tables of the skull (Figs 12–8 and 12–9). Communication exists between most of these channels. Unlike systemic veins, cerebral veins have no valves and seldom accompany the corresponding cerebral arteries.

Internal Drainage

The interior of the cerebrum drains into the single midline **great cerebral vein** (of **Galen**), which lies beneath the splenium of the corpus callosum. The internal cerebral veins (with their tributaries, the **septal, thalamostriate,** and **choroidal** veins) empty into this vein, as do the basal veins (of Rosenthal), which wind

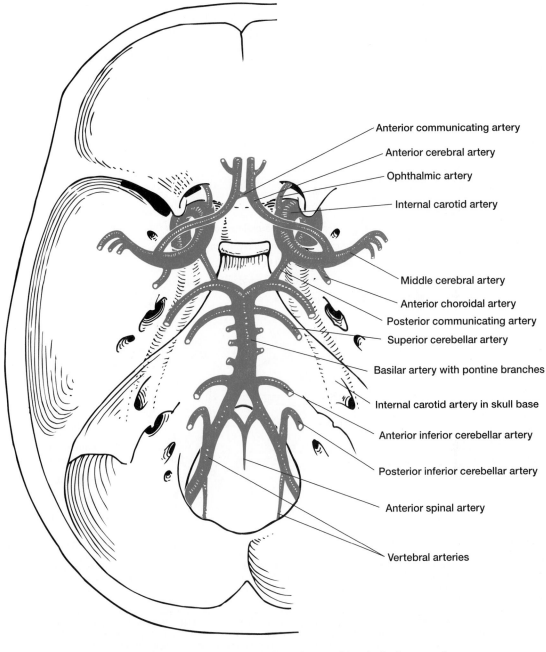

Figure 12–3. Principal arteries on the floor of the cranial cavity (brain removed).

(one right and one left) around the side of the midbrain, draining the base of the forebrain. The precentral vein from the cerebellum and veins from the upper brain stem also empty into the great vein, which turns upward behind the splenium and joins the inferior sagittal sinus to form the **straight sinus.** The venous drainage of the base of the cerebrum is also into the

deep middle cerebral vein (coursing in the lateral fissure) and then to the **cavernous sinus.**

Cortical Veins

Venous drainage of the brain surface is generally into the nearest large vein or sinus, from there to the

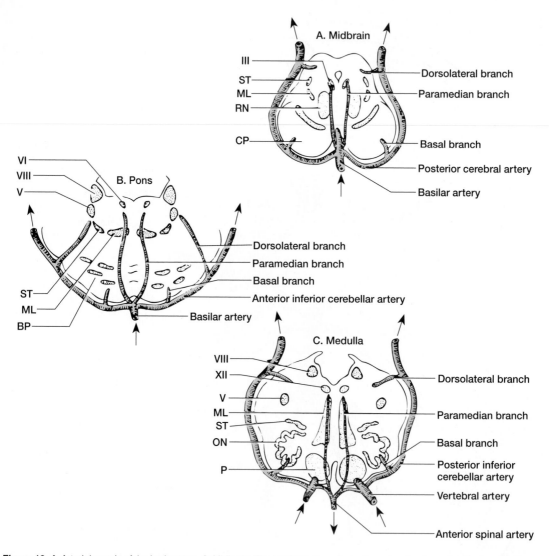

Figure 12–4. Arterial supply of the brain stem. **A:** Midbrain. The basilar artery gives off paramedian branches that supply the oculomotor (III) nerve nucleus and the red nucleus (RN). A larger branch, the posterior cerebral artery, courses laterally around the midbrain, giving off a basal branch that supplies the cerebral peduncle (CP) and a dorsolateral branch supplying the spinothalamic tract (ST), medial lemniscus (ML), and superior cerebellar peduncle. The posterior cerebral artery continues (upper arrows) to supply the thalamus, occipital lobe, and medial temporal lobe. **B:** Pons. Paramedian branches of the basilar artery supply the abducens (VI) nucleus and the medial lemniscus (ML). The anterior inferior cerebellar artery gives off a basal branch to the descending motor pathways in the basis pontis (BP) and a dorsolateral branch to the trigeminal (V) nucleus, the vestibular (VIII) nucleus, and the spinothalamic tract (ST) before passing to the cerebellum (upper arrows). **C:** Medulla. Paramedian branches of the vertebral arteries supply descending motor pathways in the pyramid (P), the medial lemniscus (ML), and the hypoglossal (XII) nucleus. Another vertebral branch, the posterior inferior cerebellar artery, gives off a basal branch to the olivary nuclei (ON) and a dorsolateral branch that supplies the trigeminal (V) nucleus, the vestibular (VIII) nucleus, and the spinothalamic tract (ST) on its way to the cerebellum (upper arrows). (Reproduced, with permission, from Greenberg DA, Aminoff MJ, Simon RP: *Clinical Neurology,* 2nd ed. Appleton & Lange, 1993.)

confluence of the sinuses, and ultimately to the **internal jugular vein** (see Fig 12–8).

The veins of the cerebral convex surfaces are divided into superior and inferior groups. The 6–12 **superior cerebral veins** run upward on the hemisphere's surface to the superior sagittal sinus, generally passing under any lateral lacunae. Most of the **inferior cerebral veins** end in the superficial middle cerebral vein. The inferior cerebral veins that do not end in this fashion terminate in the transverse sinus. **Anastomotic veins** can be found; these connect the deep middle cerebral vein with the superior sagittal sinus or transverse sinus.

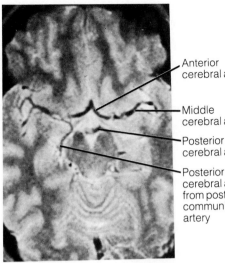

Figure 12–5. MRI of a horizontal section at the level of the circle of Willis.

Anterior cerebral artery

Middle cerebral artery

Posterior cerebral artery

Posterior cerebral artery from posterior communicating artery

Venous Sinuses

Venous channels lined by mesothelium lie between the inner and outer layers of the dura; they are called intradural (or dural) sinuses. Their tributaries come mostly from the neighboring brain substance. All sinuses ultimately drain into the internal jugular veins or **pterygoid plexus.** The sinuses may also communicate with extracranial veins via the **emissary veins.** These latter veins are important because the blood can flow through them in either direction, and because infections of the scalp may extend by this route into the intracranial structures.

Of the venous sinuses, the following are considered most important:

Superior sagittal sinus: Between the falx and the inside of the skullcap.

Inferior sagittal sinus: In the free edge of the falx.

Straight sinus: In the seam between the falx and the tentorium.

Transverse sinuses: Between the tentorium and its attachment on the skull cap.

Sigmoid sinuses: S-curved continuations of the transverse sinuses into the jugular veins. A transverse and a sigmoid sinus together form a lateral sinus.

Sphenoparietal sinuses: Drain the deep middle cerebral veins into the cavernous sinuses.

Cavernous sinuses: On either side of the sella turcica.

Inferior petrosal sinuses: From the cavernous sinus to the jugular foramen.

Superior petrosal sinus: From the cavernous sinus to the beginning of the sigmoid sinus.

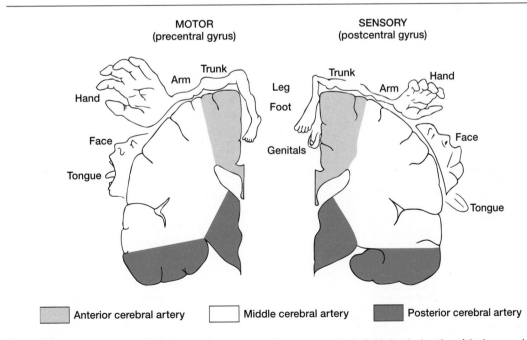

Figure 12–6. Arterial supply of the primary motor and sensory cortex (coronal view). Notice the location of the homunculus with respect to the territories of the cerebral arteries. (Reproduced, with permission, from Greenberg DA, Aminoff MJ, Simon RP: *Clinical Neurology*, 2nd ed. Appleton & Lange, 1993.)

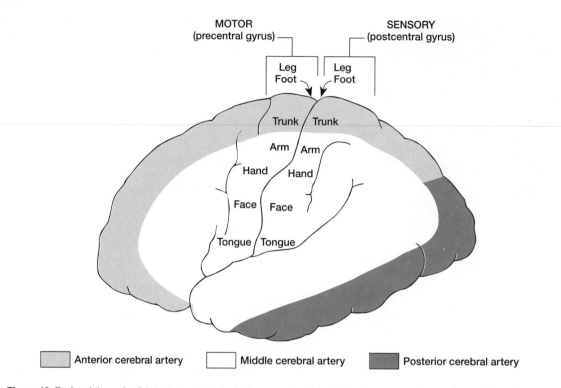

Figure 12–7. Arterial supply of the primary motor and sensory cortex (lateral view). (Reproduced, with permission, from Greenberg DA, Aminoff MJ, Simon RP: *Clinical Neurology,* 2nd ed. Appleton & Lange, 1993.)

Table 12–1. Factors affecting brain-blood flow.

Factor	Increases Flow	Decreases Flow
Physiologic		
Carotid sinus pressure	Higher	Lower
CO_2 in blood	Raised	Lowered
O_2 in blood	Lowered	Raised
Sympathetic stimulation	Decreased	Increased
Cerebrovascular tone (autonomic nervous system)	Dilatation	Constriction
CSF pressure	Decreased	Increased
Mean arterial minus venous blood pressure	Raised	Lowered
Pathologic		
Pathologic changes	Hemangioma	Arteriosclerosis
Anomalies	Arteriovenous malformation	
Drugs	Vasodilation	Vasoconstriction
Other		
	Anemia	Polycythemia
	Hyperthyroidism	Hypothyroidism

The pressure of the cerebrospinal fluid (CSF) varies directly with acute changes in venous pressure. The Queckenstedt test is used with lumbar-puncture manometry to determine whether CSF block is present (see Chapter 6).

CEREBROVASCULAR DISORDERS

Cerebrovascular disease is the most common cause of neurologic disability in adults and is the third most common cause of death in our society. About 500,000 people are disabled or killed by cerebrovascular disease each year in the United States. Cerebrovascular disease is responsible for more than one-half of the admissions to many busy acute neurologic services and accounts for about 15% of admissions to chronic care institutions.

Most authorities classify cerebrovascular disease into *ischemic* and *hemorrhagic* disorders. As a result of its high metabolic rate and limited energy reserves, the CNS is uniquely sensitive to ischemia. Ischemia results in rapid depletion of ATP stores in the CNS and because Na-K ATP-ase function is impaired, there is an accumulation of K in the extracellular space, which leads to neuronal depolarization (see Chapter 3). According to the **excitotoxic hypothesis,** within gray matter of the CNS, there is an ensuing avalanche of neurotransmitter release (including inappropriate re-

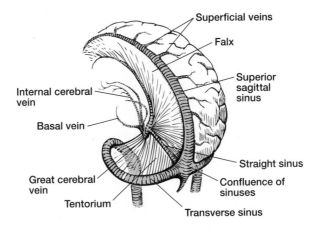

Figure 12–8. Veins and sinuses of the brain, left posterior lateral view.

lease of excitatory transmitters such as glutamate). This leads to an influx of calcium, via glutamate-gated channels as well as voltage-gated calcium channels that are activated as a result of depolarization. Within white matter of the CNS, where synapses are not present, calcium is carried into nerve cells via other routes, including the Na-Ca exchanger, a specialized molecule that exchanges calcium for sodium. It is generally thought that increased intracellular calcium represents a "final common pathway" leading to irreversible cell injury (the **calcium hypothesis** of neuronal cell death) because calcium activates a spectrum of enzymes including proteases, lipases, and endonucleases that damage the neuronal cytoskeleton and plasma membrane.

Transient ischemia, if brief enough, may produce reversible signs and symptoms of neuronal dysfunction. If ischemia is prolonged, however, death of neurons (infarction) occurs and is usually accompanied by persistent neurologic deficits.

Classification

Diseases involving vessels of the brain and its coverings have characteristic clinical profiles and can be classified as follows (Table 12–2):

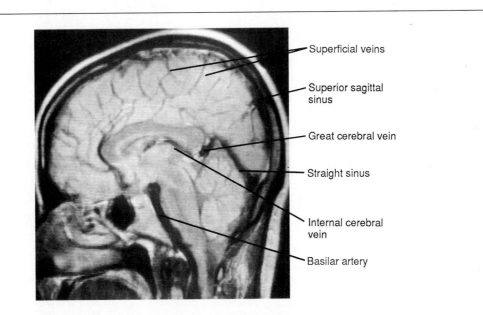

Figure 12–9. MRI (long time sequence; see Chapter 23) of a midsagittal section through the head showing venous channels.

Table 12–2. Clinical profile of cerebrovasular disorders.

	Hypertensive Intracerebral Hemorrhage	Cerebral Infarct (Thrombotic)	Cerebral Infarct (Embolic)	Subarachnoid Hemorrhage	Vascular Malformations (can include bleeding)	Subdural Hemorrhage	Epidural Hemorrhage
Pathology	Hemorrhage in deep structures (putamen, thalamus, cerebellum, pons) or lobar white matter.	Infarct in territory of large or small artery.	Infarct in territory of large or medium-sized arteries. May be located at periphery of hemisphere (gray-white matter junction).	Bleeding into subarachnoid space from aneurysm. Hemorrhage into parenchyma may occur.	Bleeding or infarct near AVM; localization variable.	Hemorrhage into subdural space, often over cerebral convexity. May see rupture of meningeal or bridging vein.	Hemorrhage into epidural space. Often seen in association with skull fracture over middle meningeal artery.
Onset and course	Rapid (minutes to hours) onset of hemiplegia or other signs and symptoms.	Sudden, gradual (or stepwise onset of focal deficits. Often preceded by TIAs (transient monocular blindness, hemiparesis, etc.).	Sudden onset (usually within seconds or minutes).	Sudden severe headache. Possible loss of consciousness. Focal neurologic signs may be present.	Can present with repeated seizures (because of ischemia), or sudden onset of deficit due to bleed.	Variable time-course. May see slow deterioration. Depressed level of consciousness, sometimes with hemiparesis. Can occur after even trivial trauma.	Rapid deterioration, often after a "lucid interval" following head trauma.
Blood pressure	Hypertension.	Hypertension often.	Normal.	Hypertension often.	Normal.	Normal at onset.	Normal at onset.
Special findings	Cardiac hypertrophy; hypertensive retinopathy.	Arteriosclerotic cardiovascular disease frequently present.	Cardiac arrhythmias or infarction (source of emboli often in heart).	Subhyaloid (preretinal) hemorrhages; nuchal rigidity.	Subhyaloid hemorrhages and retinal angioma.	Trauma, bruises may be present.	Severe trauma often present.
CT scan findings	Increased density surrounded by hypodensity from edema; may see blood in ventricles. Commonly see mass effect.	Less dense in avascular area.	Less dense in avascular area.	Increased density due to blood in basal cisterns.	Abnormal vessels, sometimes with calcifications. Dense cisterns may be seen after bleeding.	Dense (later, lighter) zone (high over convexity).	Dense segment under the skull fracture (low over convexity).
MR image	MRI very sensitive. May see blood clot. Signal characteristics change with time after bleed.	Decreased density on T_1; increased density on T_2.	Decreased density on T_1; increased density on T_2.	Often normal. Less sensitive than CT for subarachnoid blood.	May see hemorrhage.	May see hemorrhage.	May see hemorrhage.
CSF	May be bloody.	Clear.	Clear.	Grossly bloody or xanthochromic.	Bloody if hemorrhage has occurred.	May be bloody or xanthochromic.	Clear.

Occlusive cerebrovascular disorders: These result from arterial or venous thrombosis, or embolism, and can lead to infarction of well-defined parts of the brain. Because each artery irrigates a specific part of the brain, it is often possible, on the basis of the neurologic deficit, to identify the vessel that is occluded.

Transient cerebral ischemia: Transient ischemia, if brief enough, can occur without infarction. Episodes of this type are termed transient ischemic attacks **(TIAs).** As with occlusive cerebrovascular disease, the neurologic abnormalities often permit the clinician to predict the vessel that is involved.

Hemorrhage: The rupture of a blood vessel is often associated with hypertension or vascular malformations or with trauma.

Vascular malformations and developmental abnormalities: These include aneurysms or arteriovenous malformations, which can lead to hemorrhage. Hypoplasia or absence of vessels occurs in some brains.

Degenerative diseases of the arteries: These can lead to occlusion or to hemorrhage.

Inflammatory diseases of the arteries: A variety of inflammatory diseases, including systemic lupus erythematosis, giant cell arteritis, and syphilitic arteritis can result in occlusion of cerebral vessels, which, in turn, can produce infarction.

The acute onset of most types of infarcts or hemorrhages—cerebrovascular accidents **(CVAs)**—usually associated with vascular disease of the nervous system can lead to sudden, severe focal disturbances of brain function (ie, hemiplegia, aphasia). The term **stroke** is a general one and further determination of the site (Where is the lesion?) and type of disease (What is the lesion?) are essential for correct diagnosis and treatment.

Occlusive Cerebrovascular Disease

Insufficient blood supply to portions of the brain leads to infarction and swelling with necrosis of brain

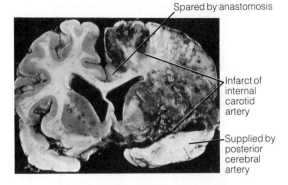

Figure 12–11. Coronal section through the cerebrum showing a large infarct caused by occlusion of the internal carotid artery.

tissue (Figs 12–10 to 12–13 and Table 12–2). If an infarcted area is later perfused with blood, it may become a red, or hemorrhagic, infarct; if not, it remains a pale, or white, infarct. Most infarcts are caused by **atherosclerosis** of the vessels, leading to narrowing, occlusion, or **thrombosis;** a **cerebral embolism,** ie, occlusion caused by an **embolus** (a plug of tissue or a foreign substance) from outside the brain; or other conditions such as prolonged hypotension, drug action, spasm, or inflammation of the vessels. Venous infarction may occur when a venous channel becomes occluded.

The extent of an infarct depends on the presence or absence of adequate anastomotic channels. Capillaries from adjacent vascular territories and corticomeningeal capillaries at the surface may reduce the size of the infarct. When arterial occlusion occurs proximal to the circle of Willis, *collateral circulation* through the anterior

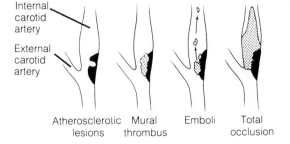

Figure 12–10. Schematic illustration of stages of occlusion of the internal carotid artery. (Modified and reproduced, with permission, from Escourolle R, Poirier J: *Manual of Basic Neuropathology.* Saunders, 1971.)

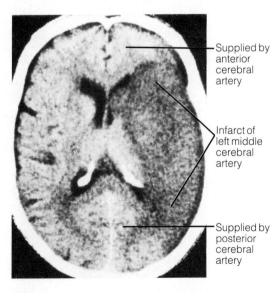

Figure 12–12. CT image of a horizontal section of the head showing an infarct caused by middle cerebral artery occlusion.

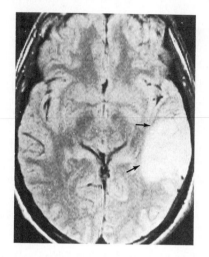

Figure 12–13. MRI of a coronal section of the head showing an infarct (arrows) caused by occlusion of a branch of the middle cerebral artery.

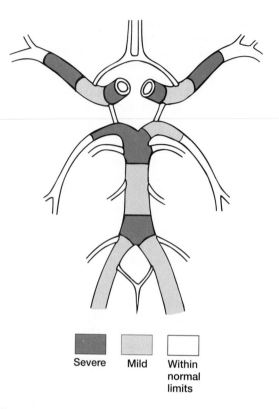

Severe   Mild   Within normal limits

Figure 12–15. Distribution of degenerative lesions in large cerebral arteries of the circle of Willis. The severity of the lesions is illustrated by the intensity of the shaded areas, with the darkest areas showing the most severe lesions.

communicating artery and posterior communicating arteries may permit blood flow that prevents infarction. Similarly, in some cases where the internal carotid artery is occluded in the neck, anastomotic flow in the retrograde direction via the ophthalmic artery, from the external carotid artery, may provide adequate circulation and prevent infarction.

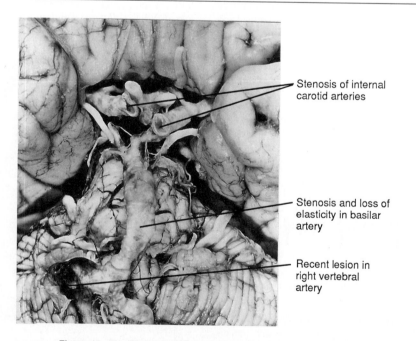

Stenosis of internal carotid arteries

Stenosis and loss of elasticity in basilar artery

Recent lesion in right vertebral artery

Figure 12–14. Atherosclerosis in arteries at the base of the brain.

Although sudden occlusion can lead to irreparable damage, slowly developing local ischemia may be compensated for by extensive anastomoses through one or more routes: the circle of Willis, the ophthalmic artery (whose branches communicate with external carotid vessels), or corticomeningeal anastomoses from meningeal vessels.

Atherosclerosis of the Brain

The principal pathologic change in the arteries of the brain occurs in the vasculature of the neck and brain, although similar changes may be present in other systemic vessels also. The disease is progressive; it is considered by many to be a manifestation of the aging process in humans. Disturbances in metabolism—especially of fats—are believed to be a prominent associated change. Hypertension accelerates the progression of atherosclerosis and is a risk factor for stroke.

Atheromatous changes in the arterial system are found relatively frequently at postmortem examination of the bodies of people who have reached middle age (Fig 12–14). Vessels of all sizes may be affected. A combination of degenerative and proliferative changes can be seen microscopically. The muscularis is the main site of proliferation; the intima may be absent. Disseminated areas of softening of the brain (infarcts) are frequently found.

Frequently the areas most often involved are near branchings or confluences of vessels (Fig 12–15 and Table 12–3). The most common and severe atherosclerotic lesions are in the carotid bifurcation. Others occur at the origin of the vertebral arteries and in the upper and lower parts of the basilar artery as well as in the internal carotid artery at its trifurcation, the first third of the middle cerebral artery, and the first part of the posterior cerebral artery. Narrowing of vessels severe enough to cause vascular insufficiency can be present in young adulthood, but it is more often present in older persons.

Table 12–3. Frequency distribution (in %) of arterial lesions causing cerebrovascular insufficiency.*

Lesion	Left	Right
Stenosis		
Brachiocephalic	—	4
Internal carotid (near bifurcation)	34	34
Anterior cerebral	3	3
Proximal vertebral	22	18
Distal vertebral	4	5
Occlusion		
Brachiocephalic	—	1
Internal carotid (near bifurcation)	8	8
Anterior cerebral	2	1
Posterior vertebral	5	4
Distal vertebral	3	3

*Figures based on Hass WK et al: Joint study of extracranial arterial occlusion. *JAMA* 1968;203:916.

Cerebral Embolism

The sudden occlusion of a brain vessel by a blood clot, a piece of fat, a tumor, a clump of bacteria, another substance—or air—interrupts the blood supply to a portion of the brain abruptly and results in necrosis or infarction (see Fig 12–12 and Table 12–2). One of the most common causes of cerebral embolism is atrial fibrillation. Other common causes of cerebral embolism include endocarditis and mural thrombus after myocardial infarction. Fracture of a long bone can produce fat emboli, and lung lesions or cuts in large superficial veins can cause an air embolism. **Artery-to-artery embolization** also occurs in some cases when there is an intra-arterial source of emboli. For example, a thrombus in a large artery can break up, yielding fragments that move distally and occlude smaller vessels; alternatively, atheromatous material can break off from a plaque in the carotid artery and after being carried distally may occlude smaller arteries.

Transient Cerebral Ischemia

Focal cerebral ischemic attacks, especially in middle-aged and older persons, may be caused by transient occlusion of an already narrow vessel. The cause is thought to be a vasospasm, a small embolus that is later carried away, or thrombosis of a diseased vessel (and subsequent anastomosis). Such **transient ischemic attacks (TIAs)** result in reversible ischemic neurologic deficits such as sudden vertigo or weakness, loss of cranial nerve function, or even brief loss of consciousness. These episodes are usually due to ischemia in the territory of an artery within the carotid or vertebrobasilar system. In TIAs, there is usually full recovery in less than 24 hours (commonly within 30 minutes). These attacks are considered warning signs of future—or imminent—occlusion and merit a rapid work-up as shown in Clinical Illustration 12–1.

Localization of the Vascular Lesion in Stroke Syndromes

It is often possible, in stroke syndromes, to identify the affected blood vessel on the basis of the neurologic signs and symptoms.

Carotid artery disease is often accompanied by contralateral weakness or sensory loss. If the dominant hemisphere is involved, there may be aphasia or apraxia. Transient blurring or loss of vision (amaurosis fugax) may occur if there is retinal ischemia. In ischemia that is limited to the territory of the middle cerebral artery, weakness predominantly affects the contralateral face and arm; this is often seen with carotid artery disease because the anterior and posterior cerebral artery territories are nourished via collateral flow from the contralateral circulation via the anterior communicating and

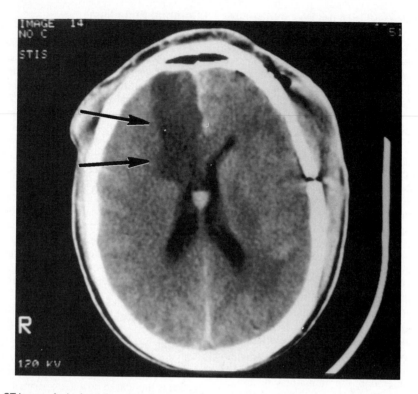

Figure 12–16. CT image of a horizontal section of the head, showing an infarct caused by a right-sided anterior cerebral artery occlusion (arrows). Notice the location of the infarct (compare to Figs 12–6 and 12–7). The patient had developed weakness and numbness of the left leg.

Table 12–4. Brain-stem syndromes resulting from vascular occlusion.

Syndrome	Artery Affected	Structure Involved	Clinical Manifestations
Medial syndromes			
Medulla	Paramedian branches	Emerging fibers of twelfth nerve	Ipsilateral hemiparalysis of tongue
Inferior pons	Paramedian branches	Pontine gaze center, near or in nucleus of sixth nerve	Paralysis of gaze to side of lesion
		Emerging fibers of sixth nerve	Ipsilateral abduction paralysis
Superior pons	Paramedian branches	Medial longitudinal fasciculus	Internuclear ophthalmoplegia
Lateral syndromes			
Medulla	Posterior inferior cerebellar	Emerging fibers of ninth and tenth nerves	Dysphagia, hoarseness, ipsilateral paralysis of vocal cord; ipsilateral loss of pharyngeal reflex
		Vestibular nuclei	Vertigo, nystagmus
		Descending tract and nucleus of fifth nerve	Ipsilateral facial analgesia
		Solitary nucleus and tract	Taste loss on ipsilateral half of tongue posteriorly
Inferior pons	Anterior inferior cerebellar	Emerging fibers of seventh nerve	Ipsilateral facial paralysis
		Solitary nucleus and tract	Taste loss on ipsilateral half of tongue anteriorly
		Cochlear nuclei	Deafness, tinnitus
Midpons		Motor nucleus of fifth nerve	Ipsilateral jaw weakness
		Emerging sensory fibers of fifth nerve	Ipsilateral facial numbness

(From Brust JC In: *Merritt's Textbook of Neurology,* 8th ed. Rowland LP (editor). Lea & Febiger, 1989. Modified, with permission, from Rowland LP In: *Principles of Neural Science,* 3rd ed. Kandel ER, Schwartz JH (editors). Elsevier, 1985.)

posterior communicating arteries. Clinical Illustration 12–1 provides an example.

As predicted from its position with respect to the motor and sensory homunculi, unilateral occlusion of the anterior cerebral artery results in weakness and sensory loss in the contralateral leg (Fig 12–16). In some patients following bilateral occlusion of the anterior cerebral arteries, there is a state of *akinetic mutism,* in which the patient is indifferent and apathetic, moving little and not speaking, even though there is no paralysis of the immobile limbs.

Vertebrobasilar artery disease often presents with vertigo, ataxia (impaired coordination), dysarthria (slurred speech), and dysphasia (impaired swallowing). Vertigo, nausea, and vomiting may be present and if the oculomotor complex is involved, there may be diplopia (double vision). The brain stem syndromes are discussed in Chapter 7 and those arising from arterial occlusion are summarized in Table 12–4.

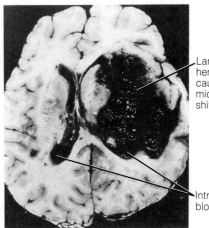
Large hematoma causing midline shift

Intraventricular blood

Figure 12–17. Horizontal section through the head showing a large intracerebral hematoma.

Hypertensive Hemorrhage

Chronic high blood pressure may result in the formation of small areas of vessel distention—**microaneurysms**—mostly in small arteries that arise from much larger vessels. A further rise in blood pressure then ruptures these aneurysms, resulting in an **intracerebral hemorrhage** (Fig 12–17 and Table 12–2). In order of frequency, the most common sites are the lentiform nucleus, especially the **putamen**, supplied by the lenticulostriate arteries (Fig 12–18); the **thalamus**, supplied by posterior perforating arteries off the posterior cerebral-basilar artery bifurcation (Fig 12–19); the **white matter** of the cerebral hemispheres (lobar hemorrhages); the **pons**, supplied by small perforating arteries from the basilar artery; and the **cerebellum**, supplied by branches of the cerebellar arter-

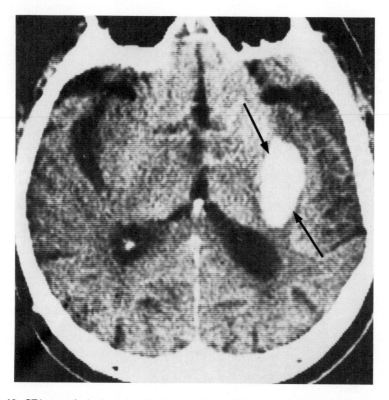

Figure 12–18. CT image of a horizontal section through the head showing a hematoma (arrows) in the putamen.

ies. Such hemorrhages may remain small and become cystic defects, or they may break through into adjacent structures or spaces including the ventricles. The blood clot compresses and may destroy adjacent brain tissue; cerebellar hemorrhages may compress the underlying fourth ventricle and produce acute hydrocephalus. Intracranial hemorrhages are thus medical emergencies and require prompt diagnosis and treatment.

Subarachnoid Hemorrhage

Often seen in normotensive persons, subarachnoid hemorrhages derive from ruptured aneurysms or vascular malformations (Figs 12–20 to 12–22; see Table 12–2). Aneurysms (abnormal distention of local vessels) may be congenital **(berry aneurysm)** or the result of infection **(mycotic aneurysm).** Loss of elasticity because of atherosclerosis **(tubular aneurysm)** may be a contributing factor. One complication of subarachnoid hemorrhage, arterial spasm, can lead to infarct formation. Venous aneurysms (eg, of the great cerebral vein) may be present in childhood.

Congenital berry aneurysms are seen most frequently in the circle of Willis or in the middle cerebral trifurcation; they are especially common at sites of arterial branching. Aneurysms are seen infrequently in vessels of the posterior fossa. A ruptured aneurysm generally bleeds into the subarachnoid space or, less frequently, into the brain substance itself.

Vascular malformations, especially arteriovenous malformations (AVMs), often occur in younger persons and are found on the surface of the brain, deep in the brain substance, or in the meninges (dural arteriovenous malformations). Bleeding from such malformations can be intracerebral, subarachnoid, or subdural. In some cases, the size of the malformation can be reduced by introducing coagulative emboli (via a catheter) into one or more of the feeder arteries prior to neurosurgical treatment.

Subdural Hemorrhage

Tearing of the bridging veins between brain surface and dural sinus is the most frequent cause of subdural hemorrhage (Figs 12–23 to 12–25; see Table 12–2). Often it occurs as the result of a relatively minor trauma and some blood may be present in the subarachnoid space. Children (because they have thinner veins) and adults with brain atrophy (because they have longer bridging veins) are at greatest risk. The bleeding may recur; the subdural blood may be reabsorbed or it may become encapsulated or even calcified.

Epidural Hemorrhage

Bleeding from a torn meningeal vessel (usually an artery) may lead to an extradural (outside the dura) accumulation of blood. Severe trauma and fracture of the

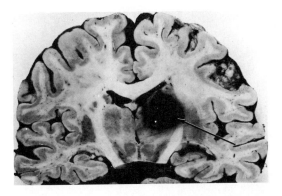

Figure 12–19. Hemorrhage in the right posterior thalamus and internal capsule in a 64-year-old woman.

skull often cause this type of epidural, or extradural, hemorrhage (Figs 12–26 and 12–27; see Table 12–2). Uncontrolled arterial bleeding may lead to compression of the brain and subsequent herniation. Immediate diagnosis and surgical drainage are essential.

Arteriovenous Shunts

Trauma can cause the rupture of adjacent vessels, allowing arterial blood to flow into nearby veins. For example, in a **carotid-cavernous fistula,** the internal carotid drains into the cavernous sinus and jugular vein causing ischemia in the cerebral arteries. There is often pulsating exophthalmos (forward protrusion of the eye in the orbit) and there may be extraocular palsies because of pressure on the oculomotor, trochlear, and abducens nerves, which run through the cavernous sinus.

Interventional methods, such as inserting a balloon into the shunt via a catheter or surgery, are usually required to correct the problem. Spontaneous correction has occurred occasionally after long air flights, presumably because of pressure changes.

CASE 15

A 44-year-old woman was admitted after having a seizure. She was lethargic, with a right facial droop, right hemiparesis, and right hyperreflexia. She complained of headache and a painful neck. A few days later, she seemed slightly more alert and made purposeful movements with her left hand—but not her right hand. She was still unresponsive to spoken commands and had a rigid neck. Other findings included bilateral papilledema, a right pupil that was smaller than the left, incomplete extraocular movements on the left side (nerve VI function was normal), decreased right corneal reflex, and right nasolabial droop. The patient's right arm was hypertonic and paretic, but the other extremities were normal. All re-

flexes appeared within normal range. The right plantar extensor response was equivocal, but the left was normal.

The blood pressure was 120/85; pulse rate 60; and temperature 38° C (100.4° F). The white blood count was 11,200/μl, and the erythrocyte sedimentation rate was 30 mm/h.

Where is the lesion? What is the cause of the lesion? What is the differential diagnosis?

A CT scan showed a high-density area in the cisterns, especially on the right side. What is the diagnosis now? Would you request a lumbar puncture with analysis of the cerebrospinal fluid?

CASE 16

A 55-year-old salesman exhibiting signs of confusion was brought to the hospital. The history gathered from his landlady disclosed that he had been separated from his family because he drank too much. Although he was apparently in good health, his landlady had entered the apartment on the day of admission because he did not respond to her calls. She found him lying on the floor, incontinent of urine and appearing bewildered; he had also bitten his lip. The landlady remembered that two months earlier he had been involved in a fight in a bar; three weeks previously he had fractured his wrist falling down stairs.

On examination, the patient was unconcerned, disheveled, and dirty. Bruises on his head and legs were consistent with recent trauma from a fall. The liver was palpable 4 cm below the right costal margin. The patient appeared to fall asleep when left alone. Neurologic examination showed normal optic fundi, normal extraocular movements, and no abnormalities that would result from dysfunction of other cranial nerves. When the left hand was extended, it showed a slow downward drift. The reflexes were normal and symmetric, and there was a left-sided plantar extensor response.

Vital signs, complete blood count, and urinalysis were within normal limits. A lumbar puncture showed an opening pressure of 180 mm of water, xanthochromia, a protein level of 80 mg/dL, and a glucose level of 70 mg/dL. Cell counts in all tubes showed red blood cells, 800/μL; lymphocytes, 20/μL; and polymorphonuclear neutrophils, 4/μL. A CT scan of the head was obtained.

Over the next 36 hours, the patient became deeply obtunded and seemed to develop a left-sided hemiparesis.

What is the differential diagnosis? What is the most likely diagnosis?

Questions and answers pertaining to Section IV (Chapters 7–12) can be found in Appendix D.

Cases are discussed further in Chapter 25.

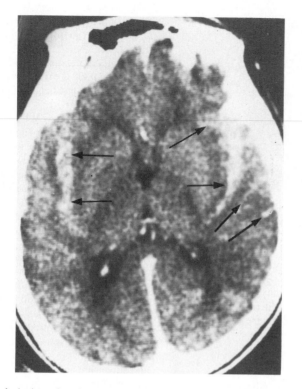

Figure 12–20. CT image of a horizontal section through the head, showing high densities, representing a subarachnoid hemorrhage (arrows) in the sulci.

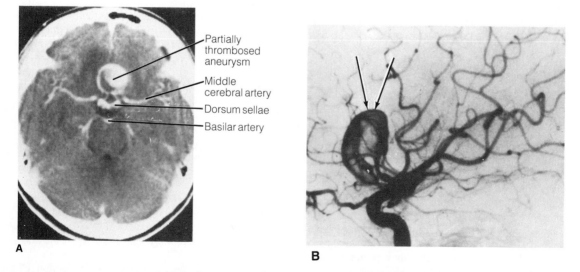

Partially
thrombosed
aneurysm

Middle
cerebral artery

Dorsum sellae

Basilar artery

A

B

Figure 12–21. *A:* CT image of a horizontal section through the head, showing a large aneurysm of the anterior communicating artery. (Reproduced, with permission, from deGroot J: *Correlative Neuroanatomy of Computed Tomography and Magnetic Resonance Imaging.* Lea & Febiger, 1984.) *B:* Corresponding angiogram showing the partially thrombosed aneurysm (arrows).

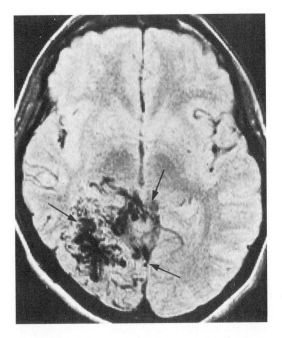

Figure 12–22. MR image of a horizontal section through the head, demonstrating an arteriovenous malformation (arrows).

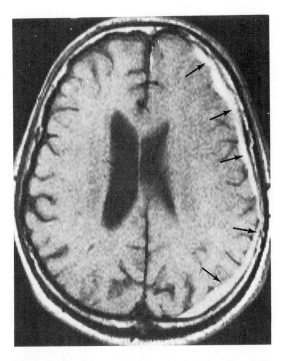

Figure 12–24. MR image of a horizontal section through the head, showing a left subdural hematoma (arrows) causing a midline shift.

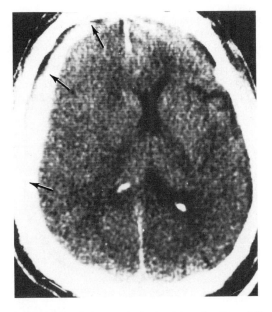

Figure 12–23. CT image of a horizontal section through the head, showing a right subdural hematoma (arrows) causing a shift away from the lesion.

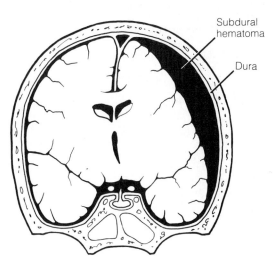

Figure 12–25. Schematic illustration of a subdural hemorrhage.

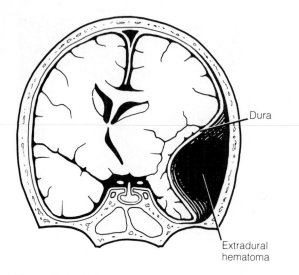

Figure 12–26. Schematic illustration of a epidural hemorrhage.

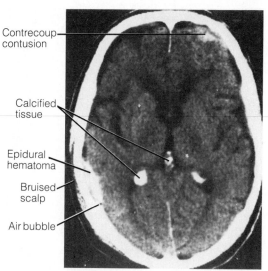

Figure 12–27. CT image of a horizontal section through the head, showing an extradural hematoma and intracerebral contrecoup lesion. (Reproduced, with permission, from deGroot J: *Correlative Neuroanatomy of Computed Tomography and Magnetic Resonance Imaging.* Lea & Febiger, 1984.)

REFERENCES

Barnett HJ et al: *Stroke-Pathophysiology, Diagnosis, and Management.* Churchill Livingston, 1985.

Choi DW: Cerebral hypoxia: some new approaches and unanswered questions. *J Neurosci* 1990;**10:**2493.

Fisher CM: Lacunar strokes and infarcts: A review. *Neurology* 1982;**32:**871.

Garcia JH: Circulatory disorders and their effects on the brain. In: *Textbook of Pathology,* 2nd ed. Davis RL, Robertson DM (editors). Williams & Wilkins, 1990.

Ross Russell RW (editor): *Vascular Disease of the Central Nervous System,* 2nd ed. Churchill Livingston, Edinburg, 1983.

Salamon G: *Atlas of the Arteries of the Human Brain.* Sandoz, 1973.

Schurr A, Rigor B: *Cerebral Ischemia and Resuscitation.* CRC Press, 1990.

Sokoloff L: Circulation and energy metabolism in the brain. In: *Basic Neurochemistry,* 4th ed. Siegel G et al. (editors). Raven, 1989.

Stephens RB, Stilwell DL: *Arteries and Veins of the Human Brain.* Thomas, 1969.

Thomas DJ, Bannister R: Preservation of autoregulation of cerebral flow in autonomic failure. *J Neurol Sci* 1980;**44:**205.

Waxman SG, Ransom BR, Stys PK: Nonsynaptic mechanisms of calcium-mediated injury in the CNS white matter. *Trends in Neurosci* 1991;**14:**461.

Section V
Functional Systems

Control of Movement

13

CONTROL OF MOVEMENT

Evolution of Movement

Movement (motion) is a fundamental property of animal life. In simple, unicellular animals, motion and locomotion (movement from one place to another) depend upon the contractility of protoplasm and the action of accessory organs: cilia, flagella, and so forth. Rudimentary multicellular animals possess primitive neuromuscular mechanisms; in more advanced forms of animal life, motion is based upon the transmission of impulses from a receptor through an afferent neuron and ganglion cell to motor neurons and muscle. This same arrangement is found in the reflex arc of higher animals, including humans, in whom the spinal cord has further developed into a central regulating mechanism. The brain is concerned with the initiation of movement and the integration of complex motions.

Control of Movement in Humans

The motor system controls a complex neuromuscular organism. Commands must be sent to many muscles (sometimes dozens), and several ipsilateral and contralateral joints must also be stabilized. The motor system includes cortical and subcortical areas of gray matter; the corticobulbar, corticospinal, corticopontine, rubrospinal, reticulospinal, vestibulospinal, and tectospinal descending tracts; gray matter of the spinal cord; efferent nerves; and input from the cerebellum and basal ganglia (Figs 13–1 and 13-5). Continuous feedback from sensory systems and cerebellar afferents further influences the motor system. The muscles that produce movement do not function continuously; they require an adequate blood supply and replenishment of glucose as they tire.

The motor system does not function in a mechanical, robot-like fashion, but dynamically, in a highly complex interaction of the afferent, efferent, metabolic, and autonomic systems. (Some aspects of motor control are, in fact, still poorly understood.)

A. Hierarchy: Movement is organized in increasingly complex and hierarchical levels.

Reflexes are controlled at the spinal or higher levels (Table 13–1; see also Chapter 5).

Stereotypical repetitious movements such as walking or swimming are governed by neural networks that include the spinal cord, brain stem, and cerebellum. Normal walking movement can be elicited in experimental animals even after transection of the upper brain stem, probably as a result of the presence of **central pattern generators,** or local circuits of neurons that can trigger simple repetitive motor activities, in the lower brain stem or spinal cord.

Specific, goal-directed movements are initiated at the level of the cerebral cortex. With repetition, even these movements (writing, playing a musical instrument) can be relearned, so that lower brain centers can take over the control functions.

B. Components: Control over movement is achieved by the functional interconnections between the major motor components of the nervous system: corticospinal and corticobulbar tracts, basal ganglia, subcortical descending systems (red nucleus, vestibular nucleus, reticular activating system), and cerebellum.

MAJOR MOTOR SYSTEMS

Corticospinal & Corticobulbar Tracts

A. Origin and Composition: The fibers of the corticospinal and corticobulbar tracts arise from the **sensorimotor cortex** around the central sulcus (Figs 13–1 and 7–10); about 55% originate in the frontal lobe (areas 4 and 6), and about 35% arise from areas 3, 1, and 2 in the postcentral gyrus of the parietal lobe (see Fig 10–12). About 10% of the fibers originate in other **frontal** or **parietal areas.** The axons arising from the large pyramidal cells in layer V **(Betz cells)** of area 4 contribute only about 5% of the fibers of the corticospinal tract and its pyramidal portion.

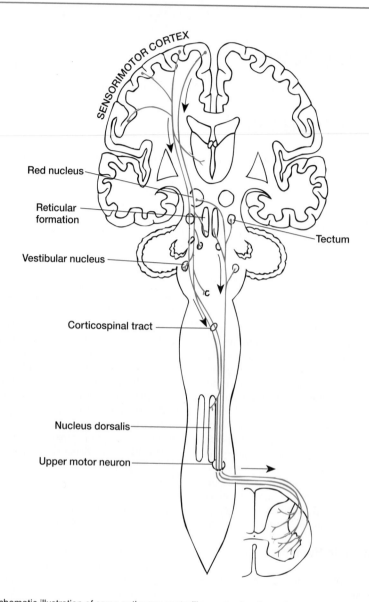

Figure 13–1. Schematic illustration of some pathways controlling motor functions. Arrows denote descending pathways.

The portion of the pyramidal tract that arises from the frontal lobe is concerned with motor function; the portion from the parietal lobe is more concerned with modulation of the ascending systems. The tracts have endings or collaterals that synapse in the thalamus (ventral nuclei), the brain stem (pontine nuclei, reticular formation, and nuclei of cranial nerves), and the spinal cord (anterior horn motoneurons and interneurons; Fig 13–2). A direct pathway to spinal cord motoneurons exists only for the musculature of the distal extremity.

B. Pathways: The **corticobulbar (corticonuclear) fibers** originate in the region of the sensorimotor cortex, where the face is represented (see Figs 10–13 and 10–14). They pass through the posterior limb of the internal capsule and the middle portion of

the crus cerebri to their targets, the somatic and brachial efferent nuclei in the brain stem. The **corticospinal tract** originates in the remainder of the sensorimotor cortex and other cortical areas; it follows a similar trajectory through the brain stem and then passes through the pyramids of the medulla (hence, the name pyramidal tract), decussates, and descends in the lateral column of the spinal cord (Figs 13–1, 13–2, and 5–13). About 10% of the pyramidal tract does not cross in the pyramidal decussation but descends in the anterior column of the spinal cord; these fibers decussate at lower cord levels, close to their destination. In addition, up to 3% of the descending fibers in the lateral corticospinal tract are uncrossed. These ipsilateral descending projections control axial musculature, ie,

Table 13–1. Summary of reflexes.

Reflexes	Afferent Nerve	Center	Efferent Nerve
Superficial reflexes			
Corneal	Cranial V	Pons	Cranial VII
Nasal (sneeze)	Cranial V	Brain stem and upper cord	Cranials V, VII, IX, X, and spinal nerves of expiration
Pharyngeal and uvular	Cranial IX	Medulla	Cranial X
Upper abdominal	T7, 8, 9, 10	T7, 8, 9, 10	T7, 8, 9, 10
Lower abdominal	T10, 11, 12	T10, 11, 12	T10, 11, 12
Cremasteric	Femoral	L1	Genitofemoral
Plantar	Tibial	S1, 2	Tibial
Anal	Pudendal	S4, 5	Pudendal
Deep reflexes			
Jaw	Cranial V	Pons	Cranial V
Biceps	Musculocutaneous	C5, 6	Musculocutaneous
Triceps	Radial	C6, 7	Radial
Periosteoradial	Radial	C6, 7, 8	Radial
Wrist (flexion)	Median	C6, 7, 8	Median
Wrist (extension)	Radial	C7, 8	Radial
Patellar	Femoral	L2, 3, 4	Femoral
Achilles	Tibial	S1, 2	Tibial
Visceral reflexes			
Light	Cranial II	Midbrain	Cranial III
Accommodation	Cranial II	Occipital cortex	Cranial III
Ciliospinal	A sensory nerve	T1, 2	Cervical sympathetics
Oculocardiac	Cranial V	Medulla	Cranial X
Carotid sinus	Cranial IX	Medulla	Cranial X
Bublocavernosus	Pudendal	S2, 3, 4	Pelvic autonomic
Bladder and rectal	Pudendal	S2, 3, 4	Pudendal and autonomics

musculature of the trunk and proximal limbs, and thus participate in the maintenance of an upright stance and in gross positioning of the limbs.

The pyramidal tract has a somatotopic organization throughout its course. (The origin, termination, and function of this tract have been described more fully in Chapter 5.)

The pyramidal corticospinal and corticobulbar tracts are not solely a system for initiating movement but also for modulating (through their origins and terminations) the function of ascending systems in the thalamus (ventroposterior nucleus), brain stem (dorsal column nuclei), and spinal cord (dorsal horn laminas).

The Extrapyramidal Motor System

The extrapyramidal system is a set of subcortical circuits and pathways, phylogenetically older than the corticospinal system, that includes the corpus striatum (caudate nucleus, putamen, and globus pallidus), together with the subthalamic nucleus, substantia nigra, red nucleus, and brain stem reticular formation (Figs 13–4 and 13–5A). Some authors include descending spinal cord tracts other than the corticospinal tracts

(such as the vestibulospinal, rubrospinal, tectospinal, and reticulospinal tracts) in the extrapyramidal motor system. Cortical subcortical components of the motor system are richly interconnected, either directly and reciprocally, or by way of fiber loops. Many of these interconnections involve the extrapyramidal system and the majority traverse the basal ganglia.

Basal Ganglia

A. Pathways and Nuclei: The anatomy of the gray masses in the forebrain that make up the basal ganglia has been described in Chapter 10 (see Figs 10–16 and 13–5). The **striatum (caudate** and **putamen)** is the major *site of input* to the basal ganglia (Fig 13–5B). The striatum receives afferents via the **corticostriate projections** from a large portion of the cerebral cortex, especially from the sensorimotor cortex (areas 4, 1, 2, and 3), the more anterior premotor cortex (area 6), and the frontal eye fields (area 8) in the frontal and parietal lobes. These corticostriatal projections are excitatory. The striatum also receives inputs from the intralaminar thalamic nuclei, substantia nigra, and midbrain raphe nuclei. Inhibitory and excitatory

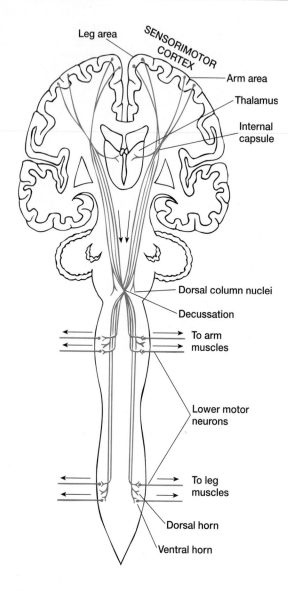

Figure 13–2. Diagram of the corticospinal tract, including descending fibers that provide sensory modulation to thalamus, dorsal column nuclei, and dorsal horn.

interneurons (the latter using ACh as a transmitter) are present within the striatum.

The caudate and putamen send inhibitory (GABAergic) axons to the **globus pallidus,** which is the *major outflow nucleus* of the corpus striatum. These projections provide a strong inhibitory input to the globus pallidus (Fig 13–5C).

The globus pallidus, in turn, sends inhibitory axons (GABAergic) to the ventral nuclei (ventral anterior, VA; and ventral lateral, VL) of the thalamus (which also receives input from the cerebellum, the subthalamic nucleus, and substantia nigra). Axons from the globus pallidus project to the thalamus by passing

through or around the internal capsule, then traveling in small bundles (the **ansa lenticularis** and the **lenticular fasciculus,** also known as the **H₂ field of Forel**) prior to entering the **thalamic fasciculus,** which leads into the thalamus (Fig 13–5C). The VA and VL thalamic nuclei complete the feedback circuit by sending axons back to the cerebral cortex (Fig 13–5D). The circuit thus traverses in order:

cortex → striatum → globus pallidus → thalamus → cortex

Another important feedback loop involves the **substantia nigra,** which is reciprocally connected with the putamen and caudate nucleus. Dopaminergic neurons in the **pars compacta** of the substantia nigra project to the striatum (the **nigrostriatal projection**) where they form inhibitory synapses (Fig 13–5B). Reciprocal projections travel from the striatum to the substantia nigra **(striatonigral projection)** and are also inhibitory (Fig 13–5C). This loop travels along the pathway:

cortex → striatum → substantia nigra → striatum → → cortex

Dopaminergic neurons in the substantia nigra also project to the thalamus (ventral anterior and ventral lateral), which, in turn, sends projections to the sensorimotor cortex; this pathway involves the following circuit:

cortex → striatum → substantia nigra → thalamus → cortex

The **subthalamic nucleus** (also called the **nucleus of Luys**) also receives inhibitory inputs from the globus pallidus and from the cortex; efferents from the subthalamic nucleus return to the globus pallidus (Fig 13–5C). Thus, the subthalamic nucleus participates in the feedback loop:

cortex → globus pallidus → subthalamic nuclei → → globus pallidus → cortex

Another loop involves the cerebellum. Portions of the thalamus project by way of the central tegmental tract to the inferior olivary nucleus; this nucleus, in turn, sends fibers to the contralateral cerebellar cortex. From the cerebellum, the loop to the thalamus is closed via the dentate and contralateral red nuclei.

Although there are no direct projections from the caudate nucleus, putamen, or globus pallidus to the spinal cord, the subthalamic region, including the prerubral field and the red nucleus, is an important relay and modifying station. Projections from the globus pallidus to the red nucleus converge with inputs from the motor cortex and the deep cerebellar nuclei. Efferent fibers from the red nucleus descend in the spinal cord as the rubrospinal tract, which modulates the tone of flexor muscles (see following section). The organizational theme for the basal ganglia appears to involve complex *loops* of neurons (including many inhibitory

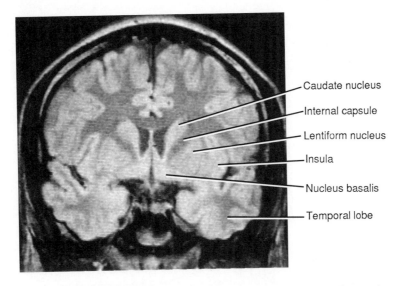

Figure 13–3. MRI of a coronal section through the head at the level of the lentiform nucleus.

neurons) feeding back to the sensorimotor cortex. These neuronal loops play an important role in motor control. Electrical engineers are well acquainted with abnormal oscillations or "ringing" that can occur when inhibitory feedback circuits are damaged. Indeed, disorders of the basal ganglia are often characterized by abnormal movements that can be repetitive or rhythmic (see section, "Basal Ganglia").

Subcortical Descending Systems

Additional pathways—important for certain types of movement—include the rubrospinal, vestibulospinal, tectospinal, and reticulospinal systems (see Fig 13–1 and Chapters 5 and 8).

A. Pathways: Subcortical descending systems originate in the red nucleus and tectum of the midbrain,

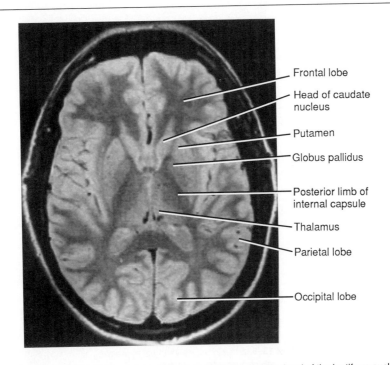

Figure 13–4. MR image of an axial section through the head at the level of the lentiform nucleus.

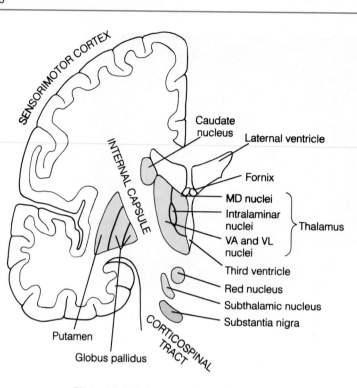

Figure 13–5. *A:* Basal ganglia—major structures.

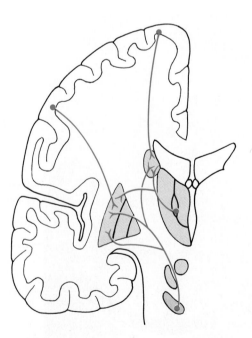

Figure 13–5. *B:* Major afferents to basal ganglia.

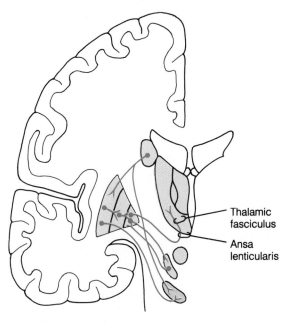

Figure 13–5. C: Intrinsic connections.

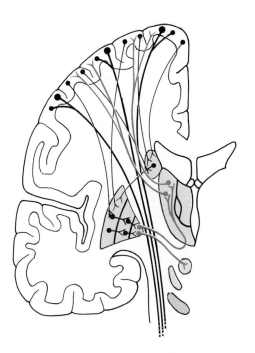

Figure 13–5. D: Efferent connections.

in the reticular formation, and in the vestibular nuclei of the brain stem.

The **rubrospinal tract** arises in the red nucleus. The red nucleus receives input from the contralateral deep cerebellar nuclei (via the superior cerebellar peduncle) and the motor cortex bilaterally. Axons descend from the red nucleus in the crossed rubrospinal tract that descends in the lateral column and then synapses on interneurons in the spinal cord.

The sensorimotor cortex projects to several nuclei in the reticular formation of the brain stem, which then sends fibers to the spinal cord in the form of the reticulospinal tract in the lateral column. Descending axons in this tract terminate on interneurons in the spinal cord and on gamma motor neurons.

The **vestibulospinal tract** arises in the vestibular nuclei, located in the floor of the fourth ventricle. The four vestibular nuclei receive afferents from the vestibular nerve and cerebellum. The vestibulospinal tract arises primarily from the lateral vestibular nucleus and medial vestibular nucleus and contains both crossed and uncrossed fibers that project to anterior horn neurons in the spinal cord (mostly interneurons that project to alpha and gamma motor neurons; extensor muscle motor neurons may be supplied directly). Activity in the vestibulospinal tract resets the gain on the gamma loop so as to facilitate the activity of motor neurons that innervate antigravity muscles; thus, the vestibulospinal tract plays an important role in maintaining an erect posture.

The **tectospinal tract** arises from cells in the superior colliculus and crosses in the midbrain at the level of the red nuclei. Descending tectospinal fibers become incorporated into the medial longitudinal fasciculus in the medulla. Other tectospinal fibers descend in the anterior funiculus of the spinal cord and terminate at cervical levels where they form synapses with interneurons that project to motor neurons. The tectospinal tract carries impulses that control reflex movements of the upper trunk, neck, and eyes in response to visual stimuli.

B. Function: Clinical observations and experiments in animals suggest that the corticospinal and rubrospinal systems cooperate to control hand and finger movement. The rubrospinal tract appears to play an important role in control of flexor muscle tone.

The reticulospinal, vestibulospinal, and tectospinal systems play a limited role in movements of the extremities (their main influence is on the musculature of the trunk). Pure unilateral lesions of corticospinal tract (ie, lesions that spare the other descending pathways) may result in relatively minor weakness, although precise movements of distal musculature (eg, movements of the individual fingers) are usually impaired; it is likely that, in these cases, descending control of motor neurons innervating proximal parts of the limbs and the trunk, is mediated by the reticulospinal, vestibulospinal, and tectospinal pathways, and by uncrossed axons in the anterior and lateral corticospinal tract.

Decerebrate rigidity occurs when the posterior part of the brain stem and spinal cord are isolated from the rest of the brain by injury at the superior border of the pons. In decerebrate rigidity, there is increased tone of the extensor muscles in all of the limbs and of the trunk and neck. When the brain stem is transected, inhibitory influences from the cortex and basal ganglia can no longer reach the spinal cord and facilitory influences, which descend in the vestibulospinal and reticulospinal tracts, dominate. This results in increased activity of alpha motor neurons innervating extensor muscles, which is due to increased gamma motor neuron discharge for these muscles (see Fig 5–20).

Cerebellum

A. Pathways: The cerebellum is interconnected with several regions of the central nervous system (Fig 13–6; see also Chapter 7): ascending tracts from the spinal cord and brain stem, corticopontocerebellar fibers from the opposite cerebral cortex and cerebellar efferent systems to the contralateral red nucleus, the reticular formation, and the ventral nuclei of the contralateral thalamus (which connects to the cerebral cortex). These have been discussed in Chapter 7.

B. Function: The cerebellum has two major functions: coordination of voluntary motor activity (fine, skilled movements and gross, propulsive movements such as walking, swimming); and control of equilibrium and muscle tone. Experimental work suggests that the cerebellum is essential in motor learning (the acquisition or learning of stereotyped movements) and memory mechanisms (the retention of such learned movements).

MOTOR DISTURBANCES

Motor disturbances, including weakness (paresis), paralysis, abnormal movements, and abnormal reflexes can result from lesions of the motor pathways in the nervous system or from lesions of the muscles themselves (Table 13–2).

Muscles

A muscle may be unable to react normally to stimuli conveyed to it by the lower motor neuron, with resulting weakness, paralysis, or tetanic contraction. Muscle tone may be decreased (hypotonia) and deep tendon reflexes may be reduced (hyporeflexia) or abolished (areflexia) as a result of muscle weakness (Fig 13–7). The cause of these disturbances may lie in the muscle itself or at the myoneural junction. Myasthenia gravis, myotonia congenita, and progressive muscular dystrophy are typical muscle disorders characterized by muscle dysfunction in the presence of apparently normal neural tissue.

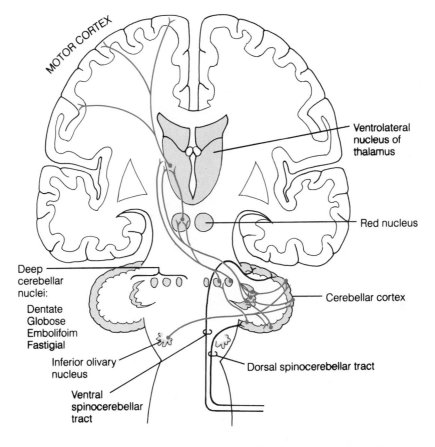

Figure 13–6. Schematic illustration of some cerebellar afferents and outflow pathways.

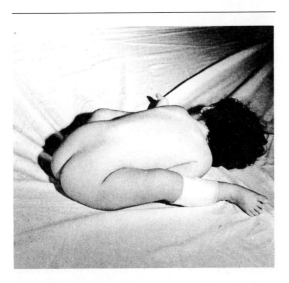

Figure 13–7. Child with hypotonia, hyporeflexia, and muscle weakness because of congenital muscular dystrophy.

Lower-Motor-Neurons

A. Description: These nerve cells in the anterior gray column of the spinal cord or brain stem have axons that pass by way of the cranial or peripheral nerves to the motor end-plates of the muscles (Fig 5–22). The lower-motor-neuron is called the "final common pathway" for two reasons. It is under the influence of the corticospinal, rubrospinal, olivospinal, vestibulospinal, reticulospinal, and tectospinal tracts as well as the segmental or intersegmental reflex neurons, and it is the ultimate pathway through which neural impulses reach the muscle.

B. Lesions: Lesions of the lower-motor-neurons can be located in the cells of the anterior gray column of the spinal cord or brain stem or in their axons, which constitute the ventral roots of the spinal or cranial nerves. Signs of lower-motor-neuron lesions include weakness, flaccid paralysis of the involved muscles, decreased muscle tone, muscle atrophy with fasciculations and degeneration of muscle fibers over time and histologic-reaction degeneration (10–14 days after injury; see Chapter 22). Reflexes of the involved muscle

Table 13–2. Signs of various lesions of the human motor system.

Location of Lesion	Voluntary Strength	Atrophy	Muscle Stretch Reflexes	Tone	Abnormal Movements
Muscle (myopathy	Weak (paretic)	Can be severe	Hypoactive	Hypotonic	None
Motor end-plate	Weak	Slight	Hypoactive	Hypotonic	None
Lower motor neuron (includes peripheral nerve, neuropathy	Weak (paretic or paralyzed)	May be present	Hypoactive or absent	Hypotonic (flaccid)	Fasciculations*
Upper motor neuron	Weak or paralyzed	Mild (atrophy of disuse)	Hyperactive (spastic). After a massive upper motor neuron lesion (as in stroke), reflexes may be absent at first, with hypotonia and spinal shock.	Hypertonic (clasp-knife), or spastic	Withdrawal spasms, abnormal reflexes (eg, Babinski extensor plantar response).
Cerebellar systems	Normal	None	Hypotonic (pendulous)	Hypotonic	Ataxia, dysmetria, dysdiadochokinesia, gait
Basal ganglia	Normal	None	Normal	Rigid (lead-pipe).	Dyskinesias (eg, chorea, athetosis, dystonia, tremors, hemiballismus)

*Fasciculations are spontaneous, grossly visible contractions (twitches) of entire motor units.

are diminished or absent and no abnormal reflexes are obtainable (Table 13–2).

Lesions of lower-motor-neurons are seen in **poliomyelitis** (a viral disorder that results in death of motor neurons) and **motor neuron disease** (including forms called **amyotrophic lateral sclerosis** and **spinal muscular atrophy,** in which there is degeneration, owing to poorly understood causes, of motor neurons). Mass lesions such as **tumors** involving the spinal cord can also damage lower-motor-neurons.

Upper-Motor-Neurons

A. Description: The upper-motor-neuron is a complex of descending systems conveying impulses from the motor areas of the cerebrum and subcortical brain stem to the anterior horn cells of the spinal cord. It is essential for the initiation of voluntary muscular activity. The term itself is used mainly for the portion of the pathway that courses through the brain stem and spinal cord (see Fig 5–22). One major component, the corticospinal tract, passes through the internal capsule, brain stem, and spinal cord to the lower-motor-neurons of the cord. Another component, the corticobulbar tract, projects to the brain stem nuclei of the cranial nerves that innervate striated muscles.

B. Lesions: Lesions in the descending motor systems can be located in the cerebral cortex, internal capsule, cerebral peduncles, brain stem, or spinal cord (Table 13–2). Signs of upper-motor-neuron le-

sions in the spinal cord include paralysis or paresis (weakness) of the involved muscles, increased muscle tone (hypertonia) and spasticity, hyperactive deep reflexes, no or little muscle atrophy (atrophy of disuse), diminished or absent superficial abdominal reflexes, and abnormal reflexes (eg, Babinski response).

These signs result from lesions that damage the corticospinal or corticobulbar tracts together with the rubrospinal and reticulospinal tracts; all these tracts course in the lateral white column of the spinal cord. Lesions limited to the corticospinal tract alone cause flaccid paralysis, especially of the distal extensor muscles of the extremities (eg, the fingers and wrists) and interfere with fine motor control of distal musculature (eg, movement of the fingers).

Damage to the cerebral cortex incurred in utero, during birth, or in early postnatal life may result in cerebral palsy. This is a heterogeneous group of disorders that often include a form of spastic paralysis; however, the disease may be characterized by other signs such as rigidity, tremor, ataxia, or athetosis. Combinations of these groups of symptoms are common and the disorder may be accompanied by such other significant defects as speech disorders, apraxia, hemangioma, and mental retardation in some (but by no means all) patients.

C. Patterns of Paralysis and Weakness: **Hemiplegia** is a spastic or flaccid paralysis of one side of the body and extremities; it is delimited by the median line of the body. **Monoplegia** is paralysis of one extremity only, while **diplegia** is paralysis of any two corresponding extremities, usually both lower extremities (but can be both upper). **Paraplegia** is a symmetric paralysis of both lower extremities. **Quadriplegia, or tetraplegia,** is paralysis of all four extremities. **Hemiplegia alternans** (crossed paralysis) is paralysis of one or more ipsilateral cranial nerves and contralateral paralysis of the arm and leg. The term **paresis** refers to weakness, rather than total paralysis and is used with the same prefixes.

Basal Ganglia

Defects in function of the basal ganglia (sometimes termed extrapyramidal lesions) are characterized by changes in muscle tone, poverty of voluntary movement **(akinesia)** or abnormally slow movements **(bradykinesia)**, or involuntary, abnormal movement **(dyskinesia).** (Features of disorders of the basal ganglia are summarized in Table 13–2.)

A. Athetosis: This disorder, which is characterized by slow, writhing movements of the extremities and neck musculature, is not associated with a specific lesion.

B. Chorea: This disorder is characterized by quick, repeated, involuntary movements of the distal-extremity muscles, face, and tongue; it is often associated with lesions in the corpus striatum.

C. Huntington's Chorea: This type of chorea is a late manifestation of a disease with an autosomal dominant pattern of inheritance. The corpus striatum, especially the caudate nucleus, becomes atrophic. Loss of GABAergic (inhibitory) neurons in the striatum results in chorea (Fig 13–9). The cerebral cortex also becomes atrophic and dementia is often present. Identification of the gene for Huntington's disease has raised hopes that it may be possible to understand the pathogenesis of this disorder and develop effective treatments for it.

D. Hemiballismus: In this unusual movement disorder, there are large, flailing movements of one extremity, or the arm and leg on one side. Hemiballismus usually results from damage to the contralateral subthalamic nucleus, which most commonly occurs as a result of small, deep infarctions. For reasons that are poorly understood, hemiballismus often resolves after several weeks.

E. Parkinson's Disease (Paralysis Agitans): This disorder, with onset usually between the ages of 50 and 65, is characterized by a triad of symptoms: *tremor, rigidity,* and *akinesia.* There are often accompanying abnormalities of *equilibrium, posture,* and *autonomic function.* Characteristic signs include slow, monotonous speech; diminutive writing (micrographia); and loss of facial expression (masked face), often without impairment of mental capacity.

This progressive disorder is associated with loss of pigmented (dopaminergic) neurons in the substantia

nigra (Figs 13–8 and 13–9). The cause of this degenerative disorder is unknown. Parkinsonian symptoms were seen as sequelae in some survivors of the epidemic of encephalitis lethargic (von Economo's encephalitis) that occurred from 1919 to 1929 (postencephalitic Parkinsonism). Some toxic agents (carbon monoxide, manganese) can damage the basal ganglia, and a rapidly developing Parkinson-like disease has recently been linked to the use of certain "designer drugs," eg, MPTP (1-methyl-4-phenyl-1,2,5,6-tetrahydropyridine), a synthetic narcotic related to meperidine. Moreover, use of some neuroleptics (eg, phenothiazines) can produce a drug-induced Parkinsonian syndrome. Most causes of Parkinson's disease, however, are idiopathic, and mechanisms leading to degeneration of neurons in the substantia nigra are not well understood.

Treatment with drugs is often effective. Some patients with early Parkinson's disease respond to treatment with *anticholinergic* agents, which reduce cholinergic (excitatory) transmission in the striatum and, thus, tend to restore the inhibitory:excitatory (dopaminergic:cholinergic) balance in the basal ganglia. *Levodopa (L-DOPA)* can be very effective in the treatment of Parkinson's disease. Presumably, L-DOPA is taken up by remaining dopaminergic neurons in the basal ganglia and converted (via dopa-decarboxylase) to dopamine, thereby, augmenting dopaminergic transmission. L-DOPA is often given together with carbidopa, a dopa decarboxylase inhibitor that breaks down L-DOPA; the combination of L-DOPA and a dopa-decarboxylase inhibitor *(Sinemet)* results in higher levels of L-DOPA, often improving the therapeutic response. Other drugs that are used to treat Parkinson's disease include *amantadine* (which may enhance dopamine release from neurons that have

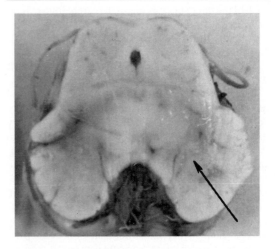

Figure 13–8. Midbrain of a 45-year-old woman with Parkinson's disease, showing depigmentation of the substantia nigra (compare with Fig 19–12).

NORMAL

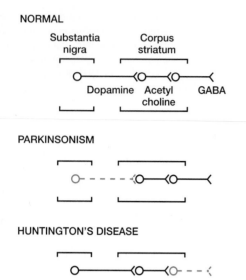

Figure 13–9. Schematic illustration of the processes underlying Parkinsonism. (Reproduced, with permission, from Katzung BG: *Basic and Clinical Pharmacology*, 5th ed. Appleton & Lange, 1992.)

not yet degenerated) and *Deprenyl* (which inhibits the metabolic breakdown of dopamine and may also have an independent, protective effect that slows the degeneration of neurons).

Cerebellum

Disorders caused by cerebellar lesions are characterized by reduced muscle tone and a loss of coordination of smooth movements (Table 13–2). Lesions in each of the three subdivisions of the cerebellum exhibit characteristic signs.

A. Vestibulocerebellum (Archicerebellum): Loss of equilibrium, often with **nystagmus,** is typical.

B. Spinocerebellum (Paleocerebellum): **Truncal ataxia** and "drunken" gait are characteristic.

C. Neocerebellum: Ataxia of extremities and **asynergy** (loss of coordination) are prominent. Decomposition of movement occurs, with voluntary muscular movements becoming a series of jerky, discrete motions rather than one smooth motion. **Dysmetria** (past-pointing phenomenon) is also seen, in which the person is unable to estimate the distance involved in muscular acts, so that an attempt to touch an object will overshoot its target. **Dysdiadochokinesia** (the inability to perform rapidly alternating movements), **intention tremor,** and **rebound phenomenon** (loss of interaction between agonist and antagonist smooth muscles) are also typical. As a result of the pattern of inputs and outputs from the cerebel-

lum, if there is a unilateral lesion of the cerebellum, these abnormalities will be present on the *same side* as the lesion.

CASE 17

A 63-year-old right-handed secretary/typist consulted her family physician when her right hand and fingers "did not want to cooperate." She also explained that her employers had become dissatisfied with her because her work habits and movements had become slow and her handwriting had become scribbly and illegible over the preceding several months. She was in danger of losing her job even though her intellectual abilities were unimpaired.

Neurologic examination showed moderate slowness of speech and mild loss of facial expression on both sides. The patient had difficulty initiating movements. Once seated, she did not move about much. Her posture was stooped and she walked with a small-stepped gait, with decreased arm-swing. There was no muscular atrophy and no weakness. Muscle tone was increased in the arms, and "cogwheel rigidity" was present. There was a fine tremor in the fingers of the right hand (frequency 3–4 times per second).

The rest of the examination and the laboratory data were within normal limits.

What is the most likely diagnosis? Where is the lesion?

CASE 18

A 49-year-old woman with known severe hypertension had a sudden loss of strength in the left leg and arm; she fell down and when brought to the emergency room seemed only partially conscious.

Neurologic examination on admission showed an obtunded woman who had difficulty speaking. There was no papilledema and no sensation on the left side of the face or body. The tongue deviated to the left when protruded. Left-central facial weakness was present. The patient complained that she could not see on the left side of both visual fields. Complete paralysis of the left upper and lower extremities was present, and there was no resistance to passive motion. Results of tests of cerebellar function were negative. Deep tendon reflexes were absent in the left upper extremity and increased in the lower extremity. There was a left extensor plantar response, but the response was equivocal on the right. Vital signs and the complete blood count were within normal limits; blood pressure was 190/100.

What is the preliminary diagnosis? Would a lumbar puncture be indicated? Would a neuroradiologic diagnostic procedure be useful?

Cases are discussed further in Chapter 25.

REFERENCES

Albin RL, Young AB, Penney JB: Functional anatomy of basal ganglia disorders. *Trends Neurosci* 1989;**12**:366.

Alexander GE, deLong MR: Central mechanisms of initiation and control of movement. In: *Diseases of the Nervous System. Clinical Neurobiology.* Asbury A et al (editors). Saunders, 1992.

Alexander J et al: Parallel organization of functionally segregated circuits linking basal ganglia and cortex. *Annu Rev Neurosci* 1986;**9**:357.

Asanuma H: *The Motor Cortex*, Raven, 1989.

Brooks VB (editor): Motor control. In: *Handbook of Physiology,* 2nd ed. Vol 2, section 1. American Physiological Society, 1981.

Grillner S, Dubue R: Control of locomotion in vertebrates: spinal and supraspinal mechanisms. In: *Functional Recovery in Neurological Disease.* Waxman SG (editor). Raven, 1989.

Kuypers HGJM, Martin GF (editors): Anatomy of descending pathways to the spinal cord. *Prog Brain Res* 1982;**57**:1–411. [Entire issue.]

Marsden CD, Fahn S (editors): *Movement Disorders 2.* Butterworth, 1987.

Mussa-Ivaldi SA, Giszter SF, Bizzi E: Motor-space coding in the central nervous system. *Cold Spring Harb Symp Quant Biol* 1990;**55**:827.

Input from the sensory systems plays a role in the control of motor function, by way of either the connections within the sensorimotor cortex or the cerebellar pathways. Conversely, impulses from the sensorimotor cortex—via the descending pathways—affect the function of sensory neurons in the spinal cord, brain stem, and thalamus.

SENSATION

Sensation can be divided into four types: superficial, deep, visceral, and special. **Superficial sensation** is concerned with touch, pain, temperature, and 2-point discrimination. **Deep sensation** includes muscle and joint position sense (proprioception), deep muscle pain, and vibration sense. **Visceral sensations** are relayed by autonomic afferent fibers and include hunger, nausea, and visceral pain (see Chapter 20). The **special senses**—smell, vision, hearing, taste, and equilibrium—are conveyed by certain cranial nerves (see Chapters 8, 15, 16, and 17).

Receptors

Receptors are specialized cells for detecting particular changes in the environment. **Exteroceptors** include receptors affected mainly by the external environment: Meissner's corpuscles, Merkel's corpuscles, and hair cells for touch; Krause's end-bulbs for cold; Ruffini's corpuscles for warmth; and free nerve endings for pain (Fig 14–1). Receptors are not absolutely specific for a given sensation; eg, strong stimuli can cause various sensations, even pain, even though the inciting stimuli are not necessarily painful. **Proprioceptors** receive impulses mainly from pacinian corpuscles, joint receptors, muscle spindles, and Golgi tendon organs. Painful stimuli are detected at the free endings of nerve fibers.

Each efferent fiber from a receptor relays stimuli that originate in a receptive field and gives rise to a component of an afferent sensory system. Note that each individual receptor fires either completely or not at all when stimulated. The greater the intensity of a stimulus, the greater the number of end-organs stimulated, the higher the rate of discharge, and the longer the duration of effect. **Adaptation** denotes the diminution in rate of discharge of some receptors upon repeated or continuous stimulation of constant intensity; the sensation of sitting in a chair or walking on even ground is suppressed.

Connections

A chain of three long neurons and a number of interneurons conducts stimuli from the receptor or free ending to the somatosensory cortex (Figs 14–1 to 14–3):

A. First-Order Neuron: The cell body of a first-order neuron lies in a dorsal root ganglion or a somatic afferent ganglion of cranial nerves.

B. Second-Order Neuron: The cell body of a second-order neuron lies within the neuraxis (spinal cord and brain stem). Its axon usually decussates and terminates in the thalamus.

C. Third-Order Neuron: The cell body of a third-order neuron, which lies in the thalamus, projects to the sensory cortex—or the thalamus itself in the case of pain. The networks of the brain process information relayed by this type of neuron; they interpret its location, quality, and intensity and make appropriate responses.

Sensory Pathways

Multiple neurons from the same type of receptor often form a bundle (tract), creating a sensory pathway. Sensory pathways ascending in the spinal cord are described in Chapter 5; their continuation within the brain stem is discussed in Chapter 7. The main sensory areas in the cortex are described in Chapter 10.

One major system—the **lemniscal (dorsal column) system** (see Fig 14–2)—carries touch, joint sensation, 2-point discrimination, and vibratory sense from re-

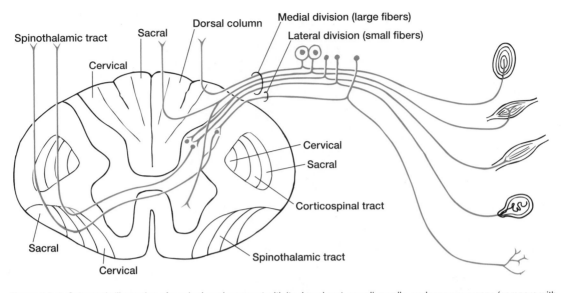

Figure 14–1. Schematic illustration of a spinal cord segment with its dorsal root, ganglion cells, and sensory organs (compare with Fig 5–6).

ceptors to the cortex. The other important system—**the ventrolateral system**—relays impulses concerning nociceptive stimuli (pain, crude touch) or changes in skin temperature (Fig 14–3). Significant anatomic and functional differences characterize these two pathways: the size of the receptive field, nerve-fiber diameter, course in the spinal cord, and function (Table 14–1). Each system is characterized by **somatotopic distribution,** with convergence in the thalamus (ventroposterior complex) and cerebral cortex (the sensory projection areas; see Figs 10–13 and 10–15). The sensory trigeminal fibers contribute to both the lemniscal and the ventrolateral systems and provide the input from the face and mucosal membranes (see Figs 7–8 and 8–12).

Cortical Areas

The **primary somatosensory cortex** (areas 3, 1, and 2) is organized in functional somatotopic columns that represent points in the receptive field. Within each column are inputs from thalamic, commissural, and associational fibers, all of which end in layers IV, III, and II (see Fig 10–10). The output is from cells in layers V and VI; however, the details of the processing occurring in each column and its functional significance (how it is felt) are largely unknown.

Additional cortical areas—secondary projection areas—also receive input from receptive fields in the columns; the somatotopic map of these areas is more diffuse, however. A separation of sensory modalities occurs within the somatosensory cortex.

Clinical Correlations

Interruption in the course of first- and second-order neurons produces characteristic **sensory deficits;** these are sometimes difficult to define in unconscious or malingering patients or in young children. Small deficits are sometimes ignored by the patient unless a sensitive area such as the fingertips is involved.

Thalamic lesions are often characterized by severe, poorly localized pain (thalamic pain) associated with weakness, ataxia, hyperkinesia, paresthesia, and loss of the ability to discriminate or localize simple crude sensations. Slight stimuli may evoke severe and disagreeable sensations (thalamic syndrome).

PAIN

Pathways

The free nerve endings in peripheral and cranial nerves are probably the specific receptors, or **nociceptors,** for pain (see Figs 14–1, 14–3, and 7–8). The pain fibers in peripheral nerves are of small diameter and are readily affected by local anesthetic. The thinly myelinated and unmyelinated fibers make up the A-delta fibers, which convey discrete, sharp, short-lasting pain, and the C fibers, which transmit chronic, burning pain.

Injured tissue may release prostaglandins, which lower the threshold of peripheral nociceptors and thereby increase the sensibility to pain **(hyperalgesia).** Aspirin and other nonsteroidal anti-inflammatory drugs inhibit the action of prostaglandins and relieve pain **(hypalgesia** or **analgesia).**

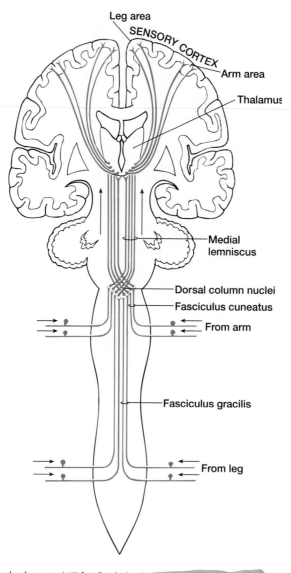

Figure 14–2. Dorsal column system for discriminative touch and position sense (lemniscus system).

Pain Systems

The central ascending pathway for sensation consists of two systems: the **spinothalamic tract** and the phylogenetically older **spinoreticulothalamic system.** The first pathway conducts the sensation of sharp, stabbing pain; the second conveys deep, poorly localized, burning pain. Both pathways are interrupted when the ventrolateral quadrant of the spinal cord is damaged by trauma or in surgery, such as a cordotomy, deliberately performed to relieve pain; contralateral loss of all pain sensation results below the lesion (Fig 14–4). Small lesions higher in the neuraxis involve one of the pathways because they course upward separately; the lesion reduces the sensation of the type of pain associated with that pathway. Isolated lesions in the spinothalamic tract in the brain stem or thalamus may, paradoxically, produce thalamic pain in some cases.

Referred Pain

The cells in lamina V of the posterior column that receive noxious sensations from afferents in the **skin** also receive input from nociceptors in the **viscera** (Fig 14–5). When visceral afferents receive a strong stimulus, the cortex may misinterpret the source. A common example is referred pain in the shoulder caused by gallstone colic: the spinal segments that relay pain from the gallbladder also receive afferents from the

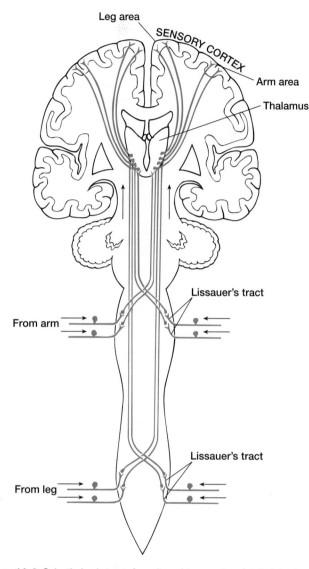

Leg area

SENSORY CORTEX

Arm area

Thalamus

Lissauer's tract

From arm

Lissauer's tract

From leg

Figure 14–3. Spinothalamic tracts for pain and temperature (ventrolateral system).

shoulder region (convergence theory). Similarly, pain in the heart caused by **acute anoxia (myocardial infarct)** is conducted by fibers that reach the same spinal cord segments where pain afferents from the ulnar nerve (lower arm area) synapse. Another theory, the facilitation theory, in which the visceral pain facilitates input from a somatic structure, has not been proved conclusively.

Relief of Pain

A. Spinal Cord Stimulation: Recent analysis of the laminar organization of the spinal cord gray matter has shown that most cells of laminas I and II and some in lamina V respond to noxious stimuli by way of small-diameter afferent fibers (see Fig 5–11). Laminas III, IV, and VI show a narrow range of response to nonnoxious stimuli via large-diameter afferents, and lamina V has a broad range of responses. The large-diameter fibers prevent the lamina V afferents from transmitting signals. Stimulating (eg, by rubbing the skin) these fibers helps to suppress the sensation of pain, especially sharp pain. (Parents of small children seem to know this instinctively: they rub the injured spot, thus activating the large-diameter fibers.) One therapeutic procedure occasionally used to inhibit pain is to stimulate the dorsal columns electrically by means of permanently implanted electrodes; this may alleviate sharp pain, but chronic, emotionally burdensome, deep, burning pain often is not relieved.

Table 14–1. Differences between lemniscal and ventrolateral systems.

	Lemniscal (Dorsal Column) Pathway	Ventrolateral Pathway
Course in spinal cord	Dorsal and dorsolateral funiculi	Ventral and ventrolateral funiculi
Size of receptive fields	Small	Small and large
Specificity of signal conveyed	Each sensation carried separately; precise localization of sensation	Multimodal (several sensations carried in one fiber system)
Diameter of nerve fiber	Large-diameter primary afferents	Small-diameter primary afferents
Sensation transmitted	Fine touch, joint sensation, vibration	Pain, temperature, crude touch, visceral pain
Synaptic chain	Two or 3 synapses to cortex	Multisynaptic
Speed of transmission	Fast	Slow
Tests for function	Vibration, 2-point discrimination, stereognosis	Pinprick, heat and cold testing

B. Endorphins: Another system of pain suppression can be activated by stimulating the endorphin receptor region in the periaqueductal gray matter of the midbrain (Fig 14–6). This region contains **opiate receptors,** membrane-bound proteins that specifically bind opiate agonists (eg, morphine) or antagonists (eg, naloxone). There are several endogenous opium-like compounds within the body: **enkephalin** and β-**endorphins** (a fragment of the pituitary hormone β-**lipotropin**), among others. These peptides bind to opiate receptors, as does morphine. In most cases, pain (especially chronic pain) is relieved. Endogenous endorphin production is empirically aided by a diet rich in **tryptophan (serotonin).**

Deep, chronic pain is relieved when periaqueductal gray cells activate serotonergic neurons in the midline pons (nucleus raphe magnus). These neurons send descending fibers to the spinal cord, ending on laminas I and V of the posterior horn, and act to inhibit pain. A method currently used to treat unbearable pain is to implant electric stimulators in the periaqueductal gray matter and connect them to a subcutaneous inductor coil. The patient can activate the stimulation with an external battery-operated induction coil as needed to provide many hours of pain relief.

C. Surgery: Various surgical procedures attempt to alleviate intolerable pain (see Fig 14–4 and Table 14–2). Although most of these are somewhat effective, a large number of patients with deep, chronic pain may not be helped.

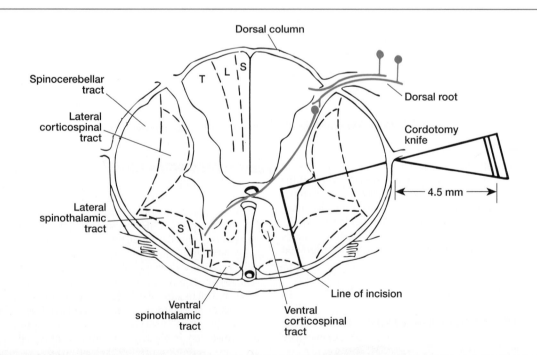

Figure 14–4. Major spinal pathways. The solid line on the right represents the line of incision in performing an anterolateral cordotomy. Notice the lamination of the tracts. S, sacral; L, lumbar; T, thoracic. (Reproduced, with permission, from Ganong WF: *Review of Medical Physiology,* 16th ed. Appleton & Lange, 1993.)

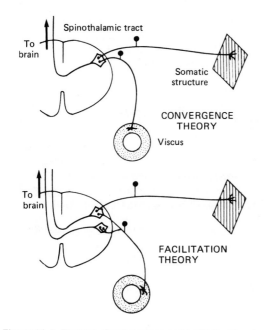

Figure 14–5. Diagram of convergence and facilitation theories of referred pain. (Reproduced, with permission, from Ganong WF: *Review of Medical Physiology,* 16th ed. Appleton & Lange, 1993.)

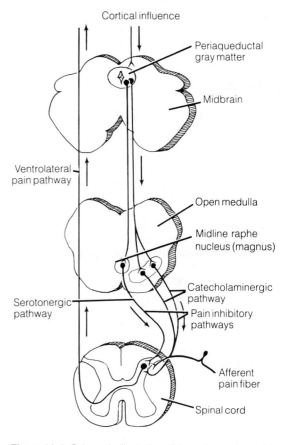

Figure 14–6. Schematic illustration of the pathways involved in pain control. (Courtesy of Al Basbaum.)

D. Placebos: People have known throughout history that treatment itself often influences the course of a disease, even if the treatment is not specific or suggestive. This placebo ("I will please") effect is defined as consistent improvement following the administration of a substance without pharmacologic effect.

CASE 19

A 41-year-old woman was referred after complaining of numbness and tingling in her right hand for more than a year. These sensations started gradually, at first only in the fingers, but ultimately extending to the entire right hand and forearm. She was unable to do fine work such as sewing, and she sometimes dropped objects because of weakness that had developed in that hand during the last year. Three weeks before her admission to the hospital, she had burned two fingers of her right hand on her electric range; she had not felt the heat.

Neurologic examination showed considerable wasting and weakness of the small muscles in the right hand. The deep tendon reflexes in the right upper extremity were absent or difficult to elicit. The knee and ankle jerks, however, were abnormally brisk, especially on the right side; the right plantar response was extensor. Abdominal reflexes were absent on both sides. Pain and temperature senses were lost in the right hand, forearm, and shoulder, and an area of the left shoulder. Touch, joint, and vibration senses were completely normal.

A plain-film radiograph of the spine was read as normal.

Table 14–2. Procedures for pain relief.

Surgery
Single nerve section
Sympathectomy (for visceral pain)
Rhizotomy (root section at 2 or more levels)
Cordotomy (see Fig 13–4)
Mesencephalic tractotomy (for trigeminal pain)
Thalamotomy
Stimulation
Dorsal column
Periaqueductal gray matter
Medial lemniscus near thalamus

Where is the lesion? What is the differential diagnosis? Which neuroadiologic procedure(s) would be helpful? What is the most likely diagnosis?

CASE 20

A 41-year-old man was admitted to the hospital with complaints of progressive weakness and unsteadiness of his legs. His disability had begun more than a year earlier with creeping and tingling feelings in his feet. Gradually, these sensations had become more disagreeable, and he developed burning pains on the soles of his feet; the rest of his feet became numb. His legs had become so weak that they felt tired if he walked more than 100 meters, and he had lately begun to stumble frequently when walking. For about six months he had had tingling feelings in his fingers and hands; his fingers felt clumsy, and he often dropped things. He had lost more than 6 kg (about 14 pounds) during the previous six months. The patient had smoked about 30 cigarettes daily for many years, and he drank 15 glasses of beer and half a bottle of whiskey or more a day. After losing his job a year before, he had worked at several unskilled jobs and was now employed as a bartender.

Neurologic examination showed a poorly muscled man with conspicuous atrophy in the calves and forearms. There was weakness of movement at both ankles and wrists and slightly weakened movement of the knees and elbows. The patient's gait was unsteady and of the high-stepping type. There was loss of touch and pain sensation on the feet and distal thirds of the legs and on the hands and distal halves of the forearms, giving a "sock-and-glove" distribution of sensory loss. The soles of the feet and the calf muscles were hyperalgesic when squeezed. Ankle and biceps reflexes were absent, and knee jerks and triceps reflex were diminished.

What is the differential diagnosis? What is the most likely diagnosis?

Cases are discussed further in Chapter 25.

REFERENCES

Basbaum AI, Fields HL: Endogenous pain control systems. *Annu Rev Neurosci* 1984;**7**:309.

Besson J-M, Chaouch A: Peripheral and spinal mechanisms of nociception. *Physiol Rev* 1987;**67**:67.

Bowker RM, et al: Descending serotonergic, peptidergic and cholinergic pathways from the raphe nuclei: A multiple transmitter complex. *Brain Res* 1983;**288**:33.

The Visual System

15

Mammals are *visual* animals: the visual system conveys more information to the brain, by far, than any other afferent system. The visual system includes the eye and its retina, the optic nerves, and the visual pathways within the brain.

THE EYE

The functions (and clinical correlations) of the cranial nerves (III, IV, VI) involved in moving the eyes have been discussed in Chapter 8, along with the gaze centers and pupillary reflexes. The vestibulo-ocular reflex is briefly explained in Chapter 17. This chapter discusses the form, function, and lesions of the optic system from the retina to the cerebrum.

Anatomy & Physiology

The optical components of the eye are the cornea, the pupillary opening of the iris, the lens, and the retina (Fig 15–1). Light passes through the first four components, the anterior chamber, and the vitreous to reach the retina; the point of fixation (direction of gaze) normally lines up with the fovea. The retina and the optic nerve (grown as a portion of the brain itself) transform light to electrical impulses (Fig 15–2).

The retina, organized into 10 layers, contains two types of photoreceptors (**rods** and **cones**) and four types of neurons (**bipolar cells, ganglion cells, horizontal cells,** and **amacrine cells**) (Figs 15–2 and 15–3). The photoreceptors (rods and cones, which are first-order neurons) synapse with bipolar cells (Fig 15–4). These in turn synapse with ganglion cells near the surface of the retina; the ganglion cells are third-order neurons whose axons converge to leave the eye within the optic nerve.

Within the outer plexiform layer of the retina, horizontal cells connect receptor cells with each other. Amacrine cells, within the inner plexiform layer, connect ganglion cells to one another (and in some cases also connect bipolar cells and ganglion cells).

Rods, which are more numerous than cones in the retina, are sensitive to low-intensity light and provide visual input when illumination is dim, eg, at twilight and at night. Cones are stimulated by relatively high-intensity light; they are responsible for sharp vision and color discrimination. Rods and cones each contain an **outer segment,** consisting of stacks of flattened disks of membrane that contain photosensitive pigments that react to light, and an **inner segment,** which contains the cell nucleus and mitochondria and forms synapses with the second-order bipolar cells. The transduction of light into neural signals occurs when photons are absorbed by photosensitive compounds (also called visual pigments) in the rods and cones.

The visual pigment within retinal rods is **rhodopsin,** a specialized membrane receptor that is linked to G-proteins. When light strikes the rhodopsin molecule, it is converted—first to **metarhodopsin II** and then to **scotopsin** and **retinene$_1$.** This light-activated reaction of rhodopsin activates a G-protein known as **transducin,** which breaks down cyclic GMP. Because cyclic GMP acts within the cytoplasm of the photoreceptors to keep sodium channels open, the light-induced reduction in cyclic GMP leads to a closing of sodium channels, which causes a hyperpolarization (see Chapter 3). Thus, as a result of being struck by light, there is hyperpolarization within the retinal rods. This, in turn, results in decreased release of synaptic transmitter onto bipolar cells, which alters their activity (Fig 15–5).

Cones within the retina also contain visual pigments, which respond maximally to light at wavelengths of 440, 535, and 565 nM (corresponding to the three primary colors, blue, green, and red). When cones are struck by light by the appropriate wavelength, a cascade of molecular events, similar to that in rods, activates a G-protein that closes sodium channels resulting in hyperpolarization.

Transmission from photoreceptors (rods and cones, first-order sensory neurons), to bipolar cells (second-order sensory neurons), and then to ganglion cells (third-order sensory neurons) is modified by horizon-

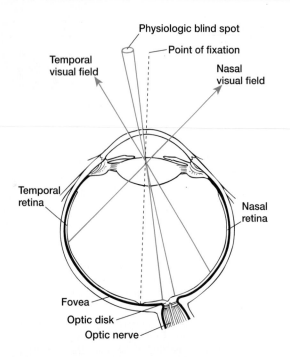

Figure 15–1. Horizontal section of the left eye; representation of the visual field at the level of the retina. The focus of the point of fixation is the fovea, the physiologic blind spot on the optic disk, the temporal (lateral) half of the visual field on the nasal side of the retina, and the nasal (medial) half of the visual field on the temporal side of the retina. (Reproduced, with permission, from Greenberg DA, Aminoff MJ, Simon RP: *Clinical Neurology,* 2nd ed. Appleton & Lange, 1993.)

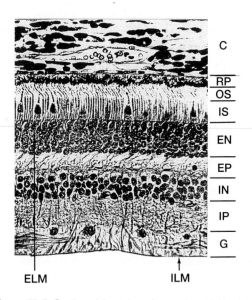

Figure 15–2. Section of the retina of a monkey. Light enters from the top and traverses the following layers: ILM, internal limiting membrane; G, ganglion cell layer; IP, internal plexiform layer; IN, internal nuclear layer (bipolar neurons); EP, external plexiform layer; EN, external nuclear layer (nuclei of rods and cones); ELM, external limiting membrane; IS, inner segments of rods (narrow lines) and cones (triangular dark structures); OS, outer segments of rods and cones; RP, retinal pigment epithelium; C, choroid. x 655.

tal cells and amacrine cells. Each bipolar cell, for example, receives input from 20–50 photoreceptor cells. The receptive field of the bipolar cell (ie, the area on the retina that influences the activity in the cell) is modified by horizontal cells. The horizontal cells form synapses on photoreceptors and nearby bipolar cells in a manner that "sharpens" the receptive field on each bipolar cell. As a result of this arrangement, bipolar cells do not merely respond to diffuse light; on the contrary, some bipolar cells convey information about small spots of light surrounded by darkness (these cells have "on"-center receptive fields), while others convey information about small, dark spots surrounded by light ("off"-center receptive fields).

Amacrine cells receive input from bipolar cells and synapse onto other bipolar cells near their sites of input to ganglion cells. They appear to play a role similar to that of horizontal cells in "sharpening" the responses of ganglion cells. Some ganglion cells respond most vigorously to a light spot surrounded by darkness, while others respond most actively to a dark spot surrounded by light.

The retinal area for central, fixated vision during good light is the **macula** (Fig. 15-6); the remainder of the retina is concerned with paracentral and peripheral

vision. The inner layers of the retina in the macular area are pushed apart, forming the **fovea centralis,** a small, central pit composed of closely packed cones, where vision is sharpest and color discrimination most acute.

Ganglion cell axons, within the retina, form the **nerve fiber layer.** The ganglion cell axons all leave the eye, forming the optic nerve, at a point located 3 mm medial to the eye's posterior pole. The point of exit is termed the **optic disc,** and can be seen through the ophthalmoscope (Fig 15–6). Because there are no rods or cones overlying the optic disc, it corresponds to a small **blind spot** in each eye.

A. Adaptation: If a person spends a considerable period of time in brightly lighted surroundings and then moves to a dimly lighted environment, the retinas slowly become more sensitive to light as the individual becomes accustomed to the dark. This decline in visual threshold, known as **dark adaptation,** is nearly maximal in about 20 minutes, although there is some further decline over longer periods. On the other hand, when one passes suddenly from a dim to a brightly lighted environment, the light seems intensely and even uncomfortably bright until the eyes adapt to the increased illumination and the visual threshold rises. This adaptation occurs over a period of about 5 minutes and is called **light adaptation.** The pupillary light reflex, which constricts the pupils, is normally a protective accompaniment to sudden increases in light intensity (see Chapter 8).

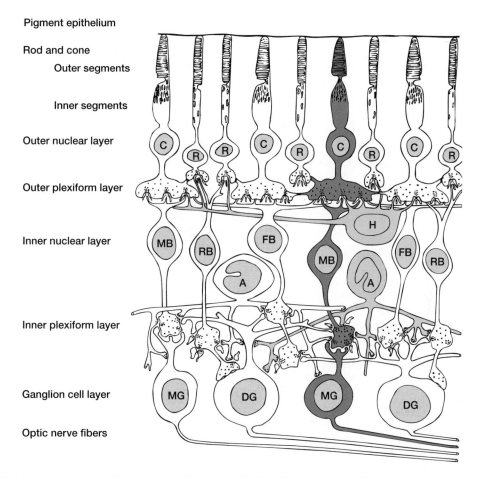

Pigment epithelium

Rod and cone
 Outer segments

 Inner segments

Outer nuclear layer

Outer plexiform layer

Inner nuclear layer

Inner plexiform layer

Ganglion cell layer

Optic nerve fibers

Figure 15–3. Neural components of the retina. C, cone; R, rod; MB, RB, FB, bipolar cells (of the midget, rod, and flat types); DG and MG, ganglion cells (of the diffuse and midget type); H, horizontal cells; A, amacrine cells. (Reproduced, with permission, from Dowling JE, Boycott BB: Organization of the primate retina: Electron microscopy. *Proc Roy Soc Lond Ser B [Biol]* 1966;**166**:80. Also from, Ganong WF: *Review of Medical Physiology*, 16th ed. Appleton & Lange, 1993.)

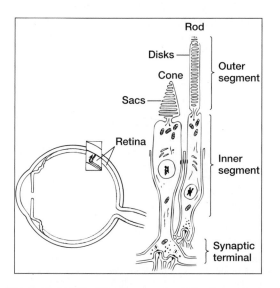

Figure 15–4. Schematic diagram of a rod and cone in the retina.

Light and dark adaptation depend, in part, on changes in the concentration of cyclic GMP in photoreceptors. In sustained illumination, there is a reduction in the concentration of calcium ions within the photoreceptor, which leads to increased guanylate cyclase activity and increased cyclic GMP levels. This, in turn, tends to keep sodium channels open so as to **desensitize** the photoreceptor.

B. Color Vision: The portion of the spectrum that stimulates the retina to produce sight ranges from 400 to 800 nm. Stimulation of the normal eye by either this entire range of wavelengths or by mixtures from certain different parts of the range produces the sensation of white light. Monochromatic radiation from one part of the spectrum is perceived as a specific color or hue. The Young-Helmholtz theory postulates that the retina contains three types of cones, each with a different photopigment maximally sensitive to one of the primary colors (red, blue, and green), and the sensation of any

Incident light

↓

Structural change in the
retinene₁ of photopigment

↓

Metarhodopsin II

↓

Activation of transducin

↓

Activation of phosphodiesterase

↓

Decreased intracellular cGMP

↓

Closure of Na⁺ channels

↓

Hyperpolarization

↓

Decreased release of
synaptic transmitter

↓

Response in bipolar cells
and other neural elements

Figure 15–5. Probable sequence of events involved in photo-transduction in rods and cones. (Reproduced, with permission, from Ganong WF: *Review of Medical Physiology,* 16th ed. Appleton & Lange, 1993.)

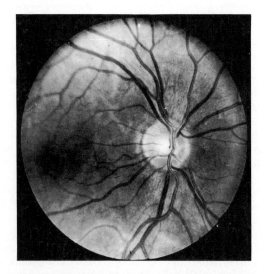

Figure 15–6. The normal fundus as seen through an ophthalmoscope. (Photo by Diane Beeston; reproduced, with permission, from Vaughan D, Asbury T, Riordan-Eva P: General *Ophthalmology,* 13th ed. Appleton & Lange, 1992.)

given color is determined by the relative frequency of impulses from each type of cone.

Each of the photopigments has been identified and characterized by recombinant DNA techniques. The amino-acid sequences of all three are about 41% homologous with rhodopsin. The green-sensitive and red-sensitive pigments are very similar—about 40% homologous with each other—and are coded by the same chromosome. The blue-sensitive pigment is only about 43% homologous with the other two and is coded by a different chromosome. The absorption spectra of these photopigments overlap somewhat.

In normal color (trichromatic) vision, the human eye can perceive the three primary colors and mix these in suitable portions to match white or any color of the spectrum. Color blindness can result from a weakness of one cone system or from dichromatic vision, in which only two cone systems are present. In the latter case, only one pair of primary colors is perceived, with the two colors being complementary to each other. Most dichromats are red-green blind and confuse red, yellow, and green. Color blindness tests use special cards or colored pieces of yarn.

C. Accommodation: The lens is held in place by fibers between the lens capsule and the ciliary body (Figs 15–1 and 15–7). In the unaccommodated state, these elastic fibers are taut and keep the lens somewhat flattened. In the accommodated state, contraction of the circular ciliary muscle slackens the tension on the elastic fibers, and the lens, which has an intrinsic capacity to become rounder, assumes a more biconvex shape. The ciliary muscle is a smooth muscle that is innervated by the parasympathetic system (cranial nerve III; see Chapter 8); it can be paralyzed with atropine or similar drugs.

D. Refraction: When viewing a distant object the normal (emmetropic) eye is unaccommodated and the object is in focus. A normal eye readily focuses an image of a distant object on its retina, 24 mm behind the cornea; the focal length of the optics and the distance from cornea to retina are well matched, a state known

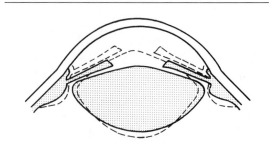

Figure 15–7. Accommodation. The solid lines represent the shape of the lens, iris, and ciliary body at rest, and the dotted lines represent the shape during accommodation. (Reproduced, with permission, from Ganong WF: *Review of Medical Physiology,* 16th ed. Appleton & Lange, 1993.)

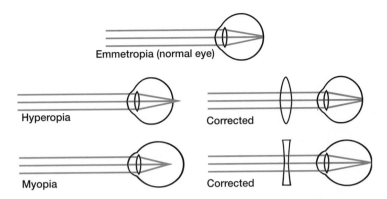

Figure 15–8. Emmetropia (normal eye) and hyperopia and myopia (common defects of the eye). In hyperopia, the eyeball is too short, and light rays come to a focus behind the retina. A biconvex lens corrects this by adding to the refractive power of the lens of the eye. In myopia, the eyeball is too long, and light rays focus in front of the retina. Placing a biconcave lens in front of the eye causes the light rays to diverge slightly before striking the eye, so that they are brought to a focus on the retina. (Reproduced, with permission, from Ganong WF: *Review of Medical Physiology,* 16th ed. Appleton & Lange, 1993.)

as **emmetropia** (Fig 15–8). To bring closer objects into focus, the eye must increase its refractive power by accommodation. The ability of the lens to do so decreases with age as the lens loses its elasticity and hardens. The effect on vision usually becomes noticeable at around the age of 40 years; by the 50s, accommodation is generally lost **(presbyopia).** Each eye is permanently focused at a constant distance, and reading becomes difficult. Holding the reading material far enough away (if possible) helps, but then the image may be too small to distinguish the letters. A positive lens helps alleviate the difficulty.

Tests of Eye Function

In assessing visual acuity, distant vision is tested with Snellen or similar cards for persons with fairly normal vision. Finger counting and finger movement tests are used for those with subnormal vision, and light perception and projection for those with markedly subnormal vision. Near vision is tested with standard reading cards.

Perimetry is used to determine the visual fields (Fig 15–9). The field for each eye (monocular field) is plotted with a device or by the confrontation method to determine the presence of a scotoma or other field defect (see section on Clinical Correlations later in this chapter). For equal-sized targets, the visual field for white is most extensive; the size of the visual fields for blue, red, yellow, and green decreases in that order. Normally the visual fields overlap in an area of binocular vision (Fig 15–10).

Clinical Correlations

A. Errors of Refraction: In **myopia** (nearsightedness), the refracting system is too powerful for the length of the eyeball, causing the image of a distant object to focus in front of, instead of at, the retina (see Fig

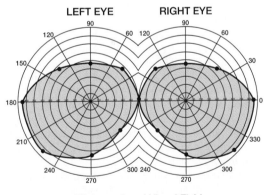

Minimum Legal Visual Field

Minimal Normal Field:

Temporally	85°
Down and temporally	85°
Down	65°
Down and nasally	50°
Nasally	60°
Up and nasally	55°
Up	45°
Up and temporally	55°
Full field	= 500°

Figure 15–9. Visual field charts. Small white objects subtending 1 degree are moved slowly to chart fields on the perimeter. The smaller the object, the more sensitive the test (with a gross error of refraction, 1 degree is reliable). Red has the smallest normal field and gives the most sensitive field test. (Reproduced, with permission, from Vaughan D, Asbury T, Riordan-Eva P: *General Ophthalmology,* 13th ed. Appleton & Lange, 1993.)

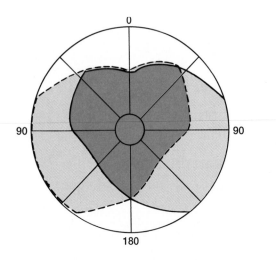

Figure 15–10. Monocular and binocular visual fields. The dotted line encloses the visual field of the left eye; the solid line, that of the right eye. The common area (heart-shaped clear zone in the center) is viewed with binocular vision. The shaded areas are viewed with monocular vision. (Reproduced, with permission, from Ganong WF: *Review of Medical Physiology*, 16th ed. Appleton & Lange, 1993.)

15–8). The object will be in focus only when it is brought nearer to the eye. Myopia can be corrected by placing an appropriate negative (minus) lens in front of the eye.

In **hyperopia** (farsightedness), the refracting power is too weak for the length of the eyeball causing the image to appear on the retina before it focuses. An appropriate positive (plus) lens placed in front of the eye provides additional refracting power.

Astigmatism, another optical problem, occurs when the curvature of either the lens or cornea is greater in one axis or meridian. For example, if the refracting power of the cornea is greater in its vertical axis than in its horizontal axis, the vertical rays will be refracted more than the horizontal rays, and a point source of light looks like an ellipse. A lens with an astigmatism that exactly complements that of the eye is used to correct the condition.

Scotomas are abnormal blind spots in the visual fields (the normal, physiologic, blind spot corresponds to the position of the optic disc, which lacks receptor cells). There are numerous types: Positive scotomas are apparent to the patient as dark spots, while negative scotomas (blank spots) may exist without the patient's knowledge. Central scotomas (loss of macular vision) are commonly seen in optic or retrobulbar neuritis (inflammation of the optic nerve close to or behind the eye, respectively); the point of fixation is involved, and central visual acuity is correspondingly impaired. Cecocentral scotomas involve the point of fixation and extend to the normal blind spot; paracentral scotomas are adjacent to the point of fixation. Ring (annular) scotomas encircle the point of fixation. Scintillating scotomas are subjective experi-

ences of bright colorless or colored lights in the line of vision. Other scotomas are caused by patchy lesions, as in hemorrhage and glaucoma.

B. Lesions of the Visual Apparatus: Inflammation of the optic nerve (**optic neuritis,** or **papillitis**) is associated with various forms of retinitis such as simple, syphilitic, diabetic, hemorrhagic, and hereditary (Fig 15–11). One form, **retrobulbar neuritis,** occurs far enough behind the optic disc so that no changes are seen on examination of the fundus; the most common cause is multiple sclerosis.

Papilledema (choked disk) is usually a symptom of increased intracranial pressure caused by a mass, eg, brain tumor (Fig 15–12). The increased pressure is transmitted to the optic disc through the extension of the subarachnoid space around the optic nerve (see Fig 15–1). Papilledema caused by a sudden increase in intracranial pressure develops within 24–48 hours. Visual acuity is not affected in papilledema although the blind spot may be enlarged. In cases where there is secondary optic atrophy, the visual fields may contract.

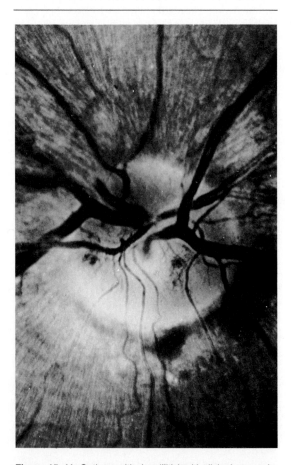

Figure 15–11. Optic neuritis (papillitis) with disk changes, including capillary hemorrhages and minimal edema (Compare with Fig 15-12). (Courtesy of WF Hoyt. Reproduced, with permission, from Vaughan D, Asbury T, Riordan-Eva P: *General Ophthalmology,* 13th ed. Appleton & Lange, 1993.)

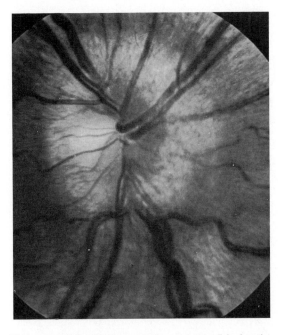

Figure 15–12. Papilledema, causing moderate disk elevation without hemorrhages. (Courtesy of WF Hoyt. Reproduced, with permission, from Vaughan D, Asbury T, Riordan-Eva P: *General Ophthalmology*, 13th ed. Appleton & Lange, 1993.)

Optic atrophy is associated with decreased visual acuity and a change in color of the optic disc to light pink, white, or gray (Fig 15–13). Primary (simple) optic atrophy is caused by a process that involves the optic nerve; it does not produce papilledema. It may be caused by tabes dorsalis, multiple sclerosis, or it may be inherited. Secondary optic atrophy is a sequel of pa-

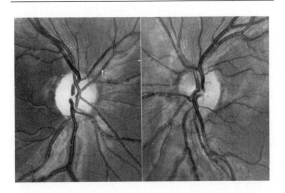

Figure 15–13. Optic atrophy. Note avascular white disk and avascular network in surrounding retina. (Courtesy of WF Hoyt. Reproduced, with permission, from Vaughan D, Asbury T, Riordan-Eva P: *General Ophthalmology*, 13th ed. Appleton & Lange, 1993.)

pilledema and may be due to neuritis, glaucoma, or increased intracranial pressure.

Holmes-Adie syndrome is characterized by a tonic pupillary reaction and the absence of one or more tendon reflexes. The pupil is said to be tonic, with an extremely slow—and almost imperceptible—contraction to light; dilatation occurs slowly upon removal of the stimulus.

VISUAL PATHWAYS

Anatomy

The **optic nerve** conveys visual impulses; it consists of about a million nerve fibers and contains axons arising from the inner, ganglion-cell layer of the retina. These fibers travel through the **lamina cribrosa** of the sclera and then course through the optic canal of the skull to form the **optic chiasm** (Fig 15–14). The fibers from the nasal half of the retina decussate within the optic chiasm; those from the lateral (temporal) half do not.

Thus, the arrangement of the optic chiasm is such that the axons from the lateral half of the left retina and the nasal half of the right retina, project centrally behind the chiasm within the left optic tract. As a result of the optics of the eye, these two halves of the left and right retina receive visual information from the right-sided half of the visual world. This anatomic arrangement permits the *left* hemisphere to receive visual information about the contralateral, ie, *right*-sided half of the visual world and vice-versa (Fig 15–14). After traveling through the optic chiasm, retinal ganglion cell axons travel centrally in the **optic tract,** which carries the axons to the **lateral geniculate body** (also termed the **lateral geniculate nucleus**) as well as the **superior colliculus.**

The lateral geniculate bodies, together with the medial geniculate bodies, constitute important relay nuclei (for vision and hearing, respectively) within the thalamus. Each lateral geniculate nucleus is a six-layered structure. Crossed fibers from the optic tract terminate within laminae 1, 4, and 6, while uncrossed fibers terminate in laminae 2, 3, and 5. The optic tract axons terminate in a highly organized manner, and their synaptic endings are organized in a map-like (retinotopic) fashion that reproduces the geometry of the retina (interestingly, the central part of the visual field has a relatively large representation in the lateral geniculate bodies, probably providing greater visual resolution, or sensitivity to detail, in this region). The receptive fields of neurons in the lateral geniculate bodies are similar to those of retinal ganglion cells and usually consist of an "on" center associated with an "off" surround or vice-versa.

From each lateral geniculate body, axons project ipsilaterally by way of the **optic radiation** to the calcarine cortex in the occipital lobe. Thus, the right

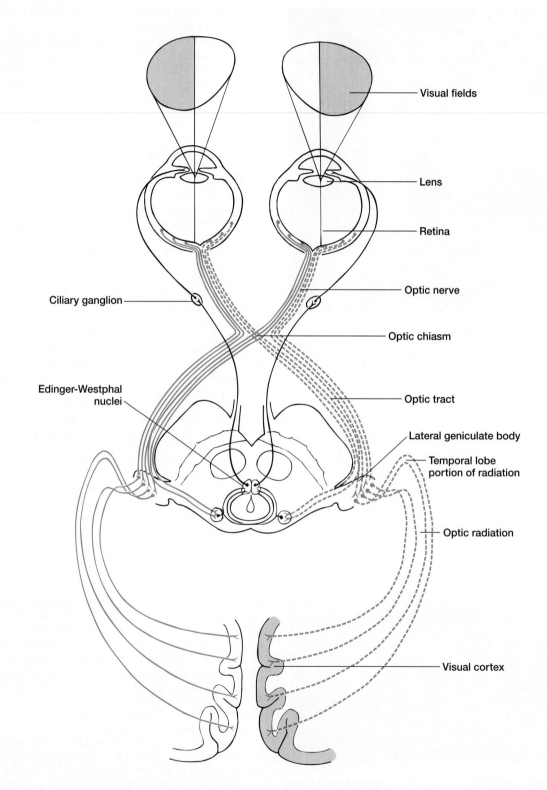

Figure 15–14. The visual pathways. The solid blue lines represent nerve fibers that extend from the retina to the occipital cortex and carry afferent visual information from the right half of the visual field. The broken blue lines show the pathway from the left half of the visual fields. The black lines represent the efferent pathway for the pupillary light reflex.

Visual fields

Lens

Retina

Optic nerve

Optic chiasm

Optic tract

Lateral geniculate body

Temporal lobe portion of radiation

Optic radiation

Visual cortex

Ciliary ganglion

Edinger-Westphal nuclei

halves of each retina (corresponding to the left halves of the visual world) project by way of the optic radiation to the right occipital lobe and vice-versa. There is a more extensive representation for the area of central vision (see Fig 15–16).

The **geniculocalcarine fibers** (optic radiations) carry impulses from the lateral geniculate bodies to the visual cortex. **Meyer's loop** is the sweep of geniculocalcarine fibers that curves around the lateral ventricle, reaching forward into the temporal lobe, before proceeding toward the calcarine cortex. Meyer's loop carries optic radiation fibers representing the *upper* part of the contralateral visual field.

In addition to projecting to the lateral geniculate bodies, retinal ganglion cell axons in the optic tract terminate in the **superior colliculus.** The superior colliculus also receives synapses from the visual cortex. As in the lateral geniculate bodies, there is an orderly map of the retina on the superior colliculus. The superior colliculus projects to the spinal cord via the tectospinal tracts, which control reflex movements of the head, neck, and eyes in response to visual stimuli (see Chapter 13).

Still other afferents from the optic tract project, via the pretectal area, to parasympathetic neurons in the **Edinger-Westphal nucleus** (part of the oculomotor nucleus). These parasympathetic neurons send axons within the oculomotor nerve and terminate in the **ciliary ganglia** (Fig 15–14). Postganglionic neurons, within the ciliary ganglia, project to the sphincter muscles of the iris. This loop of neurons is responsible for the **pupillary light reflex,** which results in constriction of the pupil in response to stimulation of the eye with light. Visual axons in each optic tract project to the Edinger-Westphal nucleus bilaterally and, as might be expected, when light is shown in one eye, there is constriction of the pupil not only in the ipsilateral eye (the direct light reflex), but also in the contralateral eye (the consensual light reflex).

Clinical Correlations

The accurate examination of visual defects in a patient is of considerable importance in localizing lesions in the eye, retina, optic nerve, optic chiasm or tracts, or visual cortex.

Impaired vision in one eye is usually due to a disorder involving the eye, retina, or the optic nerve (Fig 15–15A).

Field defects can affect one or both visual fields. If the lesion is in the optic chiasm, optic tracts, or visual cortex, both eyes will show field defects.

A chiasmatic lesion (often owing to a pituitary tumor or a lesion around the sella turcica) can injure the decussating axons of retinal ganglion cells within the optic chiasm. These axons originate in the nasal halves of the two retinas. Thus, this type of lesion produces **bitemporal hemianopia,** characterized by blindness in the lateral or temporal half of the visual field for each eye (Fig 15–15B).

Lesions behind the optic chiasm cause a field defect in the temporal field of one eye, together with a field defect in the nasal (medial) field of the other eye. The result is a **homonymous hemianopia** in which the visual field defect is on the side *opposite* to the lesion (Fig 15–15C, 15–15E).

Because Meyer's loop carries optic radiation fibers representing the upper part of the contralateral field, temporal lobe lesions can produce a visual field deficit involving the contralateral superior ("pie in the sky") quadrant (this visual field defect is called a **superior quadrantanopsia**; Fig 15–15D). An example is discussed in Clinical Illustration 15–1.

Abnormalities of pupillary size may be caused by lesions in the pathway for the pupillary light reflex (see Fig 8–9 and 15–14) or to the action of drugs that affect the balance between parasympathetic and sympathetic innervation of the eye (Table 15–1).

Argyll-Robertson pupils, usually caused by neurosyphilis, are small, sometimes unequal, or irregular pupils. The lesion is thought to be in the pretectal region, close to the Edinger-Westphal nucleus.

In **Horner's syndrome,** one pupil is small (miotic) and there are other signs of dysfunction of the sympathetic supply to the pupil and orbit (see Chapter 20 and Figs 20–5 and 20–6).

CLINICAL ILLUSTRATION 15–1

A 28-year-old physical education teacher, previously well, began to experience "spells." These began with a feeling of fear and epigastric discomfort that gradually moved upward; this was followed by a period of unresponsiveness in which the patient would stare straight ahead while making chewing movements with his mouth. Over the ensuing year, the patient had several generalized seizures. A CT scan was read as normal, but the EEG showed epileptiform activity in the right temporal lobe. A diagnosis of temporal lobe epilepsy was made and the patient was treated with anticonvulsants. The seizures stopped.

Three years later, the patient saw an ophthalmologist and complained of "poor vision in this left eye." He also complained of a left-sided headache, worse in the morning. On examination, the ophthalmologist found a homonymous quadrantanopsia ("pie in the sky" field deficit) in the left upper quadrant. The patient was referred for neurologic consultation. Examination now revealed a Babinski response and slightly increased deep tendon reflexes on the left side, in addition to the homonymous quadrantanopsia. CT scan showed a mass lesion in the right anterior temporal lobe, surrounded by edema.

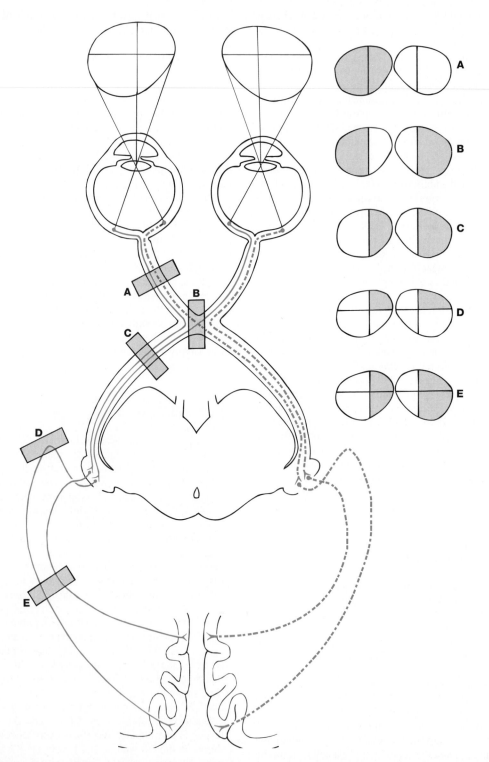

Figure 15–15. Typical lesions of the visual pathways. Their effects on the visual fields are shown on the right side of the illustration. **A:** Blindness in one eye. **B:** Bitemporal hemianopia. **C:** Homonymous hemianopia. **D:** Quadrantanopia. **E:** Homonymous hemianopia.

Table 15–1. Local effects of drugs on the eye.

Parasympathomimetics Used as miotics (to constrict pupil) for control of intraocular pressure in glaucoma	Parasympatholytics Used as mydriatics (to dilate pupil) to aid in eye examination or as cycloplegics (to relax ciliary muscles)	Sympathomimetics Used for mydriasis; do not cause cycloplegia

Pilocarpine
Carbachol
Methacholine
Cholinesterase Inhibitors
   Physostigmine (eserine)
   Isoflurophate
	Mydriatic:
	   Eucatropine
	Cyctoplegic and Mydriatic:
	   Homatropine
	   Scopolamine (hyoscine)
	   Atropine
	   Cyclopentolate
		Phenylephrine
		Hydroxyamphetamine
		Epinenephrine
		Cocaine

The patient was taken to surgery and an oligodendroglioma was found. Following surgical removal of the oligodendroglioma, the patient's visual field deficit persisted. Nevertheless, he was able to return to work.

This case illustrates the fact that patients may complain of visual loss in the right or left eye when, in fact, they have a homonymous hemianopsia or quadrantanopsia on the corresponding side. In this patient, examination revealed a left-sided upper quadrantanopsia. This was because of impingement on optic radiation axons, traveling in Meyer's loop, by a slow-growing oligodendroglioma. Recognition of the tumor at a relatively early stage facilitated its neurosurgical removal.

Examination of the visual fields is an important part of the workup of any patient with a suspected lesion in the brain. The visual pathway extends from the retina to the calcarine cortex in the occipital lobe. As outlined in Figure 15–15, lesions at a variety of sites along this pathway produce characteristic visual field defects. Recognition of these visual field abnormalities often provides crucial diagnostic information.

THE VISUAL CORTEX

Anatomy

The **primary visual cortex** (also termed **calcarine cortex; area 17**) is located on the medial surface of the occipital lobe, above and below the calcarine fissure (Figs 15–16 and 15–17); it is also called the **striate cortex** because when viewed in histologic sections, it contains a light colored horizontal stripe (corresponding to white matter containing myelinated fibers within laminae IV). Areas 18 and 19, which extend concentrically outside the primary cortex, are called the **extrastriate cortex** or the **visual association cortex.**

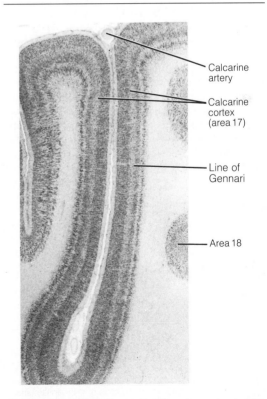

Calcarine artery

Calcarine cortex (area 17)

Line of Gennari

Area 18

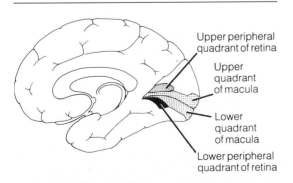

Upper peripheral quadrant of retina

Upper quadrant of macula

Lower quadrant of macula

Lower peripheral quadrant of retina

Figure 15–16. Medial view of the right cerebral hemisphere, showing projection of the retina on the calcarine cortex.

Figure 15–17. Light micrograph of the primary visual cortex (calcarine cortex) on each side of the calcarine fissure.

Visual information is relayed from the lateral geniculate body to the visual cortex via myelinated axons in the optic radiations.

The primary visual cortex receives its blood from the calcarine branch of the posterior cerebral artery. The remainder of the occipital lobe is supplied by other branches of this artery. The arterial supply can be (rarely) interrupted by emboli or by compression of the artery between the free edge of the tentorium and enlarging or herniating portions of the brain.

Histology

The primary visual cortex appears to contain six layers. It contains a line of myelinated fibers within lamina IV (the line of Gennari, or the external line of Baillarger; see Fig 15–17). The stellate cells of lamina IV receive input from the lateral geniculate nucleus, and the pyramidal cells of layer V project to the superior colliculus. Layer VI cells send a recurrent projection to the lateral geniculate nucleus.

Physiology

There is an orderly mapping (again termed retinotopic) of the visual world onto the visual cortex. The projection of the macular part of the retina is magnified within this map, a design feature that probably provides increased sensitivity to visual detail in the central part of the visual field.

As visual information is relayed from cell to cell in the cortex, it is processed in increasingly complex ways (Fig 15–18). *Simple cells* in the visual cortex have receptive fields that contain an "on" or "off" center, shaped like a rectangle with a specific orientation, flanked by complementary zones. Simple cells usually respond to stimuli at one particular location. For example, an "on"-center simple cell may respond best to a bar, precisely oriented at 45 degrees, flanked by a larger "off" area, at a particular location. If the bar is rotated slightly or moved, the response of the cell will be diminished. Thus, these cells respond to lines, at specific orientations, located in particular regions within the visual world.

Complex cells in the visual cortex have receptive fields that are usually larger than those of simple cells (Fig 15–18). These cells respond to lines or edges with a specific orientation, eg, 60 degrees, but are excited whenever these lines are present anywhere within the visual field, irrespective of their location. Some complex cells are especially sensitive to movement of these specifically oriented edges or lines.

D. Hubel and T. Wiesel, who received the Nobel Prize for their analysis of the visual cortex, suggested that the receptive fields of simple cells in the visual cortex could be built up from the simpler fields of visual neurons in the lateral geniculate and, in fact, the pattern of convergence of geniculate neurons onto visual cortical cells supports this hypothesis. Similarly, it appears that by projecting onto a complex cell in the visual cortex, a set of simple cells with appropriate receptive fields can create a higher-level response that recognizes lines and edges at a particular orientation at any of a variety of positions.

The visual cortex contains vertical *orientation columns* each about 1 mm in diameter. Each column contains simple cells whose receptive fields have almost identical retinal positions and orientations. Complex cells within these columns appear to process information so as to *generalize* by recognizing the appropriate orientation irrespective of the location of the stimulus.

About one-half of the complex cells in the visual cortex receive inputs from both eyes (the inputs are very similar for the two eyes in terms of the preferred orientation and location of the stimulus) but there is usually a preference for one eye. These cells are referred to as showing *ocular dominance,* and they are organized into another overlapping series of *ocular dominance columns* each 0.8 mm in diameter. The ocular dominance columns receiving input from one eye

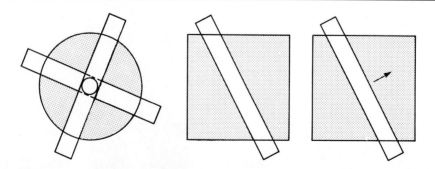

Figure 15–18. Receptive fields of cells in visual pathways. *Left:* Ganglion cells, lateral geniculate cells, and cells in layer IV of cortical area 17 have circular fields with an excitatory center and an inhibitory surround or an inhibitory center and an excitatory surround. There is no preferred orientation of a linear stimulus. *Center:* Simple cells respond best to a linear stimulus with a particular orientation in a specific part of the cell's receptive field. *Right:* Complex cells respond to linear stimuli with a particular orientation, but they are less selective in terms of location in the receptive field. They often respond maximally when the stimulus is moved laterally, as indicated by the arrow. (Modified from Hubel DH: The visual field cortex of normal and deprived monkeys. *Am Sci* 1979;**67**:532. Reproduced, with permission, from Ganong WF: *Review of Medical Physiology,* 16th ed. Appleton & Lange, 1993.)

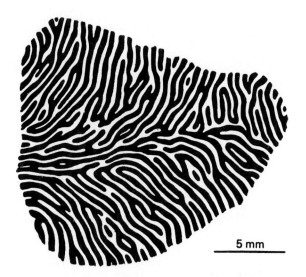

Figure 15–19. Reconstruction of ocular dominance columns in a subdivision of layer IV of a portion of the right visual cortex of a rhesus monkey. Dark stripes represent one eye, light stripes represent the other. (Reproduced, with permission, from LeVay S, Hubel DH, Wiesel TN: The pattern of ocular dominance columns in macaque visual cortex revealed by a reduced silver stain. *J Comp Neurol* 1975;**159**:559.)

alternate with columns receiving input from the other (Fig 15–19). The ocular dominance columns can be mapped by injecting radioactive amino acid in one eye. The amino acid is incorporated into protein and transported by axoplasmic flow to the ganglion cell terminals, across the geniculate synapses and along the optic radiation fibers to the visual cortex. Layer IV becomes evenly labeled. Above and below this layer, however, labeled columns alternate with unlabeled columns that receive input from the uninjected eye. Ocular dominance columns can also be demonstrated by radioautography following injection of 2-deoxyglucose into one eye while the other eye is closed.

CASE 21

A 50-year-old woman had experienced a sudden loss of consciousness three months prior to admission. She said that her husband described the incident as an epileptiform attack. The day after, she had felt much better. More recently, however, she thought that her memory was failing and her right hand had begun to feel heavy. Two weeks earlier, she began to suffer from a constant frontal headache. She felt her glasses needed changing, and the ophthalmologist referred her to the neurological service. While giving her history, the patient appeared distractable, had impaired memory, and made some inappropriate jokes about her health.

Neurologic examination showed that olfaction was totally lost on the left side but normal on the right. The right optic papilla was congested and edematous, and the left optic disc was abnormally pale. Visual acuity was normal in the right eye but impaired in the left. The muscles of facial expression were slightly weaker on the right than on the left side. Deep tendon reflexes on the right side of the body were brisker than those on the left and there was a Babinski reflex on the right. The remainder of the findings were within normal limits.

Where is the lesion? What is the differential diagnosis? Would a neuroradiologic procedure be useful? What is the most likely diagnosis?

Cases are discussed further in Chapter 25.

REFERENCES

Baylor DA: Photoreceptor signals and vision. *Invest Ophthalmol Vis Sci* 1987;**28**:34.

Dowling JE: *The Retina: An Approachable Part of the Brain.* Bellknap Press, Harvard University Press, 1987.

Dowling JE and Boycott BB: Organization of the primate retina: Electron microscopy. *Proc Roy Soc Lond Ser B* 1966;**166**:80.

Hubel DH: *Eye, Brain, and Vision.* Scientific American Library, 1988.

Hubel DH and Wiesel TN: Brain mechanisms of vision. *Scientific American* 1979;**241**:150.

Livingstone MS: Art, illusion, and the visual system. *Scientific American* 1988;**258**:78.

Shatz CJ: Impulse activity and the patterning of connections during CNS development. *Neuron* 1990;**5**:745.

Van Essen D: Functional organization of primate visual cortex. In: *Cerebral Cortex.* Peters A, Jones EG (editors). Plenum Press, 1985.

Zeki S: Parallelism and functional specialization in human visual cortex. *Cold Spring Harb Symp Quant Biol* 1990:**55**:651.

16

The Auditory System

ANATOMY & FUNCTION

The **cochlea** is the specialized organ that registers and transduces sound waves. It lies within the cochlear duct, a portion of the membranous labyrinth within the temporal bone of the skull base (Fig 16–1; see also Chapter 11). Sound waves converge through the **pinna** and **outer ear canal** to strike the **tympanic membrane** (Figs 16–1 and 16–2). The vibrations of this membrane are transmitted by way of three **ossicles (malleus, incus,** and **stapes)** in the middle ear to the oval window, where the sound waves are transmitted to the **cochlear duct.**

Two small muscles can affect the strength of the auditory signal: the **tensor tympani,** which attaches to the eardrum, and the **stapedius** muscle, which attaches to the stapes. These muscles may dampen the signal;

they also help prevent damage to the ear from very loud noises.

The **inner ear** contains the **organ of Corti** within the cochlear duct (Fig 16–3). As a result of movement of the stapes and tympanic membrane, a traveling wave is set up in the perilymph within the scala vestibuli of the cochlea. The traveling waves propagate along the cochlea, with high-frequency sound stimuli eliciting waves that reach their maximum near the base of the cochlea, ie, near the oval window. Low-frequency sounds elicit waves that reach their peak, in contrast, near the apex of the cochlea, ie, close to the round window. Thus, sounds of different frequencies tend to excite hair cells in different parts of the cochlea, which is tonotopically organized.

The traveling waves within the perilymph stimulate the organ of Corti through the vibrations of the tecto-

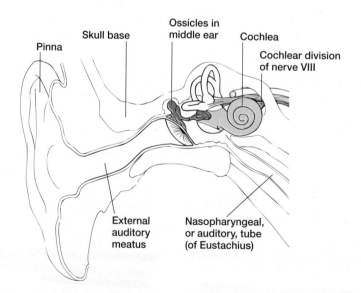

Figure 16–1. The human ear. The cochlea has been turned slightly, and the middle ear muscles have been omitted to make the relationship clear.

rial membrane against the kinocilia of the hair cells (Figs 16–3 and 16–4). The mechanical distortions of the kinocilium of each hair cell are transformed into electric signals that course into the neurons of the cochlear nerve.

AUDITORY PATHWAYS

Peripheral branches of bipolar nerve cells in the **spiral (or cochlear) ganglion** innervate the cochlear organ of Corti; central branches course in the cochlear portion of nerve VIII and terminate in the ventral and dorsal **cochlear nuclei** in the brain stem (Fig 16–5; see also Chapter 7). Second-order fibers ascend from the cochlear nuclei on both sides; the crossing fibers pass through the **trapezoid body** where some of them synapse. The ascending fibers course in the **lateral lemnisci** within the brain stem, which travel rostrally toward the inferior colliculus and medial geniculate body; these tracts therefore carry impulses derived from both ears (Fig 16–6).

Cell groups along the course of each lateral lemniscus (nuclei of the trapezoid body, lateral lemniscus, and inferior colliculus) probably receive collateral fibers, some of which end in the cerebellum or reticular formation. Others cross to the opposite nucleus; they are involved in determining the difference in signal strength or latency from each auditory input and may, thus, determine the location of the sound. Reflex connections pass to eye muscle nuclei and other motor nuclei of the cranial and spinal nerves via the **tectobulbar** and **tectospinal tracts.** These connections are activated by strong, sudden sounds; the result is reflex turning of the eyes and head toward the site of the sound. In the lower pons, the **superior olivary nuclei** receive input from both ascending pathways. Efferent fibers from these nuclei course along the cochlear nerve back to the organ of Corti. The function of this **olivocochlear bundle** is to modulate the sensitivity of the cochlear organ.

The lateral lemnisci end in the **medial geniculate bodies** by way of the **inferior colliculus** and **inferior quadrigeminal brachium**; additional fibers terminate directly in these thalamic nuclei. The third-order fibers project to the **primary auditory cortex** in the upper and medial portion of the superior temporal gyrus (area 41; Figs 16–6 and 10–11).

Tonotopia, a precise localization of high-frequency to low-frequency sound-wave transmission exists along the entire pathway from cochlea to auditory cortex.

Clinical Correlations

A. Tinnitus: Ringing, buzzing, hissing, roaring, or "paper-crushing" noises in the ear are frequently an early sign of peripheral cochlear disease (eg, hydrops or edema of the cochlea).

B. Deafness: Deafness in one ear can be caused by an impairment in the conduction of sound through the external ear canal and ossicles to the endolymph and tectorial membrane; this is called **conduction deafness. Nerve (sensoneural)** deafness can be caused by interruption of cochlear nerve fibers from the hair cells to the brain stem nuclei (Fig 16–7). Tests used to distinguish between nerve and conduction

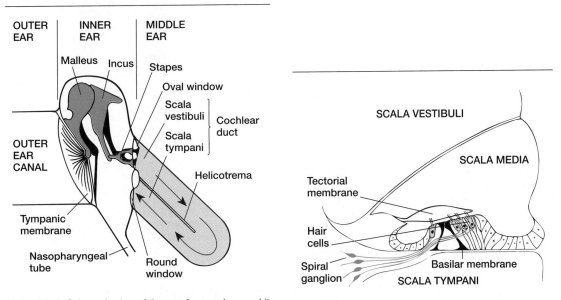

Figure 16–2. Schematic view of the ear. As sound waves hit the tympanic membrane, the position of the ossicles (which move as shown in blue and black) changes.

Figure 16–3. Cross section through one turn of the cochlea.

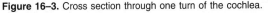

deafness are shown in Table 16–1. Nerve deafness is often located in the inner ear or in the cochlear nerve in the internal auditory meatus; conduction deafness is the result of middle or external ear disease. Progressive ossification of the ligaments between the ossicles, **otosclerosis,** is a common type of hearing loss in adults. A delicate surgical procedure, **fenestration,** exposes the cochlear duct to the outside air (a membrane is interposed), improving the air conduction of auditory signals.

A peripheral lesion in the eighth nerve with loss of hearing, such as a **cerebellopontine angle tumor,** usually involves both the cochlear and vestibular nerves (Fig 16–8). Central lesions can involve either system independently. Because the auditory pathway above the cochlear nuclei represents parts of the sound input to both ears, a unilateral lesion in the lateral lemniscus, medial geniculate body, or auditory cortex does *not* result in marked loss of hearing on the ipsilateral side. The brain stem auditory evoked response (BAER) test aids in localizing a lesion (see Chapter 24).

Hearing loss becomes a significant handicap when there is difficulty in communicating by speech. Beginning impairment has been defined as an average hearing-level loss of 16 decibels (dB) at frequencies of 500, 1000, and 2000 Hz: Sounds of these frequencies cannot be heard when their strength is 16 dB or less (a loud whisper). A person is usually considered to be deaf when the hearing level loss for these three frequencies is at or above 82 dB (the noise level of heavy traffic). Early hearing loss often appears initially at a high frequency (4000 Hz), in both children with conduction impairment and adults with **presbycusis** (lessening of hearing in old age). An artificial hearing aid may improve sound perception by amplifying the strength of the incoming sound and an experimental procedure, artificial cochlear implantation, has had promising results.

CASE 22

A 64-year-old woman was evaluated for progressive hearing loss, facial weakness, and increasing headaches, all on the right side. Her hearing loss had been present for at least five years, and two years prior to admission, she had noted the gradual development of unsteadiness in walking. During recent months, she began to experience weakness and progressive numbness of the right side of the face as well as double vision. There was no nausea or vomiting.

Neurologic examination showed beginning bilateral papilledema, decreased pain and touch sensation in the right half of the face, moderate right peripheral facial weakness, absence of both the right corneal reflex and blinking with the right eye. Tests of air and

bone conduction showed hearing was markedly decreased on the right side. Caloric labyrinthine stimulation was normal on the left; there was no response on the right. On gaze to the right, there was mild weakness of abduction of the right eye (weakness of the abducens). Examination of the motor system, reflexes, and sensations yielded normal results, with the exception of three findings: a broad-based gait, bilateral Babinski signs, and the inability to walk with feet tandem.

What is the differential diagnosis? What is the most likely diagnosis?

Cases are discussed further in Chapter 25.

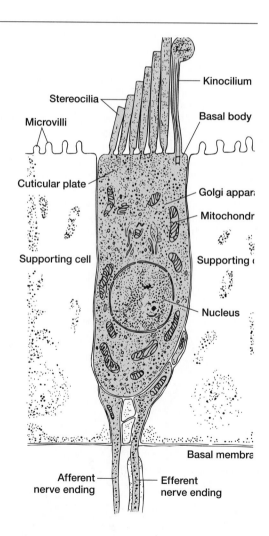

Figure 16–4. Structure of hair cell. (Reproduced, with permission, from Hudspeth AJ: The hair cells of the inner ear. *Sci Am* 1983;**248:**54.)

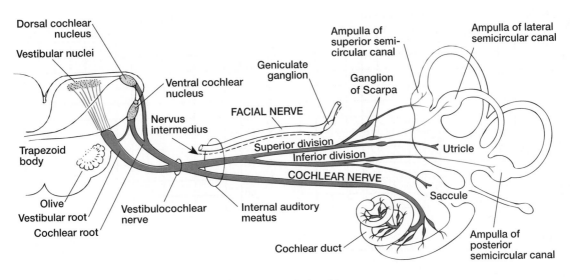
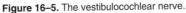

Figure 16–5. The vestibulocochlear nerve.

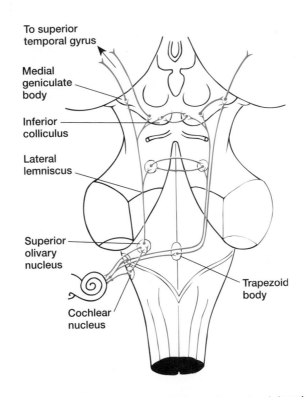

Figure 16–6. Diagram of main auditory pathways superimposed on a dorsal view of the brain stem.

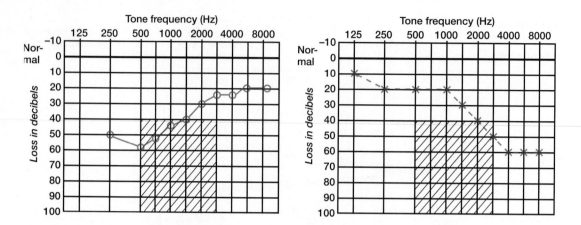

Figure 16–7. ***Left:*** Middle ear, or conduction, deafness. Representative air conduction curve shows greatest impairment of pure tone thresholds in lower frequencies. ***Right:*** Perception, or nerve, deafness. Representative bone conduction curve of pure tone thresholds shows greatest deficit at higher frequencies.

Table 16–1. Common tests with a tuning fork to distinguish between nerve and conduction hearing loss.

Method	Normal	Conduction Hearing Loss (one ear)	Nerve (sensorineural) Hearing Loss (one ear)
Weber Base of vibrating tuning fork placed on vertex of skull	Sound equal on both sides	Sound louder in diseased ear because masking effect of environmental noise is absent on diseased side.	Sound louder in normal ear
Rinne Base of vibrating tuning fork placed on mastoid process until subject no longer hears it, then held in air next to ear	Hears vibration in air after bone conduction is over	Does not hear vibrations in air after bone conduction is over	Hears vibration in air after bone conduction is over

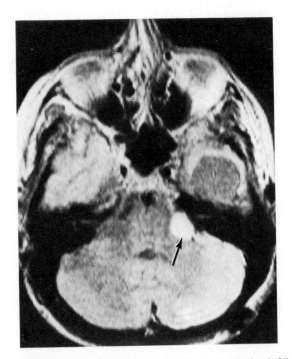

Figure 16–8. Magnetic resonance image of a horizontal section through the head at the level of the lower pons and internal auditory meatus. A left acoustic nerve schwannoma with its high intensity is shown in the left cerebellopontine angle (arrow).

REFERENCES

Hart RG, Gardner DP, Howieson J: Acoustic tumors: Atypical features and recent diagnostic tests. *Neurology* 33;**211**:1983.

Hudspeth AJ: How the ear's works work. *Nature* 1989; **341**:397.

Kim Do, Molnar CE: Cochlear mechanics. Pages 45–56 In: *The Nervous System.* Vol 3. Eagles EL (editor). Raven, 1975.

Luxon LM: Disorders of hearing. Pages 434–450 In: *Diseases of the Nervous System: Clinical Neurobiology.* Asbury AK, McKhann GM, MacDonald WI (editors). Saunders, 1992.

Morest DK: Structural organization of the auditory pathways. Pages 19–30 In: *The Nervous System.* Vol 3. Eagles EL (editor). Raven, 1975.

Patuzzi R, Robertson D: Tuning in the mammalian cochlea. *Physiol Rev* Vol 68, 1988.

Schubert ED: *Hearing: Its Function and Dysfunction.* Springer-Verlag, 1980.

Smith CA: Inner Ear. Pages 1–18 In: *The Nervous System.* Vol 3. Eagles EL (editor). Raven, 1975.

17

The Vestibular System

This system, which participates in the maintenance of stance and body posture, coordination of body, head, and eye movements, and in visual fixation, includes the peripheral vestibular receptors, vestibular component of the VIII nerves, the vestibular nuclei, and their central projections.

ANATOMY

The membranous **labyrinth,** filled with endolymph and surrounded by perilymph, lies in the bony labyrinthine space within the temporal bone of the skull base (Fig 17–1). Two special sensory systems receive their input from structures in the membranous labyrinth: the auditory system from the cochlea (see Chapter 16), and the vestibular system from the remainder of the labyrinth.

The **static labyrinth** gives information regarding the position of the head in space; it includes the specialized sensory areas located within the **saccule** and the **utricle** (Fig 17–1). Within the utricle and saccule, **otoliths** (small calcium carbonate crystals, also termed **otoconia**) are located adjacent to hair cells clustered in **macular** regions. The otoliths displace the hair cell processes and excite the utricle in response to horizontal acceleration and the utricle to verticle acceleration.

The **kinetic labyrinth** consists of the three **semicircular canals.** Each canal ends in an enlarged **ampulla,** which contains hair cells, within a receptor area called the **crista ampullaris.** A gelatinous partition **(cupula)** covers each ampulla and is displaced by rotation of the heads, thus, displacing hair cells so that they generate impulses. The three semicircular canals are oriented at 90 degrees to each other, providing a mechanism that is sensitive to rotation along any axis.

VESTIBULAR PATHWAYS

The peripheral branches of the bipolar cells in the **vestibular ganglion** course from the specialized receptors (hair cells) in the ampullae, and from the maculae of the utricle and the saccule. The central branches enter the brain stem and end in the **vestibular nuclei** (Figs 17–1 and 17–2; see also Chapter 7).

Some vestibular connections go from the superior and lateral vestibular nuclei to the cerebellum where they end in the cerebellar cortex within the flocculonodular component (see Chapter 7). Others course from the lateral vestibular nuclei into the ipsilateral spinal cord via the lateral **vestibulospinal tracts,** from the superior and medial vestibular nuclei to nuclei of the eye muscles, and to the motor nuclei of the upper spinal nerves via the **medial longitudinal fasciculi** (MLF) of the same and opposite sides (Fig 17–3). The **medial vestibulospinal tract** (the descending portion of the MLF) connects to the anterior horn of the cervical and upper thoracic cord; this tract is involved in the labyrinthine righting reflexes that adjust the position of the head in response to signals of vestibular origin. Some vestibular nuclei send fibers to the reticular formation. Some ascending fibers from the vestibular nuclei travel by way of the thalamus (ventral posterior nucleus) to the parietal cortex (area 40).

FUNCTIONS

As previously noted, the vestibular nerve conducts two types of information to the brain stem: the position of the head in space and the angular rotation of the head.

Static information about the position of the head is signaled when pressure of the otoliths on the sensitive areas in the utricle and saccule is transduced to impulses in the inferior division of the vestibular nerve (Figs 17–1 and 17–4). Dynamic information, about rotation of the head is produced by the three semicircular canals (superior, posterior, and lateral) (Fig 17–5). Within each ampulla, a flexible crista changes its shape and direction according to the movement of the endolymph within the canal, so that any rotation of the head can affect the crista and its afferent nerve fibers (Fig 17–6). Acting together, the semicircular canals

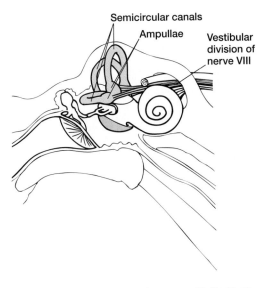

Figure 17–1. The human ear (compare with Fig 16–1).

send impulses along the superior division of the vestibular nerve to the central vestibular pathways.

The entire vestibular apparatus thus provides information that contributes to the maintenance of **equilibrium** and, together with information from the visual and proprioceptive systems, provides a complex position sense in the brain stem and cerebellum.

When the head moves, a compensatory adjustment of gaze, the **vestibulo-ocular reflex,** is required to keep the eyes fixed on one object. Clockwise rotation of the eyes is caused by counterclockwise rotation of the head. The pathways for the reflex are via the medial longitudinal fasciculus and involve the vestibular system and the motor nuclei for eye movement (see Fig 8–7).

Clinical Correlations

Nystagmus is an involuntary back-and-forth, up-and-down, or rotating movement of the eyeballs, with a slow pull and a rapid return jerk. (The name comes from the rapid jerking component, which is a compensatory adjustment to the slow reflex movement.) Nystagmus can be induced in normal individuals; if it occurs spontaneously it is a sign of a lesion. The lesions that cause nystagmus affect the complex neural mechanism that tends to keep the eyes constant in relation to their environment and is thus concerned with equilibrium.

Physiologic nystagmus can be elicited by turning the eyes far to one side or by stimulating one of the semicircular canals (usually the lateral) with cool (30 °C) or warm (40 °C) water injected into one external ear canal (Fig 17–7). Cool water produces nystagmus toward the opposite side; warm water produces nystagmus to the same side. (A mnemonic for this is COWS: cool, opposite; warm, same.) **Peripheral vestibular nystagmus** results from stimulation of the peripheral vestibular apparatus and is usually accompanied by vertigo. Fast spinning of the body, some-

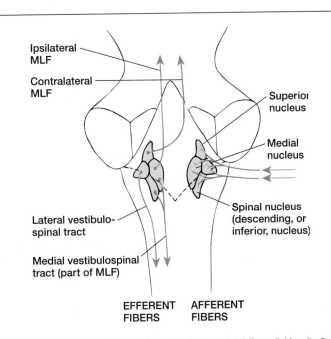

Figure 17–2. Efferent and afferent fibers of the vestibular nuclei. MLF, medial longitudinal fasciculus.

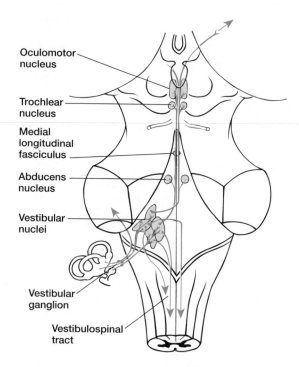

Figure 17–3. Simplified diagram of main vestibular pathways superimposed on a dorsal view of the brain stem (cerebellar connections are not shown).

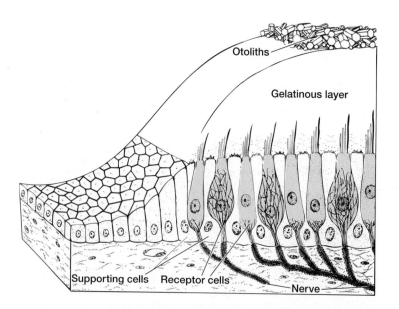

Figure 17–4. Macular structure. (Reproduced, with permission, from Junqueira LC, Carneiro J, Kelley RO: *Basic Histology*, 7th ed. Appleton & Lange, 1992.)

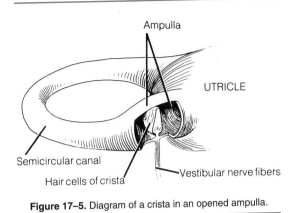

Figure 17–5. Diagram of a crista in an opened ampulla.

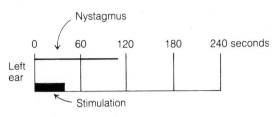
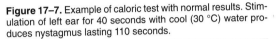

Figure 17–7. Example of caloric test with normal results. Stimulation of left ear for 40 seconds with cool (30 °C) water produces nystagmus lasting 110 seconds.

times seen on the playground, is an example: if the child is suddenly stopped, its eyes show nystagmus for a few seconds. Professional skaters and dancers learn not to be bothered by nystagmus and vertigo. **Central nervous system nystagmus** is seldom associated with vertigo; it occurs with lesions in the region of the fourth ventricle. **Optokinetic (railroad or freeway) nystagmus** occurs when there is continuous movement of the visual field past the eyes, as when traveling by train. **Nystagmus** may occur during treatment with certain drugs. For example, nystagmus is often seen in patients treated with the anticonvulsant phenytoin. Streptomycin and other drugs may even cause degeneration of the vestibular organ and nuclei.

Vertigo, an illusory feeling of giddiness with disorientation in space that usually results in a disturbance of equilibrium, is often a sign of labyrinthine disease originating in the middle or internal ear. Adjustment to peripheral vestibular damage is rapid (within a few days). Even though a labyrinth is not intact or functioning, balance is still remarkably good when vision

is present: visual information can even compensate for the loss of both labyrinths. Vertigo can also result from tumors or other lesions of the vestibular system (eg, **Meniere's syndrome,** or **paroxysmal labyrinthine vertigo**) or from reflex phenomena (eg, **seasickness**). Seasickness is caused by continuous, irregular movement of the endolymph in susceptible individuals. It is characterized by disturbances in equilibrium and by nausea and vomiting that are not related to diet. Vertigo is sometimes relieved or induced by placing the head in certain positions; it can often be prevented by medication.

Vestibular ataxia, with clumsy, uncoordinated movements, may result from the same lesions that produce vertigo. Nystagmus is often present. Vestibular ataxia must be distinguished from other types: **cerebellar ataxia** (see Chapters 7 and 13) and **sensory ataxia** (caused by lesions in the proprioceptive pathways; see Chapter 5).

Interruption of the pathway between the nuclei of nerves VIII, VI, and III (the medial longitudinal fasciculus, pathway of the vestibulo-ocular reflex) results in **internuclear ophthalmoplegia,** an inability to adduct the eye ipsilateral to the lesion.

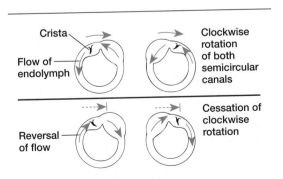

Figure 17–6. Schematic illustration of the effects of head movements (top) and the subsequent cessation of movement (bottom) on the crista and the direction of endolymph flow.

CASE 23

A 38-year-old male clerk saw his doctor because he experienced sudden episodes of nausea and dizziness. These attacks had started three weeks earlier and seemed to be getting worse. The abnormal episodes at first lasted only a few minutes, during which "the room seemed to spin." Lately they had been lasting for many hours. A severe attack caused him to vomit and to hear abnormal sounds (ringing, buzzing, paper-rolling) in the left ear. He thought that he was becoming deaf on that side.

The neurologic examination was within normal limits except for a slight sensorineural hearing loss in the left ear. CT examination of the head was unremarkable.

What is the probable diagnosis?

Cases are further discussed in Chapter 25.

REFERENCES

Baloh RW, Honrubia V: *Clinical Neurophysiology of the Vestibular System.* Davis, 1979.

Brandt T, Daroff RB: The multisensory physiological and pathological vertigo syndromes. *Ann Neurol* 1980;**7:**195.

Harada Y: *The Vestibular Organs.* Kugler & Ghedini, 1988.

Luxon LM: Diseases of the eighth cranial nerve. In: *Peripheral Neuropathy,* 2nd ed. Dyck PJ et al (editors). Saunders, 1984.

Reticular Formation

18

ANATOMY

The reticular formation consists of interconnected regions in the tegmentum of the brain stem, the lateral hypothalamic area, and the medial, intralaminar, and reticular nuclei of the thalamus (Fig 18–1). Thalamic efferents project to most of the cerebral cortex. The term itself derives from the characteristic appearance of loosely packed cells of varying sizes and shapes that are embedded in a dense meshwork of cell processes, including dendrites and axons.

FUNCTIONS

Arousal

Regulation of arousal and the level of consciousness is a generalized function of the reticular formation. The neurons of the activating portion of the reticular formation are excited by a wide variety of sensory stimuli that are conducted by way of collaterals from the somatosensory, auditory, visual, and visceral sensory systems. The reticular formation is therefore nonspecific in its response and performs a generalized regulatory function. When a novel stimulus is received, attention is focused on it while general alertness increases. This **behavioral arousal** is independent of the modality of stimulation and is accompanied by electroencephalographic changes from low-voltage to high-voltage activity over much of the cortex. The nonspecific thalamic regions project to the cortex, specifically to the distal dendritic fields of the large pyramidal cells. When the stimulus is repeated, the arousal response becomes habituated (dies down). In fact, slow repetitive stimuli, such as those in counting sheep or inducing hypnosis, will reduce cortical activity and lull a person to sleep. If the reticular formation is depressed by anesthesia or destroyed, sensory stimuli still produce activity in the specific thalamic and cortical sensory areas, but they do not produce generalized cortical arousal.

Consciousness

Many regions of the cerebral cortex produce generalized arousal when stimulated (this is the basis for the saying, "pinch yourself to see if you're dreaming"). Arousal, which is abolished by lesions in the mesencephalic reticular formation, does not require an intact corpus callosum. The cortex and the mesencephalic reticular-activating system are mutually sustaining areas involved in maintaining consciousness. Lesions that destroy a large area of the cortex, a small area of the midbrain, or both produce coma (Fig 18–2).

The loss of consciousness in **syncope** (fainting) is usually brief in duration and sudden in onset; more prolonged and profound loss of consciousness is described as **coma.** A patient in coma is unresponsive and cannot be aroused. There may be no reaction—or only a primitive defense movement such as corneal reflex or limb withdrawal—to painful stimuli. **Stupor, obtundation,** and **confusion** are still lesser grades and are characterized by variable degrees of disorientation and impaired reactivity. Acute confusional states must be distinguished from dementia (see Chapter 22). In the former case, the patient is disoriented, inattentive, and sleepy but reacts appropriately to certain stimuli.

Coma may be of intracranial or extracranial origin. **Intracranial** causes include head injuries, cerebrovascular accidents, central nervous system infections, tumors, degenerative diseases, and increased intracranial pressure. **Extracranial** causes include vascular disorders (shock or hypotension caused by severe hemorrhage or myocardial infarction), metabolic disorders (diabetic acidosis, hypoglycemia, uremia, hepatic coma, addisonian crisis, electrolyte imbalance), intoxication (with alcohol, barbiturates, narcotics, bromides, analgesics, ataractics, carbon monoxide, heavy metals), and miscellaneous disorders (hyperthermia, hypothermia, electric shock, anaphylaxis, severe systemic infections). The **Glasgow Coma Scale** offers a practical method of assessing changes in

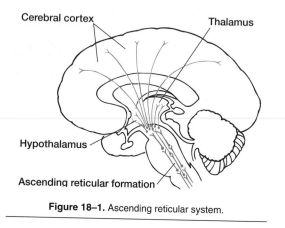

Figure 18–1. Ascending reticular system.

the level of consciousness based upon eye opening and verbal and motor responses (Table 18–1).

Sleep

A. Periodicity: The daily cycle of arousal, which includes periods of sleep and of waking, is regulated by reticular formation structures in the hypothalamus and brain stem. The sleep process of this 24-hour circadian rhythm is an active physiologic function. Nerve cells in the reticular formation of the pons begin to discharge just prior to the onset of sleep. Lesions of the pons just forward of the trigeminal nerve produce a state of hyperalertness and much less sleep than normal.

B. Stages: The sleep cycle consists of several stages that follow one another in an orderly fashion, each taking about 90 minutes (Fig 18–3). The stages can be defined by characteristic wave patterns on electroencephalograms (see Chapter 24). There are two distinct types of sleep: slow-wave sleep and rapid eye movement sleep.

Slow-wave sleep is further divided into stages. Stage 1 of **slow-wave (spindle) sleep** is characterized by easy arousal. Stages 2–4 are progressively deeper, and the electroencephalographic pattern becomes more synchronized. In stage 4, the deepest stage of slow-wave sleep, blood pressure, pulse rate, respiratory rate, and the amount of oxygen consumed by the brain are very low. The control mechanisms for slow-wave sleep are not known.

Rapid eye movement (REM) sleep is characterized by the sudden appearance of an asynchronous pattern on electroencephalograms. The sleepers make intermittent rapid eye movements, are hard to awake, show a striking loss of muscle tone in the limbs, and have vivid visual imagery and complex dreams. There is a specific need for REM sleep, which is triggered by neurons in the dorsal midbrain and pontine tegmentum.

In experiments involving cats, a waking pattern was found if a transection was made at the junction of the medulla and spinal cord (**encephale isole**); a slow-

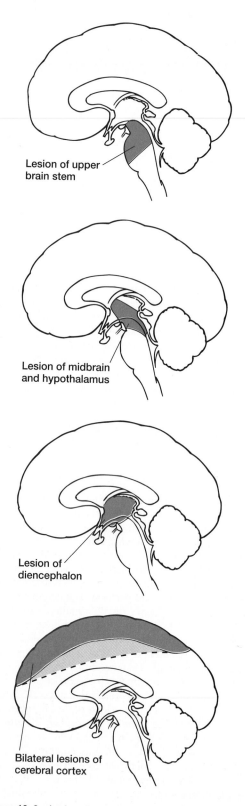

Figure 18–2. Lesions that cause coma or loss of consciousness.

Table 18–1. Glasgow Coma Scale. A practical method of assessing changes in level of consciousness, based upon eye opening and verbal and motor responses. The response can be expressed by the sum of the scores assigned to each response. The lowest score is 3, and the highest score is 15.*

	Examiner's Test	Patient's Response	Assigned Score
Eye opening	Spontaneous	Opens eyes on own	4
	Speech	Opens eyes when asked to do so in a loud voice	3
	Pain	Opens eyes when pinched	2
	Pain	Does not open eyes	1
Best motor response	Commands	Follows simple commands	6
	Pain	Pulls examiner's hand away when pinched	5
	Pain	Pulls a part of body away when pinched.	4
	Pain	Flexes body inappropriately to pain (decorticate posturing).	3
	Pain	Body becomes rigid in an extended position when pinched (decerebrate posturing).	2
	Pain	Has no motor response to pinch.	1
Verbal response (talking)	Speech	Carries on a conversation correctly and tells examiner where and who he or she is and the month and year.	5
	Speech	Seems confused or disoriented.	4
	Speech	Talks so examiner can understand words but makes no sense.	3
	Speech	Makes sounds examiner cannot understand.	2
	Speech	Makes no noise.	1

*Slightly modified and reproduced, with permission, from Rimel RN, Jane JA, Edlich RF: Injury scale for comprehensive management of CNS trauma. *JACEP* 1979;**8**:64.

wave pattern was found if the transection was at a higher midbrain level **(cerveau isole).** Studies involving cats have also suggested that REM sleep is initiated by nuclei in the brain stem. The **midline raphe system** of the pons may be the main center responsible for bringing on sleep; it may act through the secretion of serotonin, which modifies many of the effects of the reticular activating system. Paradoxic REM sleep follows when a second secretion (norepinephrine), produced by the **locus ceruleus,** supplants the raphe secretion. The effects resemble normal wakefulness.

Destruction of the rostral reticular nucleus of the pons abolishes REM sleep, usually without affecting slow-wave sleep or arousal. REM sleep is suppressed by dopa or monoamine oxidase inhibitors, which increase the norepinephrine concentration in the brain. Lesions of the raphe nuclei in the pons cause prolonged wakefulness. The raphe nuclei contain appreciable amounts of serotonin, and it has been shown that treatment with p-chlorophenylalanine (which inhibits serotonin synthesis) causes wakefulness in cats. When cats are treated with compounds that increase serotonin, there is an increase in the amount of slow-wave sleep.

C. Clinical Correlations:

1. Somnambulism and nocturnal enuresis–Somnambulism (sleepwalking) and nocturnal enuresis (bed-wetting) are particularly apt to occur during arousal from slow-wave sleep. Somnambulists walk with their eyes open and avoid obstacles, but they cannot recall the episode (which may last several minutes) when they are awakened.

2. Hypersomnia and apnea–Hypersomnia (excessive daytime sleepiness) and recurrent apnea during sleep may occur. Affected patients are apt to be obese middle-aged men who snore loudly. Functional obstruction of the oropharyngeal airway during sleep has been implicated in these patients, and symptoms in severe cases may be relieved by tracheostomy.

3. Narcolepsy–Narcolepsy is a chronic clinical syndrome characterized by intermittent episodes of uncontrollable sleep. Sudden transient loss of muscle tone in the extremities or trunk **(cataplexy)** and pathologic muscle weakness during emotional reactions may also occur. There may be **sleep paralysis,** the inability to move in the interval between sleep and arousal, and **hypnogogic hallucinations** may occur at the onset of sleep. Sleep attacks can occur several times daily under appropriate or inappropriate circumstances, with or without forewarning. The attacks last from minutes to hours.

Narcolepsy usually persists throughout life. Although the attacks of somnolence and sleep may be relieved by medical treatment, the cataplexy and attacks of muscular weakness that accompany emotional reactions (eg, laughing and crying) are usually not affected by drug therapy. The nocturnal sleep of narcoleptics is usually unremarkable.

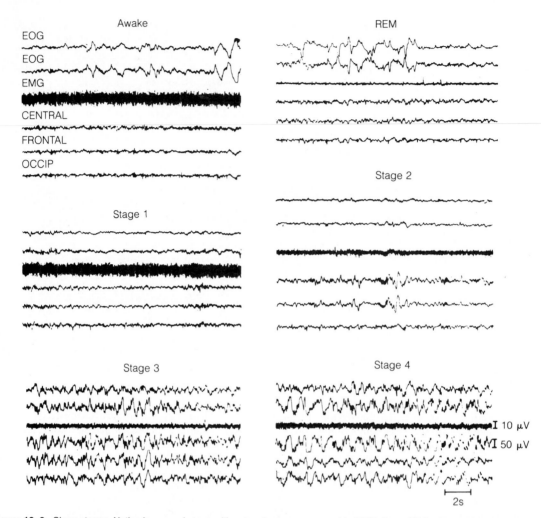

Figure 18–3. Sleep stages. Notice low muscle tone with extensive eye movement in REM sleep. EOG, electro-oculogram registering eye movements; EMG, electromyogram registering skeletal muscle activity. Central, Frontal, Occip, 3 electroencephalographic leads. (Reproduced, with permission, from Kales A et al: Sleep and dreams: Recent research on clinical aspects. *Ann Intern Med* 1968;**68**:1078.)

CASE 24

A 64-year-old right-handed man was admitted with subacute weakness and numbness of the left arm and leg. The patient was slightly confused and unable to speak clearly. In the previous several months, he had experienced a dozen or so transient episodes of unsteadiness of gait with weakness in both legs, together with dizziness and ringing in the left ear. Once or twice while walking in the park, he had to stop because of sharp pains in his left leg. These pains went away after a few minutes.

Neurologic examination showed a well-muscled, cooperative patient with barely intelligible speech **(dysarthria).** Findings included a left pupil that was slightly larger than the right, weakness of the right lateral rectus muscle, nystagmus on left and right gaze, decreased pain sensation in the right side of the face,

decreased right corneal reflex, paralysis of the right side of the lower face, decreased gag reflex, an inability to swallow on command, and the tongue in midline location but weak in lateral movement. The patient's strength was uniformly decreased in all extremities but more so on the right. Results of finger-to-nose and heel-to-shin tests were abnormal. Deep tendon reflexes were hyperactive, with clonus of the quadriceps muscle and bilateral plantar extensor responses. Pain sensation was decreased in the left leg; vibratory and position senses were decreased in both legs. There were no visual field defects. Laboratory findings were normal, but blood pressure was 200/90, and pulses in the lower extremities ranged from decreased to absent. The patient refused any radiologic tests.

What is the differential diagnosis? What is the most likely diagnosis?

Cases are discussed further in Chapter 25.

REFERENCES

Crick FC, Koch C: Some reflections on visual awareness. *Cold Spring Harb Symp Biol* 1990;**55:**953.

Globus GG, Maxwell G, Savodnik P (editors): *Consciousness and the Brain.* Plenum Press, 1976.

Plum F, Posner JB: *The Diagnosis of Stupor and Coma,* 3rd ed. Davis, 1980.

Steriade M, McCormick DA, Sejnowski TJ: Thalamocortical oscillations in the sleeping and aroused brain. *Science* 1993;**262:**679.

19

The Limbic System

The **great limbic lobe,** described by Broca in 1874, was so named because this cortical complex formed a limbus (border) between the diencephalon and the more lateral neocortex of the telencephalic hemispheres (Fig 19–1). This limbic lobe was said to consist of a ring of cortex outside the corpus callosum, largely made up of the subcallosal and cingulate gyri as well as the parahippocampal gyrus (Fig 19–2). Later anatomic studies showed that the **hippocampal formation** (a more primitive cortical complex) was situated even closer to the diencephalon, in part below, in part on top, of the neocortical corpus callosum. The formation consists of the **hippocampus (Ammon's horn)**; the **dentate gyrus**; the **supracallosal gyrus** (also termed the **indusium griseum**), which is the gray matter on top of the corpus callosum; the **fornix**; and a primitive precommisural area known as the **septal area** (Fig 19–3).

Histology. The three concentric cortical regions (hippocampal formation, great limbic lobe, and neocortex) have different cytoarchitectonic features. The most primitive cortex, which constitutes the hippocampus, also termed the **archicortex,** has three layers. The cortex of the transitional limbic lobe—the **mesocortex,** or **juxtallocortex**—has as many as five layers. The remaining cortex, known as the **neocortex,** or **isocortex,** has five or six layers and covers most of the cerebral hemispheres (see Chapter 10). In phylogenetically recent species such as humans, the extent of the neocortex is much greater than in lower forms (Fig 19–4).

The concentric architecture is more obvious in lower species; it is also present in higher species including humans and underscores the tiered arrangement of a phylogenetically advanced neocortex, which rests upon a more primitive limbic lobe and hippocampal formation. Because of their purported role in olfaction, the hippocampal formation and limbic lobe were also termed the rhinencephalon ("smell-brain"). More recent work has shown that many of the structures are only indirectly related to the sense of smell but are directly involved in primitive, vital, visceral functions.

Such names as the visceral brain, vital brain, emotional brain, and limbic brain were discontinued in favor of the more neutral **limbic system.** In general, this system includes phylogenetically ancient portions of the cerebral cortex, related subcortical structures, and fiber pathways that interconnect with the diencephalon and brain stem (Table 19–1).

The basic functions of the limbic system contribute to the continuation of the species as well as to the preservation of the individual. These functions include feeding behavior; aggression; the expression of emotion; and the autonomic, behavioral, and endocrinal aspects of sexual response. Smell plays an important role in triggering these types of behavior and sometimes recalls memories. The neocortex, on the other hand, is involved in somatic functions such as motor control and interpretation of sensation and in mental capacities for reasoning, remembering, and converting information into action.

OLFACTORY SYSTEM

The **olfactory receptors** are specialized neurons located in the **olfactory mucous membrane,** a portion of the nasal mucosa. The olfactory mucous membrane is blanketed by a thin layer of mucous, produced by Bowman's glands. The olfactory receptors are highly sensitive and respond with depolarizations when confronted with odor-producing molecules that dissolve in the mucous layer. The olfactory receptors contain, in their membranes, specialized odorant receptors that are coupled to G-protein molecules, which link these receptors to adenylate cyclase. When an appropriate odiferous molecule binds to the olfactory receptor, it activates the G-protein molecule, which via adenylate cyclase, generates cyclic AMP; this, in turn, leads to opening of Na^+ channels, generating a depolarization in the olfactory receptor.

The axons of the olfactory receptors travel within 10 to 15 **olfactory nerves** to convey the sensation of smell from the upper nasal mucosa through the cribiform

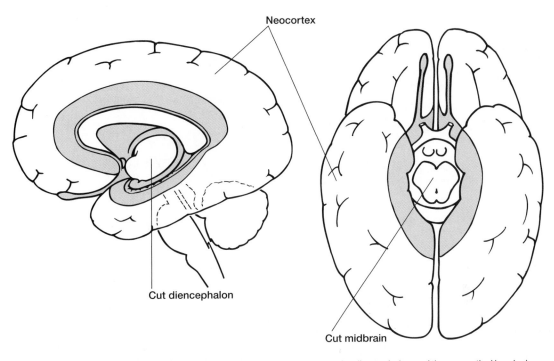

Figure 19–1. Schematic illustration of the location of the limbic system between the diencephalon and the neocortical hemispheres.

plate to the **olfactory bulb** (Figs 19–5 and 19–6). The olfactory bulb and **olfactory tract (peduncle)** lie in the **olfactory sulcus** on the orbital surface of the frontal lobe. As the tract passes posteriorly, it divides into lateral and medial olfactory striae (Fig 19–7). Within the olfactory bulb, the olfactory receptor axons terminate in specialized synaptic arrangements (termed **glomeruli**) on the dendrites of **mitral cells** (Fig 19–6). The mitral cells, in turn, send their axons posteriorly via the **olfactory tracts** (also termed the **medial** and **lateral olfactory stria**) to the olfactory cortex.

The **lateral olfactory stria** is the projection bundle of fibers that passes laterally along the floor of the lateral fissure and enters the **olfactory projection area** near the uncus in the temporal lobe (Fig 19–7). This area, which receives olfactory information, includes the **pyriform** and **entorhinal** cortex and parts of the **amygdala.** The pyriform cortex projects, in turn, via the thalamus to the frontal lobe, where conscious discrimination of odors presumably occurs.

The small **medial olfactory stria** passes medially and up toward the subcallosal gyrus near the inferior part of the corpus callosum. It carries the axons of some mitral cells to the **anterior olfactory nucleus,** which sends its axons back to the olfactory bulbs on both sides, presumably as part of a feedback circuit that modulates the sensitivity of olfactory sensation. Other olfactory fibers reach the **anterior perforated substance,** a thin layer of gray matter with many openings that permit the small lenticulostriate arteries to enter the brain; it extends from the olfactory striae to the optic tract. These fibers and the medial stria serve olfactory reflex reactions.

Clinical Correlations

Anosmia, or absence of the sense of smell, is not usually noticed unless it is bilateral. Most commonly,

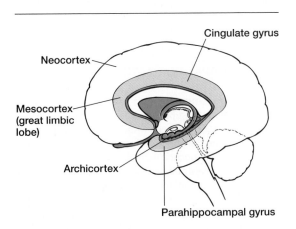

Figure 19–2. Schematic illustration of the concentric main components of the limbic system.

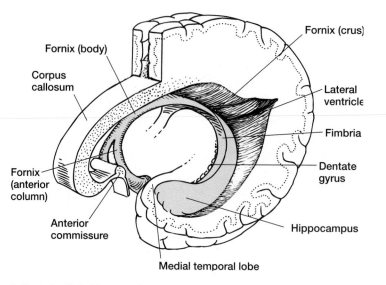

Fornix (body)

Corpus
callosum

Fornix
(anterior
column)

Anterior
commissure

Medial temporal lobe

Fornix (crus)

Lateral
ventricle

Fimbria

Dentate
gyrus

Hippocampus

Figure 19–3. Schematic illustration (left oblique view) of the position of the hippocampal formation within the left hemisphere.

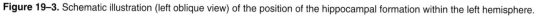

anosomia occurs as a result of **nasal infections,** including the common cold. **Head trauma** can produce anosmia as a result of injury to the cribiform plate with damage to the olfactory nerves, bulbs, or tracts. Tumors at the base of the frontal lobe **(olfactory groove meningiomas),** and frontal lobe gliomas that invade or compress the olfactory bulbs or tracts, may cause unilateral or bilateral anosmia; because damage to the frontal lobes often results in changes in behavior, it is essential in examining any patient with abnormal behavior to carefully examine the sense of smell on both sides.

Because olfactory information contributes importantly to the sense of flavor, patients with anosmia may complain of loss of taste or of loss of the ability to discriminate flavors.

Olfactory hallucinations, also termed uncinate hallucinations, may occur in patients with lesions involving the primary olfactory cortex, the uncus, or hippocampus; the patient usually perceives the presence of a pungent, often disagreeable, odor. Olfactory hallucinations may be associated with complex partial seizures (uncinate seizures). Their presence should suggest the possibility of focal pathology (including mass lesions) in the temporal lobe. An example of this is provided in Clinical Illustration 19–1.

CLINICAL ILLUSTRATION 19–1

A brilliant 38-year-old composer, who had been previously well, began to suffer from severe headaches and became increasingly irritable. He also began to experience olfactory hallucinations. A colleague noted that, "at the end of the second concert . . . he revealed that he had experienced a curious odor

of some indefinable burning smell." He was seen by several physicians, who diagnosed a "neurotic disorder," and he was referred for psychotherapy.

Several months later, the patient was seen by a physician who noticed papilledema. Several days later, he lapsed into a coma and despite emergency neurosurgical exploration, died. Postmortem examination revealed a large glioblastoma multiforme in the right temporal lobe.

The patient was George Gershwin, and this case illustrates the "George Gershwin syndrome," in which a hemispheric mass lesion (often a tumor) can remain clinically silent, although it is expanding. We now know that olfactory hallucinations should raise suspicion about a temporal lobe mass. Careful examination of this patient might have provided additional evidence of a mass lesion (eg, an upper homonymous quadrantanopsia; see Chapter 15 and Fig 15–15, lesion D) because of involvement of optic radiation fibers in Meyer's loop.

HIPPOCAMPAL FORMATION

The **hippocampal formation** consists of the dentate gyrus, the hippocampus, and neighboring subiculum.

The **dentate gyrus** is a thin, scalloped strip of cortex that lies on the upper surface of the parahippocampal gyrus. It connects with the supracallosal gyrus.

The **hippocampus,** a primitive cortical structure (also called Ammon's horn), extends the length of the floor of the inferior horn of the lateral ventricle and becomes continuous with the fornix below the splenium of the corpus callosum (see Fig 19–3). The name "hippocampus," which also means "seahorse" reflects the shape of this structure in coronal section (Fig 19–8).

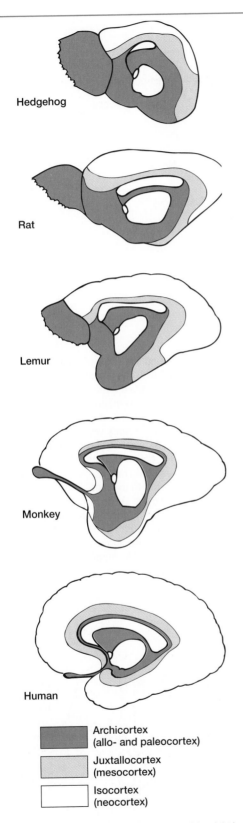

Figure 19–4. Diagrams of the medial aspect of the right hemisphere in five species. Note the relative increase in size of the human neocortex (isocortex).

The primitive cortex of the hippocampus is rolled, as seen in coronal sections, in a jelly-roll-like manner (Figs 19–9 and 19–11). At early stages in development (and in primitive mammals) the hippocampus is located anteriorly and constitutes part of the outer mantle of the brain (see Fig 19–4). However, in the fully developed human brain, the hippocampus has been displaced inferiorly and medially and is rolled inwardly, accounting for its jelly-roll-like structure.

For purposes of study, the hippocampus has been divided into several sectors, partly on the basis of fiber connections and partly because pathologic processes, such as ischemia, produce neuronal injury that is most severe in a portion of the hippocampus (H_1 [also termed CA_1 and CA_2], the Sommer sector; see Fig 19–9).

The dentate gyrus and the hippocampus itself show the histologic features of an archicortex with three layers: dendrite, pyramidal cell, and axon. The transitional cortex from the archicortex of the hippocampal to the six-layered neocortex (in this area called the subiculum) is juxtallocortex, or mesocortex, with four or five distinct cortical layers (Figs 19–8 and 19–9).

Hippocampal input and **output** have been carefully studied. The hippocampus receives input from many parts of the neocortex, especially the temporal neocortex. These cortical areas project to the entorhinal cortex within the parahippocampal gyrus (Fig 19–9). From the entorhinal cortex, axons project to the

Table 19–1. Some limbic system connections.

Structure	Connections
Dentate gyrus	From entorhinal cortex (via perforant pathway and alvear pathway) To hippocampus (via mossy fibers)
Hippocampus	From dentate gyrus (via mossy fibers), septum (via fornix), limbic lobe (via cingulum) To mamillary bodies, anterior thalamus, septal area, and tuber cinereum (via fornix); subcallosal area (via longitudinal striae)
Septal area	From olfactory bulb, amygdala, fornix To medial forebrain bundle, hypothalamus, habenula
Amygdala	From primitive temporal cortex and sensory association cortex, opposite amygdala (via anterior commissure) To hypothalamus (direct amygdalo-fugal pathway), septal area and hypothalamus (via stria terminalis)

Archicortex (allo- and paleocortex)

Juxtallocortex (mesocortex)

Isocortex (neocortex)

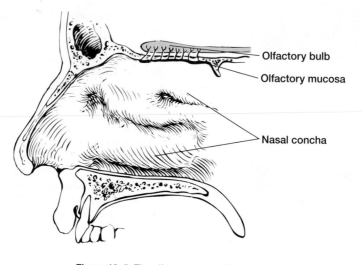

Figure 19–5. The olfactory nerves (lateral view).

dentate gyrus and hippocampus (Fig 19–10); these axons travel along the **perforant pathway** and **alvear pathways** to reach the dentate gyrus and hippocampus (Fig 19–11).

Within the dentate gyrus and hippocampus, there is an orderly array of synaptic connections (Fig 19–11). Granule cells of the dentate gyrus send axons **(mossy fibers)** that terminate on pyramidal neurons in the CA3 region of the hippocampus. These neurons, in turn, project to the fornix, which is a major efferent path-

way. Collateral branches (termed **Schaffer collaterals**) from the CA3 neurons project to the CA1 region.

The **fornix** is an arched white fiber tract extending from the hippocampal formation to the diencephalon and septal area. It constitutes the major outflow pathway from the hippocampus. Its fibers start as the **alveus,** a white layer on the ventricular surface of the hippocampus that contains fibers from the dentate gyrus and hippocampus (Figs 19–8 and 19–11). From the alveus, fibers lead to the medial aspect of the hippocampus and form the **fimbria** of the fornix, a flat band of white fibers that ascends below the splenium of the corpus callosum and bends forward to course above the thalamus, forming the crus (or beginning of the body) of the fornix. The hippocampal commissure, or commissure of the fornix, is a variable collection of

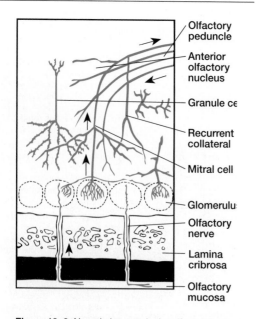

Olfactory peduncle

Anterior olfactory nucleus

Granule ce

Recurrent collateral

Mitral cell

Glomerulu

Olfactory nerve

Lamina cribrosa

Olfactory mucosa

Figure 19–6. Neural elements in the olfactory bulb.

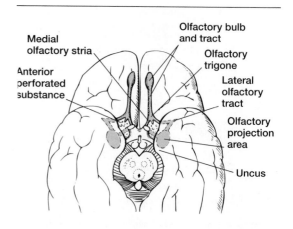

Figure 19–7. Olfactory connections projected on the basal aspect of the brain (intermediate olfactory tract not labeled).

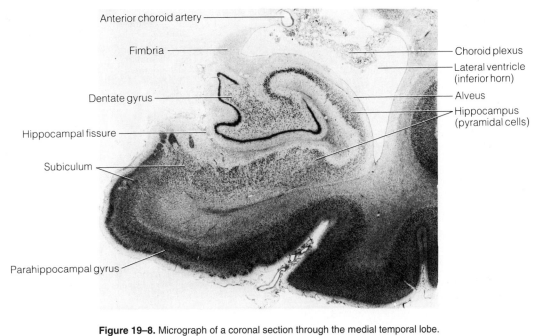

Figure 19–8. Micrograph of a coronal section through the medial temporal lobe.

transverse fibers connecting the two crura of the fornix. The two crura lie close to the undersurface of the corpus callosum and join anteriorly to form the body of the fornix. From the body, the two columns of the fornix bend inferiorly and posteriorly to enter the anterior part of the lateral wall of the third ventricle. Many axons in the fornix terminate in the **mamillary bodies** of the hypothalamus (Fig 19–10). Other axons, traveling in the fornix, terminate in other subcortical structures including the septal area and anterior thalamus.

As noted above, hippocampal efferent axons travel in the fornix and synapse on neurons in the mammillary bodies. These neurons project axons, within the **mamillo-thalamic** tract, to the anterior thalamus. The anterior thalamus projects, in turn, to the cingulate gyrus, which contains a bundle of myelinated fibers, the **cingulum** that curves around the corpus callosum to reach the parahippocampal gyrus (Fig 19–10). Thus, the following circuit is formed:

parahippocampal gyrus → hippocampus → fornix → mammillary bodies → anterior thalamic nuclei → cingulate gyrus → parahippocampal gyrus

This circuit, called the **Papez circuit** after the neuroanatomist who defined it, ties together the cerebral cortex and the hypothalamus, provides an anatomic substrate for the convergence of cognitive (cortical) activities, emotional experience, and expression.

A number of cortical structures feed into, or are part of, the Papez circuit. The **subcallosal gyrus** is the portion of gray matter that covers the inferior aspect of the rostrum of the corpus callosum. It continues posteri-

orly as the **cingulate gyrus** and **parahippocampal gyrus** (Figs 19–2 and 19–10). In the area of the genu of the corpus callosum, the subcallosal gyrus also contains fibers coursing into the supracallosal gyrus. The **supracallosal gyrus (indusium griseum)** is a thin layer of gray matter that extends from the subcallosal gyrus and covers the upper surface of the corpus callosum (Fig 19–10). The **medial** and **lateral longitudinal striae** are delicate longitudinal strands that extend along the upper surface of the corpus callosum to and from the hippocampal formation.

Anterior Commissure

The anterior commissure is a band of white fibers that crosses the midline to join both cerebral hemispheres (see Fig 19–10). It contains two fiber systems, an interbulbar system that joins both anterior olfactory nuclei near the olfactory bulbs, and an intertemporal system that connects the temporal lobe areas of both cerebral hemispheres.

Septal Area

The septal area, or septal complex, is an area of gray matter lying above the lamina terminalis, near and around the anterior commissure (Fig 19–12). A portion of it, the **septum lucidum,** is a double sheet of gray matter below the genu of the corpus callosum. In humans, the septum separates the anterior portions of the lateral ventricles.

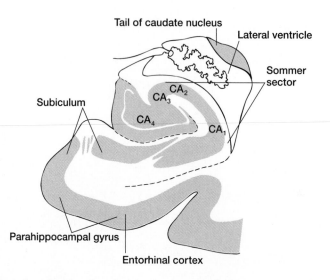

Figure 19–9. Schematic illustration of a coronal section showing the components of the hippocampal formation and subiculum (compare with Fig 19–8). CA$_1$ through CA$_4$ are sectors of the hippocampus. Much of the hippocampal input is relayed via the entorhinal cortex from the temporal neocortex.

Amygdala & Hypothalamus

The amygdala **(amygdaloid nuclear complex)** is a gray matter mass that lies in the medial temporal pole, between the uncus and the parahippocampal gyrus (Figs 19–12 and 19–13). It is situated just anterior to the tip of the anterior horn of the lateral ventricle. Its fiber connections include the semicircular **stria terminalis** to the septal area and anterior hypothalamus and a direct **amygdalofugal pathway** to the middle portion of the hypothalamus (Fig 19–12). Some fibers of the stria pass across the anterior commissure to the opposite amygdala. The stria terminalis courses along the inferior horn and body of the lateral ventricle to the septal and preoptic areas and the hypothalamus.

Two distinct groups of neurons, the large **basolateral nuclear group** and the smaller **corticomedial nuclear group,** can be differentiated. The basolateral nuclear group receives higher-order sensory information from association areas in the frontal, temporal, and insular cortex. Axons run back from the amygdala to the association regions of the cortex, suggesting that activity in the amygdala may modulate sensory information processing in the association cortex. The basolateral amygdala is also connected, via the stria terminalis and the amygdalofugal pathway, to the ventral striatum and the thalamus.

The corticomedial nuclear group of the amygdala, located close to the olfactory cortex, is interconnected with it as well as the olfactory bulb. Connections also run, via the stria terminalis and amygdalofugal pathway, to and from the brain stem and hypothalamus.

Because of its interconnections with the sensory association cortex and hypothalamus, it has been sug-

gested that the amygdala plays an important role in establishing associations between sensory inputs and various affective states. The amygdala also appears to participate in regulating endocrine activity, sexual behavior, and food and water intake, possibly by modulating hypothalamic activity. As described below, because of bilateral damage to the amygdala and neighboring temporal cortex, the Klüver-Bucy syndrome is produced.

The fornix and **medial forebrain bundle,** coursing within the hypothalamus, are also considered part of the limbic system.

FUNCTIONS & DISORDERS

A variety of experimental studies in both animals and humans indicate that stimulating or damaging some components of the limbic system causes profound changes. Stimulation alters somatic motor responses, leading to bizarre eating and drinking habits, changes in sexual and grooming behavior, and defensive postures of attack and rage. There are changes in autonomic responses, altering cardiovascular or gastrointestinal function, and in personality, with shifts from passive to aggressive behavior. Damage to some areas of the limbic system may also affect memory or olfactory function.

Autonomic Nervous System

The hierarchical organization of the autonomic nervous system (see Chapter 20) includes the limbic system; most of the limbic system output connects to the hypothalamus, in part via the **medial forebrain bun-**

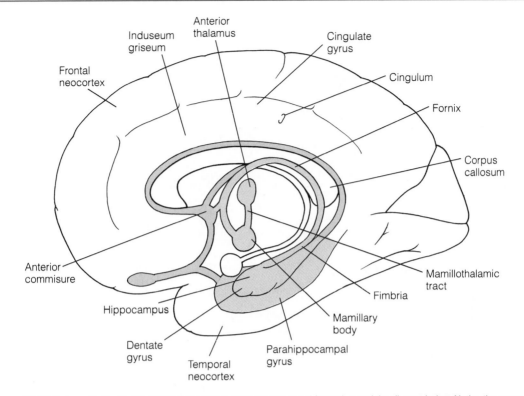

Figure 19–10. Schematic illustration of pathways between the hippocampal formation and the diencephalon. Notice the presence of a loop (Papez circuit) including the parahippocampal gyrus, hippocampus, mammillary bodies, anterior thalamus, and cingulate gyrus. Notice also that the neocortex feeds into this loop.

dle. The specific sympathetic or parasympathetic aspects of autonomic control are not well localized in the limbic system, however.

Stimulation of various limbic system structures produces changes in cardiovascular or gastrointestinal functions, and there are reports of gastric ulcer formation and emotional changes.

Septal Area

The septal area, or complex, is relatively large in such animals as the cat and rat. Because it is a pivotal region with afferent fibers from the olfactory and limbic systems and efferent fibers to the hypothalamus, epithalamus, and midbrain, no single function can be ascribed to the area. Experimental studies have shown the septal area to be a substrate mediating the sensations of self-stimulation or self-reward. Test animals will press a bar repeatedly, even endlessly, to receive a (presumed) pleasurable stimulus in the septal area. Additional areas of pleasure have been found in the hypothalamus and midbrain; the stimulation of yet other areas reportedly evokes the opposite response. Recent studies in humans indicate that antipsychotic drugs may act by modifying dopaminergic inputs from the midbrain to the septal area. Other studies suggest that an ascending pathway to the septal area may be involved in the euphoric feelings described by narcotics addicts.

Behavior

Several of the hypothalamic regions associated with typical patterns of behavior such as eating, drinking, sexual behavior, and aggression receive input from limbic system structures, especially the amygdaloid and septal complexes. Lesions in these areas can modify, inhibit, or unleash these behaviors. Some of the behavioral patterns are quite different; for example, lesions in the lateral amygdala induce unrestrained eating (bulemia), while those in the medial amygdala induce anorexia, accompanied by hypersexuality (Fig 19–14). Electrical stimulation of the amygdala in humans may produce fear, anxiety, or rage and aggression. Amygdalectomy, which in some cases has been performed to suppress these antisocial traits in patients, has sometimes been followed by hypersexuality.

Memory

The three types of memory are **immediate recall, short-term memory,** and **long-term memory.** The hippocampus is involved in converting short-term memory (up to 60 minutes) to long-term memory (several days or more). The anatomic substrate for long-term memory probably includes the temporal lobes. Patients with bilateral removal of the hippocampus (as

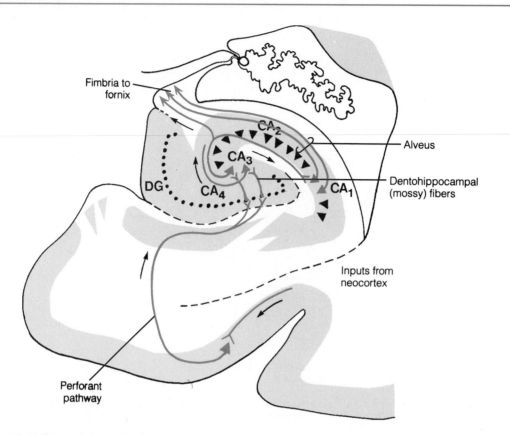

Figure 19–11. Schematic illustration of the major connections to, within, and from the hippocampal formation. (Compare with Fig 19–8.) Dentate granule cells (DG) project to pyramidal neurons in the hippocampus.

part of a bilateral temporal lobectomy for epilepsy) demonstrate **anterograde amnesia,** in which events prior to surgery are retained but no new long-term memories can be established. This lack of memory storage is also present in patients with bilateral interruption of the fornices (eg, by removal of a colloid cyst at the interventricular foramen). Memory processes also involve other structures including the dorsomedial nuclei of the thalamus and the mammillary bodies of the hypothalamus as discussed in Chapter 21.

The occurrence of **long-term potentiation,** a process whereby synaptic strength is increased when specific efferent inputs to the hippocampus are excited in a paired manner, provides a cellular/molecular basis for understanding the role of the hippocampus in memory and learning.

Other Disorders of the Limbic System

A. Klüver-Bucy Syndrome: This disturbance of limbic system activities occurs in patients with bilateral temporal lobe lesions. The major characteristics of this syndrome are **hyperorality,** characterized by a tendency to explore objects by placing them in the mouth together with the indiscriminate eating or chewing of objects and all kinds of food; **hypersexuality,** sometimes described as a lack of sexual inhibition; **psychic blindness,** or visual agnosia, in which objects are no longer recognized; and **personality changes,** usually with the development of abnormal passivity or docility. The psychic blindness observed in the Klüver-Bucy syndrome presumably results from damage to the amydalae, which normally functions as a site of transfer of information between sensory association cortex and the hypothalamus; after damage to the amygdala, visual stimuli can no longer be paired with affective (pleasurable or unpleasant) responses.

B. Temporal Lobe Epilepsy: The temporal lobe (especially the hippocampus and amygdala) has a lower threshold for epileptic seizure activity than do the other cortical areas. The seizures, called **psychomotor (complex partial) seizures,** differ from the jacksonian seizures that originate in or near the motor cortex (see Chapter 21). Temporal lobe epilepsy may include abnormal sensations, especially bizarre olfactory sensations, sometimes called uncinate fits; repeated involuntary movements such as chewing, swallowing, and lip smacking; disorders of consciousness; memory loss; hallucinations; and disorders of recall and recognition.

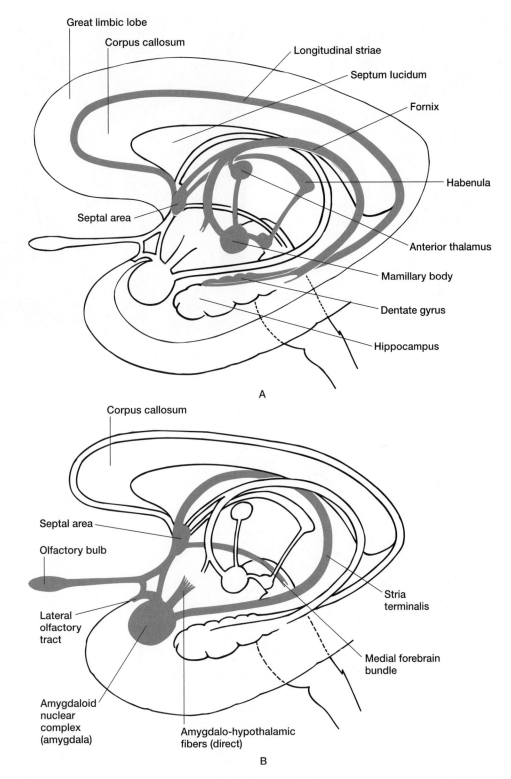

Figure 19–12. Diagram of the principal connections of the limbic system. **A:** Hippocampal system and great limbic lobe. **B:** Olfactory and amygdaloid connections.

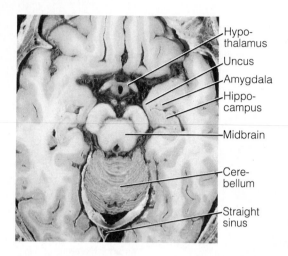

Figure 19–13. Horizontal section through the head at the level of the midbrain and amygdala. (Reproduced, with permission, from DeGroot, J: *Correlative Neuroanatomy of Computed Tomography and Magnetic Resonance Imaging*, Lea & Febiger, 1984.)

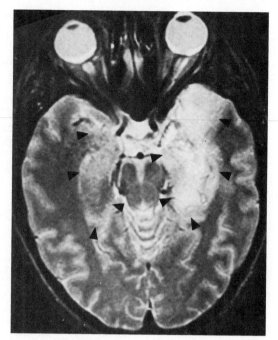

Figure 19–15. MR I of horizontal section through the head at the level of the temporal lobe. The large lesion in the left temporal lobe and a smaller one on the right side are indicated by arrowheads. CT scanning confirmed the presence of multiple small hemorrhagic lesions in both temporal lobes.

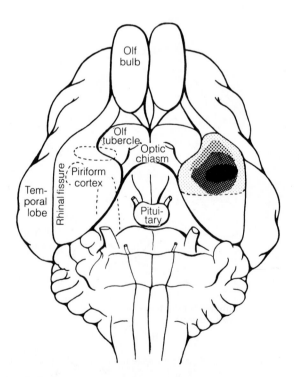

Figure 19–14. Site of lesions producing hypersexuality in male cats. Destroying the black area always produced hypersexuality. The incidence of hypersexuality in animals with lesions in the surrounding lighter zones was not as high. Olf = olfactory. (Reproduced, with permission, from Green J et al: Rhinencephalic lesions and behavior in cats. *J Comp Neurol* 1957;**108**:505.)

The underlying cause of the seizures may sometimes be difficult to determine. A tumor (eg, astrocytoma or oligodendroglioma) may be responsible, or glial scar formation after trauma to the temporal poles may trigger seizures. Small hamartomas or areas of temporal sclerosis have been found in patients with temporal lobe epilepsy. Although anticonvulsant drugs are often given to control the seizures, they may be ineffective. In these cases, neurosurgical removal of the seizure focus in the temporal lobe may provide excellent seizure control.

CASE 25

A 59-year-old unemployed male was brought to the hospital by his wife because of the display of bizarre behavior for nearly a week. During the prior two days he had been confused and had suffered two shaking "fits." His wife said that he did not seem to be able to remember things. Twenty-four hours prior to admission, he had developed a severe headache, generalized malaise, and a temperature of 102 °F (38.8 °C) and refused to eat. Examination showed the patient was lethargic and confused, had dysphasia, and was generally in poor health. He could only remember one of three objects after 3 minutes. There was no stiffness of the neck. The serum glucose level was 165 mg/dL. Lumbar puncture findings showed pressure, 220 mm of water; white blood count 153/μL, mostly lymphocytes; red blood cells, 1450/μl, with xanthochromia; protein, 71 mg/dL; and glucose, 101 mg/dL. An electroencephalogram showed focal slowing over the temporal region on both sides, with some sharp periodic bursts. Brain biopsy revealed the features of an active granuloma, without pus formation. Results of CT scanning are shown in Figure 19–15.

What is the differential diagnosis?

Over the next eight days, the patient became increasingly drowsy and dysphasic. A repeat scan showed extensive defects of both temporal lobes. The patient died on the tenth day after admission, despite appropriate drug treatment.

Cases are discussed further in Chapter 25.

REFERENCES

Ben-Ari Y (editor): *The Amygdaloid Complex.* Elsevier, 1981.

Cofer CN (editor): *The Structure of Human Memory.* Freeman, 1976.

deGroot J: The limbic system: An anatomical and functional orientation. Chap 6, pp 89–106, In: *American Handbook of Psychiatry.* Vol 6. Arieti S (editor). Basic Books, 1975.

Doty RL: *Mammalian Olfaction, Reproductive Processes, and Behavior.* Academic Press, 1976.

Eslinger PJ, Damasio AR, Van Hoesen GW: Olfactory dysfunction in man: A review of anatomical and behavioral aspects. *Brain Cogn* 1982;**2**:259.

Isaacson RL: *The Limbic System,* 2nd ed. Plenum, 1982.

Livingston KE, Hornykiewicz O (editors): *Limbic Mechanisms.* Plenum, 1978.

Moulton DG, Beidler LM: Structure and function in the peripheral olfactory system. *Physiol Rev* 1987;**47**:1.

20

The Autonomic Nervous System

The autonomic (visceral) nervous system (ANS) is concerned with control of the target tissues: the cardiac muscle, the smooth muscle in viscera, and the glands. It also helps maintain a constant internal body environment (homeostasis). The autonomic nervous system consists of efferent pathways, afferent pathways, and groups of neurons in the brain and spinal cord that regulate the system's functions. Autonomic reflex activity in the spinal cord is modulated by brain centers, so that there is a hierarchical organization within the central nervous system itself.

AUTONOMIC OUTFLOW

The efferent components of the autonomic system are the sympathetic and parasympathetic divisions, which arise from preganglionic cell bodies in different locations. A two-neuron chain characterizes the structure of the autonomic outflow. The cell body of the primary neuron (the **presynaptic,** or **preganglionic,** neuron) within the central nervous system is located in the lateral gray column of the spinal cord or in the brain stem nuclei (see Chapter 8). It sends its axon out to synapse with the secondary neuron (the **postsynaptic,** or **postganglionic,** neuron) located in one of the autonomic ganglia. From there, the postganglionic axon passes to its terminal distribution in a target organ. Since the postganglionic fibers outnumber the preganglionic neurons by a ratio of about 32:1, a single preganglionic neuron may control the autonomic functions of a rather extensive terminal area.

Sympathetic Division

The sympathetic **(thoracolumbar)** division of the autonomic nervous system arises from preganglionic cell bodies located in the lateral cell columns of the 12 thoracic segments and the upper two lumbar segments of the spinal cord (Fig 20–1).

A. Preganglionic Efferent Fiber System: Preganglionic fibers are mostly myelinated. Coursing with the ventral roots, they form the **white communicating rami** of the thoracic and lumbar nerves, through which they reach the ganglia of the sympathetic chains or trunks (Fig 20–2). These **trunk ganglia** lie on the lateral sides of the bodies of the thoracic and lumbar vertebrae. Upon entering the ganglia, the fibers may synapse with a number of ganglion cells, pass up or down the sympathetic trunk to synapse with ganglion cells at a higher or lower level, or pass through the trunk ganglia and out to one of the collateral (intermediary) sympathetic ganglia (eg, the **celiac** and **mesenteric ganglia**).

The **splanchnic nerves** arising from the lower seven thoracic segments pass through the trunk ganglia to the **celiac** and **superior mesenteric ganglia.** There, synaptic connections occur with ganglion cells whose postganglionic axons then pass to the abdominal viscera via the **celiac plexus.** The splanchnic nerves arising from spinal cord segments in the lowest thoracic and upper lumbar region convey fibers to synaptic stations in the **inferior mesenteric ganglion** and to small ganglia associated with the **hypogastric plexus** through which postsynaptic fibers are distributed to the lower abdominal and pelvic viscera.

B. Postganglionic Efferent Fiber System: The mostly unmyelinated postganglionic fibers form the **gray communicating rami.** The fibers may course with the spinal nerve for some distance or go directly to their target tissues.

The gray communicating rami join each of the spinal nerves and distribute the vasomotor, pilomotor, and sweat gland innervation throughout the somatic areas. Branches of the **superior cervical sympathetic ganglion** enter into the formation of the sympathetic plexuses about the internal and external carotid arteries for distribution of sympathetic fibers to the head (Fig 20–3). The superior **cardiac nerves** from the three pairs of cervical sympathetic ganglia pass to the **cardiac plexus** at the base of the heart and distribute ac-

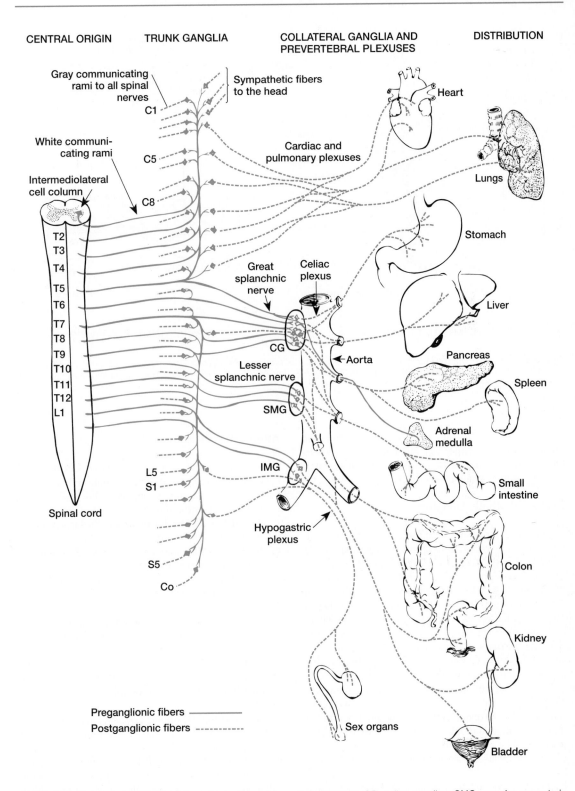

Figure 20–1. Sympathetic division of the autonomic nervous system (left half). CG, celiac ganglion; SMG, superior mesenteric ganglion; IMG, inferior mesenteric ganglion.

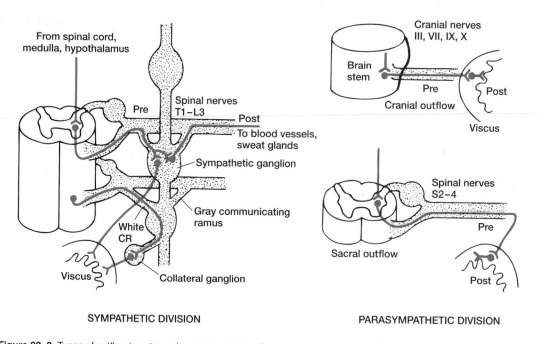

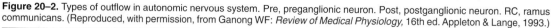

Figure 20–2. Types of outflow in autonomic nervous system. Pre, preganglionic neuron. Post, postganglionic neuron. RC, ramus communicans. (Reproduced, with permission, from Ganong WF: *Review of Medical Physiology,* 16th ed. Appleton & Lange, 1993.)

celerator fibers to the myocardium. Vasomotor branches from the upper five thoracic ganglia pass to the thoracic aorta and to the posterior **pulmonary plexus,** through which dilator fibers reach the bronchi.

Parasympathetic Division

The parasympathetic (craniosacral) division of the autonomic nervous system arises from preganglionic cell bodies in the gray matter of the brain stem and the middle three segments of the sacral cord (S2–S4) (Figs 20–2 and 20–4). Most of the preganglionic fibers run without interruption from their central origin either to the wall of the viscus they supply or to the site where they synapse with terminal ganglion cells associated with the **plexuses of Meissner** and **Auerbach** in the wall of the intestinal tract. The parasympathetic distribution is confined entirely to visceral structures.

Four cranial nerves convey preganglionic parasympathetic (visceral efferent) fibers: The **vagus nerve** (cranial nerve X) distributes its autonomic fibers to the thoracic and abdominal viscera via the **prevertebral plexuses.** The **pelvic nerve (nervus erigens)** distributes parasympathetic fibers to most of the large intestine and to the pelvic viscera and genitals via the **hypogastric plexus;** the **oculomotor, facial,** and **glossopharyngeal nerves** (cranial nerves III, VII, and IX) distribute parasympathetic or visceral efferent fibers to the head (Fig 20–3; see also Chapters 7 and 8).

Autonomic Plexuses

The autonomic plexuses are large networks of nerves that serve as areas of redistribution for the sympathetic and parasympathetic (and afferent) fibers that enter into their formation (Figs 20–1 and 20–4).

The **cardiac plexus,** located about the bifurcation of the trachea and roots of the great vessels at the base of the heart, is divided into superficial and deep parts. It is formed from the cardiac sympathetic nerves and cardiac branches of the vagus nerve, which it distributes to the myocardium and walls of the vessels leaving the heart.

The right and left **pulmonary plexuses** are intimately joined with the cardiac plexus and are located about the primary bronchi and pulmonary arteries at the roots of the lungs. They are formed from both the vagus and the upper thoracic sympathetic nerves and are distributed mainly to the vessels and bronchi of the lung.

The **celiac (solar) plexus** is located in the epigastric region of the abdomen over the abdominal aorta near the origin of the celiac and superior mesenteric arteries. It is formed from vagal fibers reaching it via the esophageal plexus, sympathetic fibers arising from celiac ganglia, and sympathetic fibers coursing down from the thoracic aortic plexus. The distribution of the celiac plexus includes most of the abdominal viscera, which it reaches by way of numerous subplexuses

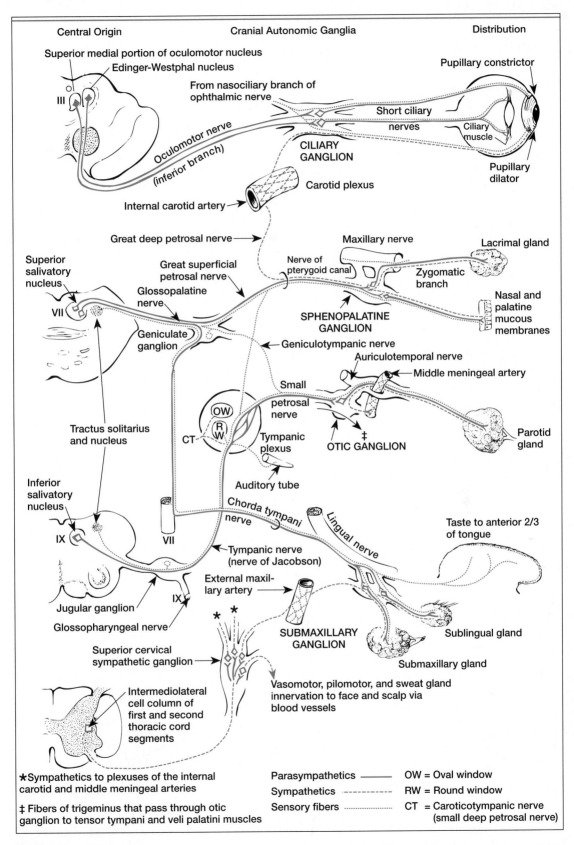

Figure 20–3. Autonomic nerves to the head. OW, oval window; RW, round window; CT, caroticotympanic (small deep petrosal) nerve.

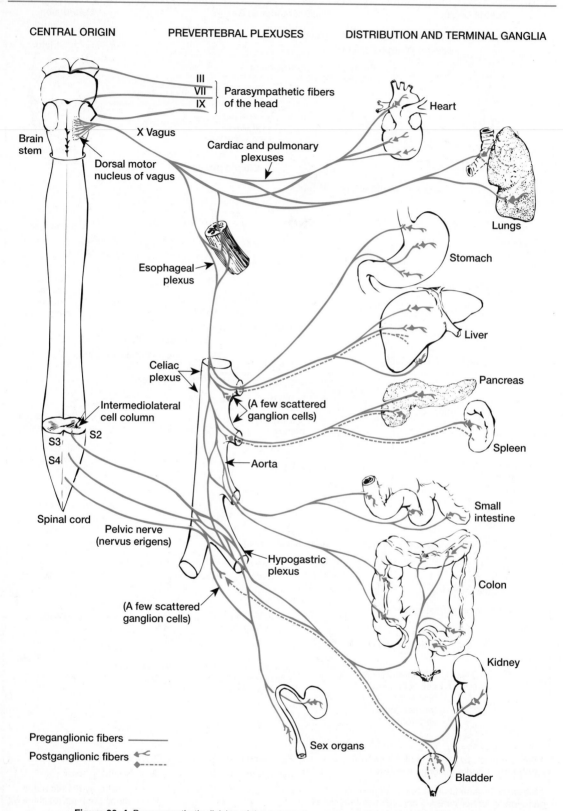

CENTRAL ORIGIN   PREVERTEBRAL PLEXUSES   DISTRIBUTION AND TERMINAL GANGLIA

Figure 20–4. Parasympathetic division of the autonomic nervous system (only left half shown).

along the various visceral branches of the aorta. These subplexuses include the phrenic, hepatic, splenic, superior gastric, suprarenal, renal, spermatic or ovarian, abdominal aortic, and superior and inferior mesenteric plexuses.

The **hypogastric plexus** is located in front of the fifth lumbar vertebra and the promontory of the sacrum. It receives sympathetic fibers from the aortic plexus and lumbar trunk ganglia and parasympathetic fibers from the pelvic nerve. Its two lateral portions, the **pelvic plexuses,** lie on either side of the rectum. Distribution to the pelvic viscera and genitals is effected by subplexuses that extend along the visceral branches of the hypogastric artery. These subplexuses of the hypogastric plexus include the middle hemorrhoidal plexus, to the rectum; the vesical plexus, to the bladder, seminal vesicles, and ductus deferens; the prostatic plexus, to the prostate, seminal vesicles, and penis; the vaginal plexus, to the vagina and clitoris; and uterine plexus, to the uterus and uterine tubes.

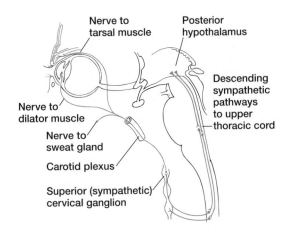

Figure 20–6. Sympathetic pathways to the eye and orbit. Interruption of these pathways inactivates the dilator muscle and thereby produces miosis, inactivates the tarsal muscle and produces the effect of enophthalmos, and reduces sweat secretion in the face (Horner's syndrome).

Clinical Correlations

Horner's syndrome consists of unilateral enophthalmos, ptosis, miosis, and loss of sweating over the ipsilateral half of the face or forehead (Fig 20–5). It is caused by ipsilateral involvement of the sympathetic pathways in the carotid plexus, the cervical sympathetic chain, the upper thoracic cord, or the brain stem (Fig 20–6).

Raynaud's disease affects the toes, the fingers, the edges of the ears, and the tip of the nose and spreads to involve large areas. Beginning with local changes when the parts are pale and cold, it may progress to local asphyxia characterized by a blue-gray cyanosis and, finally, symmetric dry gangrene. It is a disorder of the peripheral vascular innervation. **Scleroderma,** a thickening of the skin, that can be diffuse or circumscribed may be accompanied by or follow Raynaud's disease or other disturbances of peripheral vessel innervation.

Causalgia, a painful condition of the hands or feet, is caused by irritation of the median or sciatic nerve through injury. It is characterized by severe burning pain, glossy skin, swelling, redness, sweating, and trophic nail changes. Causalgia may be relieved by sympathetic blocks or sympathectomy of the involved areas.

Hirschsprung's disease (megacolon) consists of a tremendous dilatation of the colon, accompanied by chronic constipation. It is associated with congenital lack of parasympathetic ganglia and the existence of abnormal nerve fibrils in an apparently normal segment of large bowel wall.

AUTONOMIC INNERVATION OF THE HEAD

The autonomic supply to visceral structures in the head deserves special consideration (see Fig 20–3). The skin of the face and scalp (smooth muscle, glands, and vessels) receives postsynaptic sympathetic innervation only, from the superior cervical ganglion via a plexus that extends along the branches of the external carotid artery. The deeper structures (intrinsic eye muscles, salivary glands, and mucous membranes of the nose and pharynx), however, receive a dual autonomic supply from the sympathetic and parasympathetic divisions. The supply is mediated by the internal carotid plexus (postganglionic sympathetic innervation from the superior cervical plexus) and the visceral efferent fibers in four pairs of cranial nerves (parasympathetic innervation).

There are four pairs of autonomic ganglia—ciliary, pterygopalatine, otic, and submaxillary—in the head (see Fig 20–3). Each ganglion receives a sympathetic, a parasympathetic, and a sensory root (a branch of the trigeminal nerve). Only the parasympathetic fibers make synaptic connections within these ganglia, which

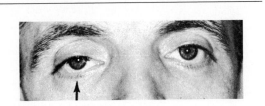

Figure 20–5. Horner's syndrome in the right eye, associated with a tumor in the superior sulcus of the right lung.

contain the cell bodies of the postganglionic parasympathetic fibers. The sympathetic and sensory fibers pass through these ganglia without interruption.

The **ciliary ganglion** is located between the optic nerve and the lateral rectus muscle in the posterior part of the orbit. Its parasympathetic root originates from cells in or near the Edinger-Westphal nucleus of the oculomotor nerve; its sympathetic root is composed of postganglionic fibers from the superior cervical sympathetic ganglion via the carotid plexus of the internal carotid artery. The sensory root comes from the nasociliary branch of the ophthalmic nerve. Distribution is through 10–12 short ciliary nerves that supply the ciliary muscle of the lens and the constrictor muscle of the iris. The dilator muscle of the iris is supplied by sympathetic nerves.

The **pterygopalatine ganglion,** located deep in the pterygopalatine fossa, is associated with the maxillary nerve. Its parasympathetic root arises from cells of the superior salivatory nucleus via the glossopalatine nerve and the great petrosal nerve. The ganglion's sympathetic root comes from the internal carotid plexus by way of the deep petrosal nerve, which joins the great superficial petrosal nerve to form the vidian nerve in the pterygoid (vidian) canal. Most of the sensory root fibers originate in the maxillary nerve, but a few arise in cranial nerves VII and IX via the tympanic plexus and vidian nerve. Distribution is through the **pharyngeal rami** to the mucous membranes of the roof of the pharynx; via the **nasal** and **palatine rami** to the mucous membranes of the nasal cavity, uvula, palatine tonsil, and hard and soft palates; and by way of the **orbital rami** to the periosteum of the orbit and the lacrimal glands.

The **otic ganglion** is located medial to the mandibular nerve just below the foramen ovale in the infratemporal fossa. Its parasympathetic root fibers arise in the inferior salivatory nucleus in the medulla and course via cranial nerve IX, the tympanic plexus, and the lesser superficial petrosal nerve; the sympathetic root comes from the superior cervical sympathetic ganglion via the plexus on the middle meningeal artery. Its sensory root probably includes fibers from cranial nerve IX and from the geniculate ganglion of cranial nerve VII via the tympanic plexus and the lesser superficial petrosal nerve. The otic ganglion supplies secretory and sensory fibers to the **parotid gland.** A few somatic motor fibers from the trigeminal nerve pass through the otic ganglion and supply the **tensor tympani** and **tensor veli palatini** muscles.

The **submaxillary ganglion** is located on the medial side of the mandible between the lingual nerve and the submaxillary duct. Its parasympathetic root fibers arise from the superior salivatory nucleus of nerve VII via the glossopalatine, chorda tympani, and lingual nerves, its sympathetic root from the plexus of the external maxillary artery, and its sensory root from the geniculate ganglion via the glossopalatine, chorda tympani, and lingual nerves. It is distributed to the **submaxillary** and **sublingual glands.**

VISCERAL AFFERENT PATHWAYS

Visceral afferent fibers have their cell bodies in **sensory ganglia** of some of the cranial and spinal nerves. Although a few of these fibers are myelinated, most are unmyelinated and have slow conduction velocities. The pain innervation of the viscera is summarized in Table 20–1.

Pathways to the Spinal Cord

Visceral afferent fibers to the spinal cord enter by way of the **middle sacral, thoracic,** and **upper lumbar nerves.** The sacral nerves carry sensory stimuli from the pelvic organs, and the nerve fibers are involved in reflexes of the sacral parasympathetic outflow that control various sexual responses, micturition, and defecation. Axons carrying visceral pain impulses from the heart, upper digestive tract, kidney, and gall bladder travel with the thoracic and upper lumbar nerves. These visceral afferent pathways are associated with sensations such as hunger, nausea, and poorly localized, dull visceral pain (Table 20–1). Pain impulses from a viscus may converge with pain impulses arising in a particular region of the skin causing referred pain. Typical examples of the phenomenon are the shoulder pains associated with gallstone attacks and the pains of the left arm or throat associated with myocardial ischemia (see also Chapter 14).

Table 20–1. Pain innervation of the viscera.

Division	Nerve(s) or segment(s)	Structures
Parasympathetic	Vagus	Esophagus, larynx, trachea
Sympathetic	Splanchnic (T7–L1)	Stomach, spleen, small viscera, colon, kidney, ureter, bladder, (upper part), uterus (fundus), ovaries, lungs
	Somatic (C7–L1)	Parietal pleura, diaphragm, parietal peritoneum
Parasympathetic	Pelvic (S2–S4)	Rectum, trigone of the bladder, prostate, urethra, cervix of the uterus, upper vagina

Pathways to the Brain Stem

Visceral afferent axons in the **glossopharyngeal nerve** and (especially) the **vagus nerve** carry a variety of sensations to the brain stem from the heart, great vessels, and respiratory and gastrointestinal tracts. The ganglia involved are the inferior glossopharyngeal nerve ganglion and the inferior vagus nerve ganglion (formerly called the nodose ganglion). The afferent fibers are also involved in reflexes that regulate blood pressure, respiratory rate and depth, and heart rate through specialized receptors or receptor areas. These **baroreceptors,** which are stimulated by pressure, are located in the aortic arch and carotid sinus (Fig 20–7).

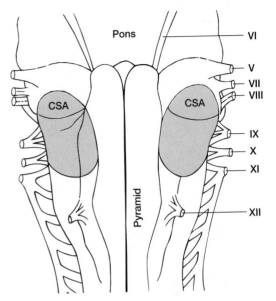

Figure 20–8. Chemosensitive areas (CSA) on the ventral surface of the medulla. (Modified and reproduced, with permission, from Mitchell RA, Severinghaus JW: Cerebrospinal fluid and regulation of respiration. *Physiol Physicians* 1965;**3**[3].)

The chemoreceptors are located in the aorta and carotid bodies, and the chemosensitive area is located in the medulla (Figs 20–7 and 20–8).

ORGANIZATION OF THE AUTONOMIC NERVOUS SYSTEM

There is a functional hierarchy in certain regions of the brain and spinal cord; through a complex interplay of connections, this hierarchy exerts its influence on visceral reflexes.

Spinal Cord

Autonomic reflexes such as peristalsis and micturition are mediated by the spinal cord, but descending pathways from the brain modify, inhibit, or initiate the reflexes (Fig 20–9). This can be demonstrated in patients who have suffered a transection of the spinal cord. A state of spinal shock develops, with hypotension and loss of reflexes governing micturition and defecation. Although the reflexes return after a few days or weeks, they may be incomplete or abnormal. For example, often the bladder cannot be completely emptied, which may result in cystitis, and voluntary initiation of micturition may be absent (**autonomic** or **neurogenic bladder**). Depending on the level of the transection, the neurogenic bladder may be spastic or flaccid (Figs 20–10 and 20–11).

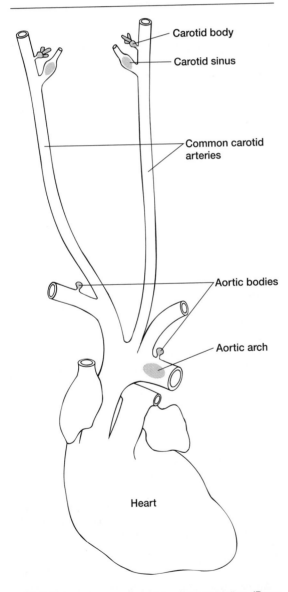

Figure 20–7. Location of carotid and aortic bodies. (Reproduced, with permission, from Ganong WF: *Review of Medical Physiology,* 14th ed. Appleton & Lange, 1989.)

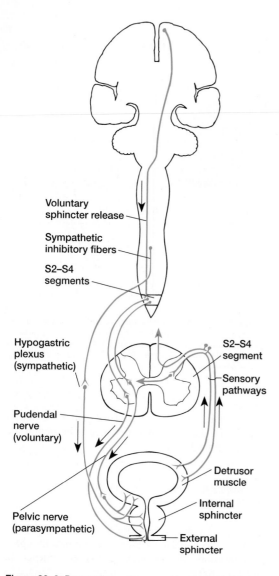

Voluntary
sphincter release

Sympathetic
inhibitory fibers

S2–S4
segments

Hypogastric
plexus
(sympathetic)

S2–S4
segment

Sensory
pathways

Pudendal
nerve
(voluntary)

Detrusor
muscle

Internal
sphincter

Pelvic nerve
(parasympathetic)

External
sphincter

Figure 20–9. Descending pathway and innervation of the urinary bladder.

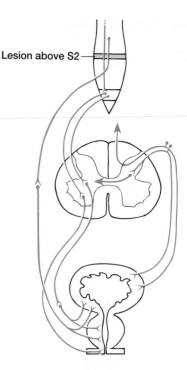

Lesion above S2

Figure 20–10. Spastic neurogenic bladder, caused by a more or less complete transection of the spinal cord above S2.

salivation, micturition, vomiting, sneezing, coughing, and gagging. The medulla is therefore an important link in the hierarchic chain of autonomic function control.

Pons

The **nucleus parabrachialis** consists of a group of neurons that are located near the superior cerebellar peduncle and that modulate the medullary neurons responsible for rhythmic respiration. This **pneumotaxic center** continues to control periodic respiration if the brain stem is transected between the pons and the medulla.

Midbrain

Accommodation, pupillary reactions to light, and other reflexes are integrated in the midbrain, near the nuclear complex of nerve III. Pathways from the hypothalamus to the visceral efferent nuclei in the brain stem course through the dorsal longitudinal fasciculus in the periaqueductal and periventricular gray matter.

Hypothalamus

An important area of coordination, the hypothalamus integrates autonomic activities in response to changes in the internal and external environments

Medulla

Medullary connections to and from the spinal cord are lightly myelinated fibers of the **tractus proprius** around the gray matter of the cord. Visceral afferent fibers of the glossopharyngeal and vagus nerves terminate in the solitary tract nucleus and are involved in control of respiratory, cardiovascular, and alimentary functions (see also Chapters 7 and 8). The major reflex actions have connections with visceral efferent nuclei of the medulla and areas of the reticular formation. These areas may contribute to the regulation of blood glucose levels and to other reflex functions, including

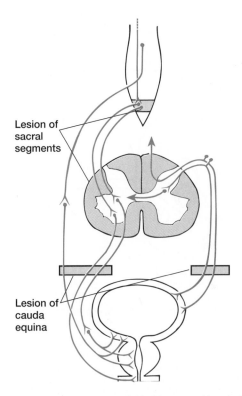

Lesion of sacral segments

Lesion of cauda equina

Figure 20–11. Flaccid neurogenic bladder, caused by a lesion of either the sacral portion of the spinal cord or the cauda equina.

(thermoregulatory mechanisms; see also Chapter 9). The posterior portion of the hypothalamus is involved with sympathetic function, and the anterior portion is involved with parasympathetic function. The descending pathway is the dorsal longitudinal fasciculus, and the connections with the hypophysis aid in the influence of the hypothalamus on visceral functions.

Limbic System

The limbic system has been called the visceral brain and has close anatomic and functional links with the hypothalamus (see also Chapter 19). Various portions of the limbic system exert control over the visceral manifestations of emotion and drives such as sexual behavior, fear, rage, aggression, and eating behavior. Electrical stimulation of limbic system areas elicits such autonomic reactions as cardiovascular and gastrointestinal responses, micturition, defecation, piloerection, and pupillary changes. These reactions are probably channeled through the hypothalamus.

Cerebral Neocortex

The cerebral neocortex may initiate autonomic reactions such as blushing or blanching of the face in response to receiving unexpected information or bad or good news. These widely known anecdotal observations are confirmed by the findings that destruction or stimulation of neocortical areas in humans can interfere with the normal regulation of many autonomic responses.

TRANSMITTER SUBSTANCES

Types

Autonomic neurotransmitters mediate all visceral functions; the principal transmitter agents are acetylcholine and norepinephrine (see also Chapter 4).

Acetylcholine is liberated at all preganglionic endings. High concentrations of acetylcholine, choline acetyltransferase, and acetylcholinesterase are found in cholinergic nerve endings.

Norepinephrine (levarterenol), a catecholamine, is the chemical transmitter at most sympathetic postganglionic endings. Norepinephrine and its methyl derivative, **epinephrine,** are secreted by the adrenal medulla. Although many viscera contain both norepinephrine and epinephrine, the latter is not considered to be a mediator at sympathetic endings; only the norepinephrine content can be related to the number of sympathetic nerve endings in the organ. Drugs that block the effects of epinephrine but not norepinephrine have little effect on the response of most organs to stimulation of their adrenergic nerve supply.

Substance P, somatostatin, vasoactive intestinal peptide (VIP), adenosine, and adenosine triphosphate (ATP) may also function as visceral neurotransmitters.

Functions

The autonomic nervous system can be divided into **cholinergic** and **adrenergic** divisions, based on the chemical mediator released. Cholinergic neurons include preganglionic and parasympathetic postganglionic neurons, sympathetic postganglionic neurons to sweat glands, and sympathetic vasodilator neurons to blood vessels in skeletal muscle. There is usually no acetylcholine in circulating blood, and the effects of localized cholinergic discharge are generally discrete and short-lived because of high concentrations of cholinesterase at the cholinergic nerve endings (Figs 20–12 and 20–13; Table 20–2). In the adrenal medulla, the postganglionic cells have lost their axons and become specialized for secreting catecholamine directly into the blood; the cholinergic preganglionic neurons to these cells act as the secretomotor nerve supply to the adrenal gland. Sympathetic postganglionic neurons are generally considered adrenergic except for the sympathetic vasodilator neurons and sweat gland neurons. Notice that norepinephrine has a more prolonged and wider action than does acetylcholine.

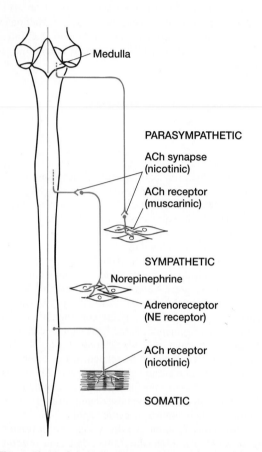

Figure 20–12. Schematic diagram showing some anatomic and pharmacologic features of autonomic and somatic motor nerves.

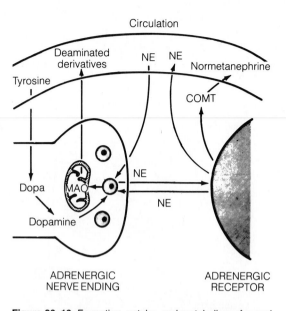

Figure 20–13. Formation, uptake, and metabolism of norepinephrine at adrenergic nerve endings. Norepinephrine in the granulated vesicles is released from the endings mainly by action potentials in the sympathetic nerves. Some of the norepinephrine constantly diffuses from the granules to the mitochondria, however, where it is oxidized to deaminated derivatives. Norepinephrine in the vesicles is formed from dopamine, taken up from the circulation, and taken up again after its release from the endings (reuptake). NE, norepinephrine; COMT, catechol-O-methyltransferase; MAO, monomine oxidase. (Reproduced, with permission, from Ganong WF: *Review of Medical Physiology,* 16th ed. Appleton & Lange, 1993.)

Receptors

The target tissues on which norepinephrine acts can be separated into two categories, based on their different sensitivities to certain drugs. This is related to the existence of two types of catecholamine receptors—α and β—in the target tissues. The α **receptors** mediate vasoconstriction, and the β **receptors** mediate such actions as the increase in cardiac rate and the strength of cardiac contraction. There are two subtypes of α receptors (α_1 and α_2) and two subtypes of β receptors ($\beta_1 1$ and β_2). The α and β receptors occur in both preganglionic endings and postganglionic membranes. The preganglionic β-adrenergic endings are of the β_1 type; the postganglionic receptors are of the β_2 type (Fig 20–14 and Table 20–2).

Effects of Drugs on the Autonomic Nervous System

Certain drugs affect the autonomic nervous system by mimicking or blocking cholinergic or adrenergic discharges (Table 20–3; see also Fig 20–12). Drugs can also alter other activities such as synthesis, storage in nerve endings, release near effector cells, action on effector cells, and termination of transmitter activity. Sometimes, a drug may affect two transmitter systems rather than one.

Despite apparent similarities in the transmitter chemistry of preganglionic and postganglionic cholinergic neurons, agents can act differently at these sites. **Muscarine** has little effect on autonomic ganglia, for example, but stimulates visceral cholinergic postganglionic neurons. Drugs with muscarine action include acetylcholine, acetylcholine-related substances, and inhibitors of cholinesterase (certain nerve gases, etc). Atropine, belladonna, and other natural and synthetic

Table 20–2. Responses of effector organs to autonomic nerve impulses and circulating catecholamines.*

Effector Organs	Cholinergic Response	Noradrenergic Impulses	
		Receptor Type	Response
Eye			
Radial muscle of iris	. . .	α	Contraction (mydriasis)
Sphincter muscle of iris	Contraction (miosis)	. . .	. . .
Ciliary muscle	Contraction for near vision	β	Relaxation for far vision
Heart			
S-A node	Decrease in heart rate; vagal arrest	β_1	Increase in heart rate
Atria	Decrease in contractility and (usually) increase in conduction velocity	β_1	Increase in contractility and conduction velocity
A-V node and conduction system	Decrease in conduction velocity; A-V block	β_1	Increase in conduction velocity
Ventricles	. . .	β_2	Increase in contractility and conduction velocity
Arterioles			
Coronary, skeletal muscle, pulmonary, abdominal viscera, renal	Dilation	α	Constriction
		β_2	Dilation
Skin and mucosa, cerebral, salivary glands	. . .	α	Constriction
Systemic veins	. . .	α	Constriction
		β_2	Dilation
Lung			
Bronchial muscle	Contraction	β_2	Relaxation
Bronchial glands	Stimulation	?	Inhibition(?)
Stomach			
Motility and tone	Increase	α, β_2	Decrease (usually)
Sphincters	Relaxation (usually)	α	Contraction (usually)
Secretion	Stimulation	. . .	Inhibition(?)
Intestine			
Motility and tone	Increase	α, β_2	Decrease
Sphincters	Relaxation (usually)	α	Contraction (usually)
Secretion	Stimulation	. . .	Inhibition(?)
Gallbladder and ducts	Contraction	. . .	Relaxation
Urinary bladder			
Detrusor	Contraction	β	Relaxation (usually)
Trigon and sphincter	Relaxation	α	Contraction
Ureter			
Motility and tone	Increase(?)	α	Increase (usually)
Uterus	Variable†	α, β_2	Variable†
Male sex organs	Erection	α	Ejaculation
Skin			
Pilomotor muscles	. . .	α	Contraction
Sweat glands	Generalized secretion	α	Slight localized secretion‡
Spleen capsule	. . .	α	Contraction
		β_2	Relaxation
Adrenal medulla	Secretion of epinephrine and norepinephrine	. . .	. . .
Liver	. . .	α, β_2	Glycogenolysis

(continued)

Table 20–2 (cont'd). Responses of effector organs to autonomic nerve impulses and circulating catecholamines.*

Effector Organs	Cholinergic Resonse	Novadrenergic Impulses	
		Receptor Type	Response
Pancreas Acini	Increase secretion	α	Decreased secretion
Islets	Increased insulin and glucagon secretion	α	Decreased insulin and glucagon secretion
		β₂	Increased insulin and glucagon secretion
Salivary glands	Profuse watery secretion	α	Thick secretion
		β₂	Amylase secretion
Lacrimal glands	Secretion	. . .	. . .
Nasopharyngeal glands	Secretion	. . .	. . .
Adipose tissue	. . .	β₁	Lipolysis
Juxtaglomerular cells	. . .	β₁	Increased renin secretion
Pineal gland	. . .	β	Increased melatonin synthesis and secretion

*Modified from Gilman AG et al (editors): *Goodman and Gilman's The Pharmacological Basis of Therapeutics,* 8th ed. Macmillan, 1990. Reproduced, with permission, from Ganong WF: *Review of Medical Physiology,* 16th ed. Appleton & Lange, 1993.
†Depends on stage of menstrual cycle, amount of circulating estrogen and progesterone, pregnancy, and other factors.
‡On palms of hands and in some other locations (adrenergic sweating).

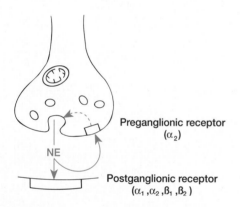

Preganglionic receptor
(α_2)

NE

Postganglionic receptor
(α_1 , α_2 , β_1 , β_2)

Figure 20–14. Preganglionic and postganglionic receptors at the ending of a noradrenergic neuron. The preganglionic receptor shown is α; the postganglionic receptors can be α_1, α_2, β_1, or β_2. (Reproduced, with permission, from Ganong, WF: *Review of Medical Physiology,* 16th ed. Appleton & Lange, 1993.)

belladonna-like drugs block the muscarine effects of acetylcholine by preventing the mediator from acting on visceral effector organs.

Some actions of acetylcholine, including the transmission of impulses from pre- to postganglionic neurons, are not affected by atropine. Because **nicotine** produces the same actions, the actions of acetylcholine in the presence of atropine are called its nicotine effects.

Curariform agents, hexamethonium, and mecamylamine act principally by blocking transmission at the cholinergic motor neuron endings on skeletal muscle fibers; they were used in the past in the treatment of hypertension.

Drugs that block the effects of norepinephrine on visceral effectors are often called adrenergic-neuron-blocking agents, adrenolytic agents, or sympatholytic agents.

Sensitization

Autonomic effectors (smooth muscle, cardiac muscle, and glands) that are partially or completely separated from their normal nerve connections become more sensitive to the action of the neurotransmitters that normally impinge on them; this has been termed **denervation hypersensitivity.** Known as Cannon's law of denervation, the effect is more pronounced after postganglionic interruption than after preganglionic interruption.

CASE 26

A 55-year-old male clerk consulted his physician about drooling, difficulty in swallowing, and a "funny-sounding" voice. Indirect laryngoscopy showed decreased motility of the right vocal cord. Findings in all other examinations and tests were within normal limits. Drugs were given to control the patient's hypersalivation.

Eight months later, the patient returned with a 10-day history of lightheadedness and fainting. He was referred to a hospital for observation and examination. The only additional abnormal findings were fasciculations in the right side of the tongue and changes in blood pressure with postural changes (lying down,

Table 20–3. Some chemical agents that affect sympathetic activity, listing only the principal actions of the agents.*

Site of Action	Agents That Augment Sympathetic Activity	Agents That Depress Sympathetic Activity
Sympathetic ganglia	**Stimulate postganglionic neurons** Nicotine Dimethphenylpiperazinium **Inhibit acetylcholinesterase** Physostigmine (eserine) Neostigmine (Prostigmin) Parathion	**Block conduction** Chlorisondamine† Hexamethonium† Mecamylamine (Inversine) Pentolinium† Tetraethylammonium† Trimethaphan (Arfonad) Acetycholine and anticholinesterase drugs in high concentrations
Endings of postganglionic neurons	**Release norepinephrine** Tyramine Ephedrine Amphetamine	**Block norephrine synthesis** Metyrosine **Interfere with norepinephrine storage** Reserpine Guanethidine (Ismelin)‡ **Prevent norepinephrine release** Bretylium tosylate Guanethidine (ismelin)‡ **Form false transmitters** Methyldopa (Aldomet)
α Receptors	**Stimulate α_1 receptors** Methoxamine (Vasoxyl) Phenylephrine (Neo-Synephrine) **Stimulate α_2 receptors** Clonidines§	**Block α receptors** Phenoxybenzamine (Dibenzyline) Phentolamine (Regitine) Prazosin (blocks α_1) Yohimbine (blocks α_2)
β Receptors	**Stimulate β receptors** Isoproterenol (Isuprel)	**Block β receptors** Propranolol (Inderal) and others (block β_1 and β_2) Metoprolol and others (block β_1) Butoxamine† (blocks β_2)

*Modified and reproduced, with permission, from Ganong WF: *Review of Medical Physiology,* 16th ed. Appleton & Lange, 1993.
†Not available in the USA.
‡Note that guanethidine is believed to have 2 principal actions.
§Clonidine stimulates α_2 receptors in the periphery, but along with others α_2 agonists that cross the blood-brain barrier, it also stimulates α_2 receptors in the brain which decrease sympathetic output. Therefore, the overall effect is decreased sympathetic discharge.

140/90; sitting up, 100/70; and standing up, too low to read). Lumbar puncture analysis showed a protein level of 95 mg/dL. While in the hospital, the patient had one episode of rotatory vertigo. After four days, he went back to work.

Three months later, the patient returned with complaints of dizziness, fainting, and increased problems in swallowing; his speech was difficult to understand. His drop in blood pressure with postural changes was still present. Neurologic examination showed a normal mental status; flat optic discs; visual fields full, with pupils normal and reactive to light; normal extraocu-

lar movements; bilateral neural hearing deficits; dysarthria; midline palate location with normal gag reflex; and a weak tongue that deviated to the right when protruded. The patient's gait was wide-based and unsteady. The heel-to-shin test showed ataxia on the right and other cerebellar tests results were normal. The deep tendon reflexes were also normal. A CT scan showed moderate ventricular enlargement.

Where is the lesion? What is the nature of the lesion? What is the explanation for the autonomic dysfunctions?

Cases are discussed further in Chapter 25.

REFERENCES

Appenzeller O: *The Autonomic Nervous System,* 3rd ed. Elsevier, 1982.

Bannister R (editor): *Autonomic Failure: A Textbook of Clinical Disorders of the Autonomic Nervous System,* 2nd ed. Oxford Univ Press, 1988.

Brooks CM, Koizumi K, Sato AY (editors): *Integrative Functions of the Autonomic Nervous System.* Elsevier, 1979.

deGroat WC: Central neural control of the lower urinary tract. In: *Neurobiology of Incontinence.* Bock G, Whelan J (editors). Wiley, 1990.

Gershon MD: The enteric nervous system. *Annu Rev Neurosci* 1981;**4:**227.

McLeod JG, Tuck RR: Disorders of the autonomic nervous system. 1. Pathophysiology and clinical features. *Ann Neurol* 1987;**21:**419.

Miller NR: *Walsh and Hoyt's Clinical Neuro-ophthalmology,* 4th ed. Williams and Wilkins, 1985.

Swanson LW, Mogensen GJ: Neural mechanisms for the functional coupling of autonomic, endocrine and somatomotor responses in adaptive behavior. *Brain Res Rev* 1981;**3:**1.

Higher Cortical Function

21

The cerebral cortex contains components of the functional systems related to the initiation of movement and to sensation from the body and the special sensory organs. The cortex is also the substrate for functions that convey comprehension, cognition, and communication.

LANGUAGE & SPEECH

Language, the comprehension and communication of abstract ideas, is a cortical function that is separate from the neural mechanisms related to primary visual, auditory, and motor function.

The motor cortex (area 4), which is connected to the motor nuclei of the brain stem (cranial nerves V, VII, IX, X, and XII), is involved in the production of audible speech. The supplementary motor cortex (area 6) is involved in mechanisms for sequencing and coordinating sounds. The ability to think of the right words, to program and coordinate the sequence of muscle contractions necessary to produce intelligible sounds, and to assemble words into meaningful sentences depends on the frontal association cortex (**Broca's area,** areas 44 and 45) within the inferior frontal gyrus, located just anterior to the motor cortex controlling the lips and tongue.

The ability to comprehend language, including speech, is dependent upon **Wernicke's area,** which is located in the posterior part of the superior temporal gyrus within the auditory association cortex (area 22).

The **arcuate fasciculus** provides a crucial association pathway within the hemisphere white matter, connecting Wernicke's and Broca's areas (Fig 21–1). Because the arcuate fasciculus connects the speech comprehension area (Wernicke's area) with the area responsible for production of speech (Broca's area), damage to this white matter tract produces impairment of repetition.

Dysarthria

Dysarthria is a speech disorder in which the mechanism for speech is damaged by lesions in the corticobulbar pathways; in one or more cranial nerve nuclei or nerves V, VII, IX, X, and XII; in the cerebellum; or in the muscles that produce speech sounds. Dysarthria is characterized by dysfunction of the phonation, articulation, resonance, or respiration aspects of speech.

Aphasia

Aphasia, as the term is generally used, refers to loss or impairment of language function as a result of brain damage. There are a number of distinct types of aphasia and most of these result from lesions in specific regions of the cerebral hemispheres (Table 21–1). In testing for aphasia, the clinician first listens to the patient's spontaneous speech output and then explores the patient's speech during conversation. The patient's speech may be categorized as *fluent* (more than 50 words per minute, effortless, absence of dysarthria, normal phrase length and normal intonation). In contrast, *nonfluent* aphasia is characterized by decreased verbal output less than 50 words per minute, poor articulation, degradation of inflection and melodic aspects of speech, agrammatism (ie, tendency to omit small, grammatical words, verb tenses and plurals, and to use only nouns and verbs), and is effortful. Naming (which is usually examined by asking the patient to name objects presented to him), repetition of phrases such as "dog," "automobile," "President Kennedy," "no ifs, ands, or buts," and comprehension of spoken language are also tested.

Aphasia with Impaired Repetition

In most common forms of aphasia, the ability to repeat spoken language is impaired. Broca's, Wer-

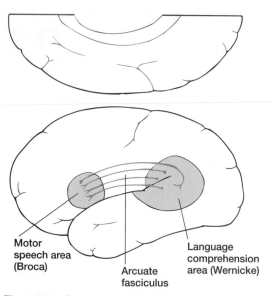

Motor
speech area
(Broca)

Arcuate
fasciculus

Language
comprehension
area (Wernicke)

Figure 21–1. Central speech areas of the dominant cerebral hemisphere. Notice that Broca's and Wernicke's areas are interconnected via fibers that travel in the arcuate fasciculus, subjacent to the cortex.

nicke's, and global aphasia are frequently seen in clinical practice.

A. Broca's Aphasia: Broca's aphasia is usually caused by a lesion in the inferior frontal gyrus in the dominant hemisphere (Broca's area; Figs 21–1 and 21–2). The patient usually has difficulty naming even simple objects. Repetition is impaired but comprehension of spoken language is normal. The patient is usually aware of the deficit and appropriately concerned about it.

Most lesions that involve Broca's area also involve the neighboring motor cortex. Thus, patients are often hemiplegic, with the arm more affected than the leg. Broca's aphasia often occurs as a result of strokes, most commonly affecting the middle cerebral artery territory.

B. Wernicke's Aphasia: This type of aphasia is caused by a lesion in or near the superior temporal gyrus, in Wernicke's area (Figs 21–1 and 21–2). Because this part of the cortex is not located adjacent to the motor cortex, there is usually no hemiplegia.

Patients with Wernicke's aphasia have fluent speech, but repetition and comprehension are impaired. The patient usually has difficulty naming objects and produces both *literal paraphasias* (eg, "wellow" instead of "yellow") and *verbal paraphasias* (eg, "mother" instead of "wife"). **Neologisms** (meaningless, nonsensical words, eg, "baffer") are used commonly and speech may be circumlocutory (ie, wordy but meaningless). Patients with Wernicke's aphasia usually do not appear concerned about, or even aware of, their speech disorder. These patients may be given a mistaken diagnosis of a psychiatric disorder. Wernicke's aphasia commonly occurs as a result of embolic strokes.

C. Global Aphasia: The *central speech area* consists of Broca's area in the frontal lobe, Wernicke's area in the temporal lobe, and the interconnecting arcuate fasciculus. Large lesions in the dominant hemisphere, which involve all three of these areas, can produce global aphasia (Fig 21–3). In this nonfluent aphasia, both repetition and comprehension are severely impaired.

Global aphasia most commonly occurs as a result of large infarctions in the dominant hemisphere, often because of occlusion of the carotid or middle cerebral artery.

D. Conduction Aphasia: In this unusual aphasia, verbal output is fluent and paraphasic. Comprehension of spoken language is intact, but repetition is severely impaired. Naming is usually impaired, although the patient often is able to select the correct name from a list. Conduction aphasia is often a result of a lesion involving the arcuate fasciculus, in the white

Table 21–1. The aphasias.

Aphasias with impaired repetition:					
Type	**Naming**	**Fluency**	**Auditory Comprehension**	**Repetition**	**Location of Lesion**
Broca's	±	−	+	−	Broca's area (area 44 and 45)
Wernicke's	−	+	−	−	Wernicke's area (area 22)
Global	−	−	−	−	Large left hemispheric lesions
Conduction	±	+	+	−	Arcuate fasciculus

	Aphasias with preserved repetition:					
	Type	**Naming**	**Fluency**	**Auditory Comprehension**	**Repetition**	**Location of Lesion**
Isolation aphasias	Motor transcortical	−	−	+	+	Surrounding Broca's area
	Sensory transcortical	−	+	−	+	Surrounding Wernicke's area
	Mixed transcortical	−	−	−	+	Surrounding Broca's and Wernicke's areas
	Anomic	−	+	+	+	Anywhere within left (or right) hemisphere

− = significantly impaired
+ = intact

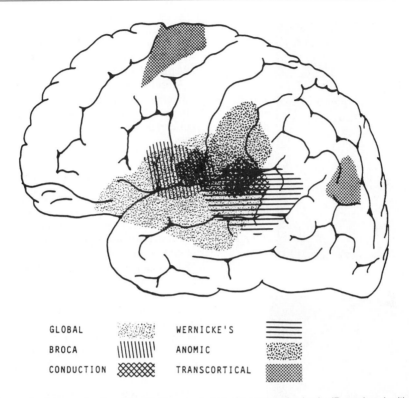

GLOBAL		WERNICKE'S	
BROCA		ANOMIC	
CONDUCTION		TRANSCORTICAL	

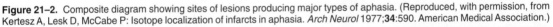

Figure 21–2. Composite diagram showing sites of lesions producing major types of aphasia. (Reproduced, with permission, from Kertesz A, Lesk D, McCabe P: Isotope localization of infarcts in aphasia. *Arch Neurol* 1977;**34**:590. American Medical Association.)

matter underlying the temporal-parietal junction; this lesion disconnects Wernicke's area from Broca's area.

Aphasias with Intact Repetition

A. Isolation Aphasias: In these unusual aphasias, repetition is spared, but comprehension is impaired. These aphasias are also referred to as *transcortical* aphasias because the lesion is usually in the cortex surrounding Wernicke's or Broca's area, or both. Depending on the precise location of the lesion, these aphasias may be fluent or nonfluent and comprehension may be impaired or preserved.

B. Anomic Aphasia: Anomia (difficulty finding the correct word) can occur in a variety of conditions including toxic and metabolic encephalopathies. When anomia occurs as an aphasic disorder, speech may be fluent but devoid of meaning as a result of word-finding difficulty. The patient has difficulty naming objects. Comprehension and repetition are relatively normal. The presence of anomic aphasia is of little value in localizing the area of dysfunction. Many patients with anomic aphasia have lesions in the dominant hemisphere, close to the angular gyrus or parietal-temporal junction. However, focal lesions throughout the dominant hemisphere, or, in some cases, in the nondominant hemisphere, can produce anomic aphasia, and anomia is also commonly present in toxic and metabolic encephalopathies.

Agraphia—an inability to write—is another type of expressive aphasia. Because writing involves the use of symbols for speech (symbolic sounds), it is a more difficult and complex function than speech. Writing ability can be affected by lesions in various locations, including the descending motor pathways and the cerebral cortex. In primary agraphia, there is an inability to construct letters, but there are no disturbances in the spheres of speech and vision. The lesion causing primary agraphia is usually in the posterior frontal cortex, excluding Broca's area. Agraphia can also occur as a result of temporal-parietal lesions or as a result of problems with visual-spatial orientation because of lesions in the nondominant hemisphere.

Alexia

Alexia (the inability to read) can occur as part of aphasic syndromes or as an isolated abnormality. **Aphasic alexia** is the term referring to impaired reading in Broca's, Wernicke's, global, and isolation aphasias.

A. Alexia with Agraphia: This disorder, in which there is impairment of reading and writing, is seen most commonly with pathology at the parietal-temporal junction area, particularly the angular gyrus. Because lesions of the angular gyrus also produce the Gerstmann syndrome (see below) and anomia, the constellation of agraphia, the Gerstmann syndrome, and anomia may occur together.

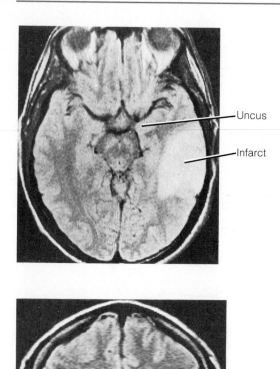

Figure 21–3. MR images of sections through the head. ***Top:*** Horizontal section with a large high-intensity area in the temporal lobe, representing an infarct caused by occlusion of a middle cerebral artery branch. ***Bottom:*** Coronal section showing the same area of infarction. (Parallel lines on the periphery of the brain represent artifacts caused by patient motion.) Large infarcts of this type, in the dominant cerebral hemisphere, can produce global aphasia that is accompanied by hemiparesis.

B. Alexia Without Agraphia: Alexia without agraphia is a striking disorder, in which the patient is unable to read although writing is not impaired. Patients with this disorder are capable of writing a paragraph but, when asked to read it, cannot do so.

This syndrome occurs when there is damage to the left (dominant) visual cortex and to the splenium of the corpus callosum (Fig 21–4). As a result of damage to the left visual cortex, there is a right-sided homonymous hemianopsia and written material in the right half of the visual world is not processed. Written material presented to the left visual field is processed in the visual cortex on the right side. However, neurons in the visual cortex on the two sides are normally interconnected via axons that project through the splenium; as a result of damage to the splenium, visual information

in the right visual cortex cannot be transmitted to the visual cortex in the left (dominant) hemisphere and, thus, is disconnected from the speech comprehension (Wernicke's) area.

Most commonly, this disorder occurs as a result of infarctions in the territory of the posterior cerebral artery on the left, which damage both the left-sided visual cortex and the posterior part of the corpus callosum.

Agnosia

Agnosia—difficulty in identification or recognition—is usually considered to be caused by disturbances in the association functions of the cerebral cortex. **Astereognosis** is a failure of tactile recognition of objects and is usually associated with parietal lesions of the contralateral hemisphere. **Visual agnosia,** the inability to recognize things by sight (eg, objects, pictures, persons, spatial relationships) can occur with or without hemianopia on the dominant side. It is a result of parieto-occipital lesions or the interruption of fibers in the splenium of the corpus callosum.

Prosopagnosia is a striking syndrome in which the patient loses the ability to recognize familiar faces. The patient may be able to describe identifying features such as eye color, length and color of hair, presence or absence of mustache, etc. However, even spouses, friends, or relatives may not be recognized. Although the anatomic basis for this syndrome remains controversial, in some patients there are lesions in the temporal and occipital lobes, often bilaterally.

Unilateral neglect is a syndrome in which the patient fails to respond to stimuli in one half of space, contralateral to a hemispheric lesion. The patient may fail to respond to visual, tactile, and auditory stimuli. In its full-blown form, the syndrome is very striking: The patient may bump into things in the neglected visual field, will fail to dress or shave the neglected half of the body, and will be unaware of motor or sensory deficits on the neglected side. The unilateral neglect may be especially apparent when the patient is asked to draw a flower or fill in the numbers on a clock (Fig 21–5).

Unilateral neglect is commonly seen as a result of parietal lobe damage, but is also found after injury to other parts of the cerebral hemispheres (frontal lobe, cortical white matter, deep structures such as basal ganglia, etc). Unilateral neglect is most severe following injury to the right cerebral hemisphere (left-sided unilateral neglect), but can also occur following injury to the left hemisphere.

Anosognosia

Anosognosia, the lack of awareness of disease or denial of illness, may occur as part of the unilateral neglect syndrome. For example, patients with left hemiparesis often neglect the paralyzed limbs and may even deny that they are part of their body, attributing them

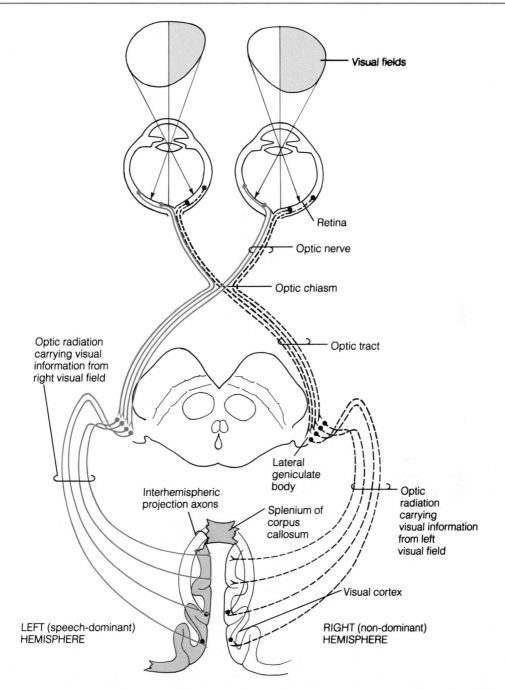

Figure 21–4. Neuroanatomic basis for the syndrome of alexia without agraphia. Damage to two regions (the visual cortex in the left, speech-dominant hemisphere and the splenium of the corpus callosum, which carries interhemispheric axons connecting the two visual cortices) is required. These regions are both irrigated by the posterior cerebral artery. Thus, occlusion of the left posterior cerebral artery can produce this striking syndrome.

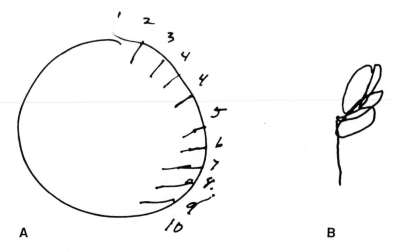

Figure 21–5. Unilateral (left-sided) neglect in a patient with a right hemispheric lesion. The patient was asked to fill in the numbers on the face of a clock (A) and to draw a flower (B).

to a doll or another patient. Even when the patient is aware of the deficit, he may not be appropriately concerned about it.

Apraxia

Apraxia, the inability to carry out motor acts correctly despite intact motor and sensory pathways, intact comprehension, and full cooperation, can occur following injury to a variety of cortical and subcortical sites. **Ideomotor apraxia** is the inability to perform motor responses upon verbal command, which were previously carried out spontaneously. For example, the patient may fail to show his teeth on command, although he can do this spontaneously. Introducing objects to be used (eg, giving the patient a hairbrush and asking him or her to demonstrate how to brush the hair) leads to improvement of the performance. Damage to a variety of sites, including Broca's area, the corpus callosum, and the arcuate fasciculus, can cause ideomotor apraxia. **Ideational apraxia** is characterized by an abnormality in the conception of movements, so that the patient may have difficulty doing anything at all, or may have problems sequencing the different components of a complex act although each separate component can be performed correctly. In ideational apraxia, introduction of objects to be used does not improve performance. Ideational apraxia may be seen after lesions of the left temporal-parietal-occipital area.

Gerstmann's Syndrome

This tetrad of clinical findings includes right-left disorientation, finger agnosia (difficulty identifying or recognizing the fingers), impaired calculation, and impaired writing. The presence of this tetrad suggests dysfunction in the angular gyrus of the left hemisphere. As previously mentioned, Gerstmann's syndrome may occur together with anomic aphasia and alexia.

CEREBRAL DOMINANCE

Clinical findings and experimental work have established that the two cerebral hemispheres are not equal in certain functions. Although the projection systems of motor and sensory pathways are alike, left and right, each hemisphere is specialized and dominates the other in some specific functions. The left hemisphere controls language and speech in most people; the right hemisphere leads in interpreting 3-dimensional images and spaces. Other distinctions have been postulated, such as music understanding in the left hemisphere, arithmetic and design in the right.

Cerebral dominance is related to handedness. Most right-handed people are left-hemisphere dominant; so are 70% of left-handed people, while the remaining 30% are right-hemisphere dominant. This dominance is reflected in anatomic differences between the hemispheres. The slope of the left lateral fissure is less steep, and the upper aspect of the left superior temporal gyrus (the planum temporale) is broader in people with left-hemisphere dominance.

When neurosurgery is contemplated in a patient, it can be useful to establish which cerebral hemisphere is dominant for speech. Typically, amobarbital or thiopental sodium is injected into a carotid artery while the patient is counting aloud and making rapidly alternating movements of the fingers of both hands. When the carotid artery of the dominant side is injected, a much greater and longer interference with speech function occurs than with injection of the other side.

MEMORY & LEARNING

The three types of memory are immediate recall, short-term memory, and long-term (or remote) memory.

Immediate recall is the phenomenon that allows people to remember and repeat a small amount of information shortly after reading or hearing it. In tests, most people can repeat, parrot-like, a short series of words or numbers for up to 10 minutes. The anatomic substrate is thought to be the auditory association cortex.

Short-term memory can last up to an hour. Tests usually involve short lists of more complicated numbers (eg, telephone numbers) or sentences for a period of an hour or less. This type of memory is associated with intactness of the deep temporal lobe. If a patient's temporal lobe is stimulated during surgery or irritated by the presence of a lesion, he or she may experience **déjà vu,** characterized by sudden flashes of former events or by the feeling that new sensations are old and familiar ones. (Occasionally, the feeling of déjà vu occurs spontaneously in normal, healthy persons.)

Long-term memory allows people to remember words, numbers, other persons, events, and so forth for many years. The formation of memories appears to involve the strengthening of certain synapses. **Long-term potentiation** (LTP), a process triggered by the accumulation of calcium in postsynaptic neurons following high-frequency activity, appears to play an important role in the processes underlying memory. Experimental and clinical observations suggest that the encoding of long-term memory involves the hippocampus and adjacent cortex in the medial temporal lobes. The medial thalamus and its target areas in the frontal lobes are also involved, together with the basal forebrain nucleus of Meynert (Fig 21–6).

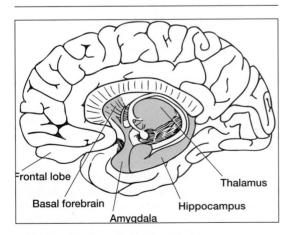

Figure 21–6. Brain areas concerned with encoding long-term memories (Reproduced, with permission, from Ganong WF: *Review of Medical Physiology,* 16th ed. Appleton & Lange, 1993.)

Clinical Correlations

If both temporal lobes are removed or bilateral temporal lobe lesions destroy the mechanism for consolidation, new events or information will not be remembered—but previous memories may remain intact. This unusual disorder, called **anterograde amnesia** is often seen as a result of bilateral limbic lesions. An example is provided by herpes simplex encephalitis, which preferentially affects the temporal lobes and by bilateral posterior cerebral infarcts, which may damage both temporal lobes. Lesions of the medial thalamus (particularly the dorsomedial nuclei) can also cause anterograde amnesia; this can occur as a result of tumor and infarctions. Memory deficit is also a common occurrence in the **Wernicke-Korsakoff syndrome** in which hemorrhagic lesions develop in the medial thalamic nuclei, hypothalamus (especially mammillary bodies), the periaquaductal gray matter, and tegmentum of the midbrain in alcoholic, thiamine-deficient patients. In all of the above disorders, **retrograde amnesia,** ie, the loss of memory for events prior to the lesion, can also occur.

EPILEPSY

Dysfunction of the cerebral cortex, alone or together with dysfunction of deeper structures, can lead to some forms of epilepsy (Table 21–2). Epilepsy is characterized by sudden, transient alterations of brain function, usually with motor, sensory, autonomic, or psychic symptoms; it is often accompanied by alterations in consciousness. Coincidental pronounced brain-wave alterations in the electroencephalogram may be detected during these episodes (see Chapter 24).

The epilepsies are a heterogeneous group of disorders. In the broadest sense, they can be categorized into disorders characterized by **generalized** or **partial (focal, local)** seizures. Some of the major types of seizures are as follows:

Generalized Seizures

A. Absence (Petit Mal) Seizures: In petit mal seizures, the patient may have a minor or abortive attack with no falling or convulsive movements of the body. Instead, there will be a momentary or transient loss of consciousness, so fleeting or camouflaged in ordinary activity that neither the patient nor anyone else may be entirely aware of it. The classic absence seizure is characterized by a sudden vacant expression (brief absence) and cessation of motor activity, sometimes with loss of muscle tone. This is followed by the abrupt return of consciousness and resumption of mental and physical activity. As many as 100 attacks may occur in a day.

Patients with petit mal seizures may appear to be day-dreaming, especially when attacks are frequent.

Table 21–2. Classification of epilepsies.*

Primary generalized epilepsies
  Absence (petit mal) seizures
  Tonic-clonic (grand mal) seizures
  Myoclonic seizures
  Atonic seizures
Partial epilepsies
  Simple partial (focal, local) epilepsy (consciousnes not
    impaired):
    With motor signs (often frontal lobe epilepsy)
    With somatosensory symptoms (parietal lobe
     epilepsy)
    With special sensory symptoms (eg, olfactory or gus-
     tatory: temporal lobe epilepsy; visual: occipital or
     temporal lobe epilepsy)
    With autonomic symptoms and signs (eg, flushing,
     pupillary dilation, epigastric sensations: temporal or
     frontal lobe epilepsy)
    With psychic symptoms (eg, fear, *déjà vu,* complex
     visual or auditory hallucinations: temporal)
  Complex partial epilepsy:
    Simple partial epilepsy at onset followed by impair-
     ment of consciousness and automatisms
    Impairment of consciousness at onset:
     Motionless stare and impaired consciousness fol-
      lowed by oroalimentary and other automatisms
      (temporal lobe epilepsy)
     Complex motor automatisms at start of impaired
      consciousness (frontal lobe epilepsy)
Secondary generalized epilepsies
  Simple partial epilepsy evolving to tonic-clonic (sec-
    ondary tonic-clonic) seizures
  Chronic partial epilepsy evolving to tonic-clonic seizures
**Myoclonic astatic or atonic epilepsies in children with
  mental retardation**
**Progressive myoclonic epilepsies in adolescents and
  adults with dementia**
Unclassified epilepsies

*Modified from the classification of the International League
Against Epilepsy and the World Health Organization.

Staring and blank spells often occur without the patient's knowledge. This type of epilepsy is especially common in children. If the correct diagnosis is not reached, teachers and others may inappropriately attribute the child's problem to impaired learning ability, short attention span, or restlessness.

The EEG usually shows regular and symmetrical three-per-second spike-and-wave complexes. It is generally thought that petit mal seizures represent the responses of abnormal cerebral cortex to the synchronized input of cells projecting from the thalamus and brain stem.

Treatment with anticonvulsant drugs such as ethosuximide or valproate can provide excellent seizure control.

B. Tonic-Clonic (Grand Mal) Seizures: An aura may signal an impending attack. The aura is usually specific for the individual patient and may consist of a sensation of nausea or numbness, an odor, a visual image, or a flash of memory. Loss of consciousness usually ensues, and the patient falls to the floor. The patient may cry out and frequently incurs some bodily injury. Convulsions usually follow, with the patient lying stiff and mildly rigid for as long as 1–2 minutes and the muscles of the body in a state of mild tonic contraction. A clonic stage follows in which rhythmic, severe, synchronous, convulsive movements of the body occur. Control of the bowel and bladder is frequently lost and biting injuries to the tongue are common. Following a grand mal episode or a series of brief seizures, patients may remain confused for several minutes (or hours). Disorientation, anxiety, hallucinations, paranoid delusions, excitement, and aggressive activity may be overwhelming. A variable period of sleep or stupor, usually lasting 1–4 hours, may follow this phase. Later, there is little recollection of events occurring during this period. Abnormal, high-amplitude discharges ("spikes") are usually seen in the EEG during tonic-clonic seizures and a generalized polyspike or polyspike-and-wave discharge is common.

The response to treatment with anticonvulsant drugs, including valproate, phenytoin, and carbamazepine, is excellent, and many patients obtain virtually complete control of seizures with these drugs.

C. Status Epilepticus: This serious disorder consists of a train of severe seizures with relatively short—or no—intervals between. The patient becomes exhausted and, frequently, hyperthermic. Death may occur as a result of status epilepticus (mortality rates of 3–25% have been reported). Status epilepticus is a medical emergency and requires prompt airway management, placement of an intravenous line (usually with administration of glucose), and treatment with intravenous anticonvulsants such as diazepam or phenytoin.

D. Myoclonic Seizures: This unusual form of epilepsy is characterized by sudden simple, bilateral jerking movements. Patients report that they are unaware of the attack itself and that they simply find themselves in an unusual position afterward, often on the floor. This disorder differs from hemiballismus and ballismus, which are caused by destruction of one or both subthalamic nuclei (see Chapter 13). Myoclonic seizures also differ from myoclonic jerks of the limbs or muscles. The latter are usually not considered epileptic and can occur either without evident alteration of consciousness or in association with a typical absence seizure. Myoclonic jerks tend to occur more frequently in the morning and upon falling asleep; normal individuals may have rare myoclonic jerks in drowsiness or light sleep. Valproate may be useful in the treatment of this form of epilepsy.

E. Partial (Focal, Local) Seizures: In partial seizures, the initial clinical and EEG changes indicate activation of a *focal* system of neurons limited to part of one cerebral hemisphere. If consciousness is not impaired as a result of the seizure, it is classified as a **simple partial seizure.** In contrast, if consciousness is impaired, the seizure is termed a **complex partial seizure.**

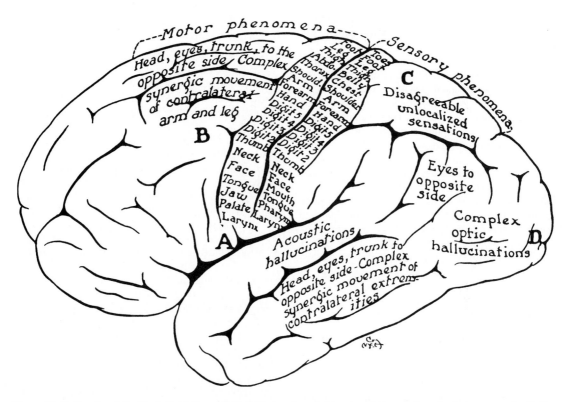

Figure 21–7. Results of electrical stimulation of the cerebral cortex. **A:** Chewing, licking, and swallowing movements. **B:** Eyes turned toward the opposite side, without visual aura. **C:** Sensory aura in the opposite leg, followed by complex synergistic movements. **D:** Unformed optical phenomena such as flames and lights. (After Foerster. Reproduced, with permission, from Bailey P: *Intracranial Tumors.* Thomas, 1933.)

F. Simple Partial (Jacksonian) Epilepsy:
Seizures resulting from focal irritation of a portion of the motor cortex may be confined to the appropriate peripheral area. These are sometimes termed **focal motor seizures.** For example, if the motor cortex for the hand is involved, the seizure may be confined to the hand. Consciousness may be retained, and the seizure may spread over the rest of the adjacent motor cortex to involve adjacent peripheral parts. The spread of seizure activity, as it extends over the homunculus on the motor cortex, may take the form of an orderly "march" over the body (see Fig 10–14). Focal motor seizures can occur with or without a march. This type of seizure is most commonly associated with structural lesions such as brain tumor, cerebral edema, or glial scar. Electrical stimulation of the exposed cortex during neurosurgery has aided in mapping the cortex and in understanding localized, partial seizures (Fig 21–7).

In some cases seizures arise as a result of focal epileptiform activity within the sensory cortex. These are termed **focal sensory seizures** or **partial sensory seizures.** Any sensory modality can be involved. **Somatosensory seizures** are usually a result of abnormal activity in the precentral cortex and, as with focal motor seizures, reflect the somatotopic organization of the

primary sensory cortex (see Fig 10–15). The patient experiences abnormal sensations (parathesias) or numbness in the part of the body corresponding to the area of abnormal activity on the sensory homunculus. **Visual seizures** and **auditory seizures** can also occur, as a result of epileptic activity in the contralateral occipital lobe and lateral temporal lobe, respectively.

G. Complex Partial Epilepsy: There are several types of complex partial epilepsy, as outlined in Table 21–2. In **temporal lobe epilepsy,** the seizure may begin with psychic or complex sensory symptoms (eg, a feeling of excitement or fear, an abnormal feeling of familiarity—déjà vu; complex visual or auditory hallucinations) or autonomic symptoms (eg, unusual epigastric sensations). Olfactory or gustatory sensations are often reported. These may be followed by automatisms, simple or complex patterned movements, incoherent speech, turning of the head and eyes, smacking of the lips or chewing, twisting, and writhing movements of the extremities, clouding of consciousness, and amnesia. Complex acts and movements such as walking, fastening or unfastening buttons may occur for periods of several seconds or as long as ten minutes. Temporal lobe foci (spikes, sharp waves, or combinations of these) are frequently associated with this type of epilepsy. These complex partial seizures may, in some patients, generalize so that the patient has tonic-clonic seizures.

H. Febrile Seizures: The occurrence of febrile seizures, in otherwise healthy children between the ages of three months and 4–5 years, is well-known. In this syndrome, generalized tonic-clonic seizures occur during the rising phase of fever. These seizures occur in 2–5% of children. Epilepsy in later life occurs in only 2–8% of children who experience febrile seizures and occurs more commonly in those with pre-existing neurologic abnormalities and multiple febrile seizures occurring in clusters. Thus, for most children the occurrence of febrile seizures does not suggest a poor prognosis and the term *benign febrile convulsions* has been used. It is of course essential to differentiate benign febrile seizures from secondary seizures due to disorders such as meningitis and encephalitis; this requires careful neurologic evaluation including, in many cases, lumbar puncture.

Causes

Epilepsy is caused by abnormal activity of brain tissue that can result from an injury, infection, damage as a result of cerebrovascular disease, tumors, etc. In many cases (idiopathic epilepsy) no cause can be identified; idiopathic epilepsy tends to run in families. Metabolic disorders such as uremia, hypoglycemia, hypocalcemia, and excessive hydration may also give rise to seizures.

The most common causes of symptomatic epilepsy in children are birth injury and anoxia, inflammatory brain lesions, cerebrovascular accidents, head injuries, and congenital brain malformations.

In susceptible individuals, physical stimuli such as sound, touch, or stroboscopic light may precipitate seizures. Other factors—excessive alcohol intake, emotional tension, fatigue, or lack of food and sleep—may indirectly affect the susceptibility of a particular patient to seizures.

Diagnosis

Epilepsy can be diagnosed on the basis of a history of recurrent seizures and observation of a typical seizure. Physical, neurologic, and neuroradiologic examinations may be helpful. Electroencephalography provides a most important objective tool in the diagnosis of epilepsy (see Chapter 24).

Treatment

The objective of therapy is the complete suppression of seizures. Most epileptic patients benefit from treatment with anticonvulsant drugs. In some patients neurosurgery can eliminate the epileptic focus that gives rise to seizures. Clinical Illustration 21–1 provides an example.

CLINICAL ILLUSTRATION 21–1

This 44-year-old woman had a generalized tonic-clonic seizure associated with fever at the age of three but was otherwise well until the age of 12 when complex partial seizure activity began. Her seizures were characterized by an aura consisting of a rising sensation in her gut, followed by loss of consciousness, tonic activity of the left hand and turning of the head to the left. Sometimes she would fall if standing. Her seizures were particularly troublesome in the premenstrual period and averaged five to 10 per month despite treatment with anticonvulsant drugs. On examination, no neurologic abnormalities were observed. Because of the failure of traditional medical therapy to control her seizures, the patient was hospitalized and extensive evaluation was performed. EEG monitoring revealed slowing and abnormal spike activity in the right anterior temporal lobe. During her seizures there was abnormal discharge of the right temporal lobe. An intracarotid amobarbital test, in which an anesthetic was injected into her carotid arteries, demonstrated left hemisphere dominance for speech and a marked disparity of memory function between the left and right hemispheres; the left hemisphere showed perfect memory and the right showed significantly impaired memory. MRI scanning showed severe atrophy of the hippocampus on the right (Fig 21–8).

The concordance of the EEG findings, together with MRI demonstration of right hippocampal atrophy, indicated right medial temporal lobe epilepsy. Because the patient's seizures had not been controlled by anticonvulsant medications, she underwent neurosurgical resection of the right medial temporal lobe (Figs 21–9 and 21–10). Subsequent to surgery, she has had no seizures with the exception of one that occurred when her anticonvulsant drug levels were very low.

This patient illustrates a classical history and findings for the most common form of epilepsy treated by surgery, medial temporal lobe epilepsy. The pathologic changes of neuronal cell loss in CA1 and CA3 hippocampal subfields are predictive of the reduced hemisphere-specific memory function, and were clearly demonstrated by MRI. At surgery, recording from intracranial electrodes confirmed seizure onset in the medial temporal, hippocampal structures. The response to neurosurgical resection of these areas can be dramatic, with nearly 90% of patients being cured of seizures. The correlation of anatomic localization by electrical, structural, and cognitive studies preoperatively and the subsequent response to resection of a circumscribed cerebral area provide a dramatic demonstration of anatomic-clinical correlation.

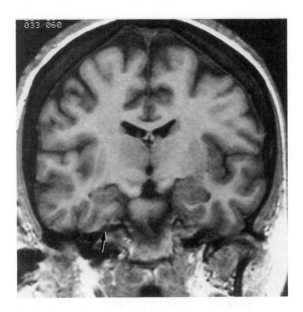

Figure 21–8. MR I of frontal section through the head, showing hippocampal atrophy (arrow) in the patient described in Clinical Illustration 21–1.

CASE 27

A 60-year-old right-handed widow had been experiencing intermittent, brief episodes of blurred vision in the right eye for a year or so. One month prior to admission to the hospital, she had a 5-minute episode of numbness and tingling in the left arm and hand, accompanied by loss of movement in the left hand. Two days before admission, she fell to the floor while taking a shower and lost consciousness. She was found by a neighbor who put her to bed. The patient was unable to move her left arm and leg, and her speech—although slurred and slow—made sense.

Neurologic examination on admission showed a blood pressure of 180/100 with a regular heart rate of 84 beats per minute. The patient was slow to respond but roughly oriented with regard to person, place, and time. She ignored stimuli in the left visual field. The

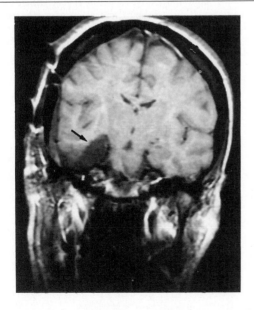

Figure 21–9. Postoperative MR image of frontal section through the head, showing anteromedial temporal lobectomy (arrow).

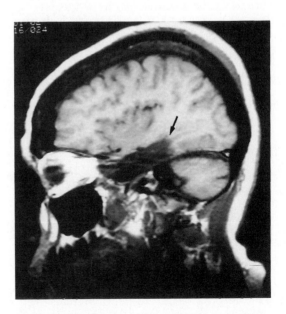

Figure 21–10. MR image in the sagittal plane, showing anteromedial temporal lobe resection (anterior to the arrow).

pupils responded to light and there was slight, but definite, bilateral papilledema. Other findings included decreased appreciation of pain on the left side of the face, complete paralysis of the left central face, and complete flaccid paralysis of the left arm and left leg. Reflexes were more pronounced on the left than on the right, and there was a left plantar extensor response. Responses to all sensory stimuli were decreased on the left side of the body. CT scanning produced an image similar to Figure 12–12, but in the opposite hemisphere.

What is the diagnosis?

CASE 28

A 63-year-old clerk suddenly experienced a strange feeling over his body, which he characterized as an electric shock, with flashes of blue light. He said the flashes looked like a stained glass window with very strong sun behind it on the right. During this episode he felt confused. When he recovered shortly after-wards, he felt tired and went to bed. The next day when he got up he inadvertently walked into the right door-jamb. He did not notice his wife bringing him a cup of coffee as she approached from his right side. During the next two weeks, he continued to bump into people and objects on his right side and complained of poor vision, which he attributed to a cataract in his right eye. His wife urged him to see a doctor. When asked about his medical history, the patient indicated that he had rheumatic heart disease that had been completely under control for the past three years.

General physical examination revealed cataracts in both eyes, which were not severe enough to compromise vision significantly. Neurologic examination showed normal visual acuity and normal optic discs, but there was right hemianopia. No other neurologic abnormality was found.

Where is the lesion? What further tests would be helpful in confirming the site? What is the most likely diagnosis?

Cases are discussed further in Chapter 25.

REFERENCES

Benson DF: *Aphasia, Alexia, and Agraphia.* Churchill-Livingstone, 1979.

Cummings JL: *Clinical Neuropsychiatry.* Grune & Stratton, 1985.

Damasio AR, Geschwind N: The neural basis of language. *Ann Rev Neurosci* 1985;**7**:127.

Engel J: *Seizures and Epilepsy.* FA Davis, 1989.

Geschwind N: The Apraxias: Neural Mechanisms of Disorders of Learned Movement. *Amer Sci* 1975;**63**:188.

Heilman KM, Valenstein E, Watson RT: Neglect. In: *Diseases of the Nervous System,* 2nd ed. Asbury AK, McKhann GM, McDonald WI (editors). Saunders, 1992.

Mesulam MM: *Principles of Behavioral Neurology,* FA Davis, 1985.

Porter RJ: Classification of epileptic seizures and epileptic syndromes. In: *A Textbook of Epilepsy.* Laidlaw J, Richens A, Chadwick D (editors). Churchill-Livingstone, 1993.

Raichle ME: Cortical information processing in the normal human brain. In: *Diseases of the Nervous System,* 2nd ed. Asbury AK, McKhann GM, McDonald WI (editors). Saunders, 1992.

Seeck M, Mainwaring N, Ives J, Blume H et al: Differential neural activity in the human temporal lobe evoked by faces of family members and friends. *Ann Neurol* 1993;**34**:369.

Springer SP, Deutch G: *Left Brain, Right Brain.* Freeman, 1987.

Aging, Degeneration, & Regeneration

22

NEUROBIOLOGY OF AGING

Although the human life span has not increased significantly, average life expectancy has lengthened markedly in this century. This increase is mainly because of medical advances: antibiotics, vaccination, a reduction in infant mortality, and a decrease in the incidence of heart disease and stroke. The increase in life expectancy may well be paralleled by an increased incidence of dementia, however, and the deterioration of intellectual function in aged persons as a result of organic disease is often associated with a decrease in the quality of life. The elderly constitute a growing fraction of the population of the USA. The burgeoning development of research in this area, **gerontology** and of the clinical specialty of **geriatrics** is recognized by scientists and medical practitioners alike.

Normal Aging

A. Gross Changes in the Brain: A number of anatomic differences between the brains of elderly people and those of young adults have been consistently noted (Figs 22–1 and 22–2).

By age 80, the brain has lost 15% of its weight. Many cortical gyri have decreased in bulk and the sulci are wider. The spaces containing cerebrospinal fluid are enlarged. The finding of big ventricles, however, does not necessarily mean that the patient is demented. In addition, arterial disease affecting both large and small vessels is usually present in older people, with a concomitant reduction of blood flow and oxygen consumption. In some elderly individuals, multiple small infarcts (in both gray and white matter) in the distribution of small penetrating arteries produce **multi-infarct dementia.**

B. Histologic Changes in the Brain: Some characteristics of the aging process are the reverse of growth changes in the young; others are present solely in elderly people. However, the significance of any of these findings and their cause and effect are not clear.

In normal older people, the number of **neurons** in various cortical regions is significantly lower than in young adults. One study reported that only 50% of the small neurons remained in the most severely affected regions. The **dendrites** of cortical pyramidal cells are also found to be much shorter, thicker, and fewer in old people than in young adults (Fig 22–3).

Synaptic density in the cortex decreases with age, and **neurofibrillary tangles** are found in the cerebral cortices (especially in the hippocampus) of elderly people (Fig 22–4). These tangles consist of knot-like clusters of abnormal fibrils that accumulate within the cytoplasm, thereby injuring neurons. The neurofibrillary tangles contain paired helical filaments that are similar in size to neurofilaments but that apparently share at least one antigenic determinant (termed the **tau protein**) with neurotubules.

Neuritic (senile) plaques consist of amyloid deposits surrounded by a web of astrocytic processes, swollen neurites, and neuron rests in the cortex (Fig 22–5). Intracellular **eosinophilic inclusions (Hirano bodies)** are seen in the brain cells of older people and **granulovascular organelles** are seen, especially in hippocampal neurons. **Lipofuscin,** a yellow, insoluble material in the cell bodies, is more abundant in old people than in young adults; however, this substance is apparently harmless to the cells.

C. Biochemical and Physiologic Changes: By age 80, there is a 30% reduction in the amount of total brain protein. There is a concomitant progressive increase in total DNA, presumably caused by proliferation of glial cells (gliosis). Lipid constituents (neural fats, cerebrosides, and phosphatides) show a minimal decrease with age, and there is only a slight increase in water content. A reduction in blood flow and oxygen consumption occurs with age.

Changes in neurotransmitter systems (enzymes, receptors, transmitters, and their metabolites) occur with aging. The synthesis and degradation of neurotransmitters are carried out by enzymes. Changes in the amount of these enzymes produced or a reduction in

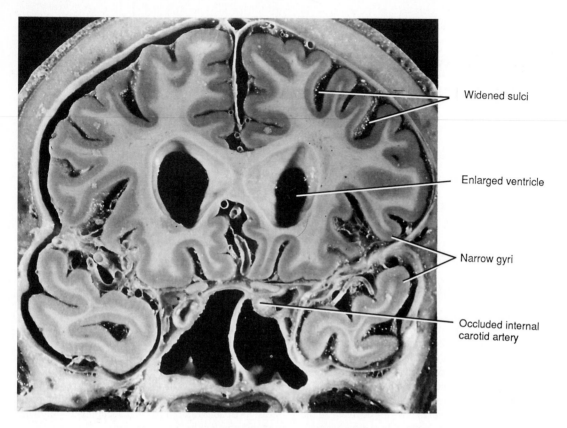

Widened sulci

Enlarged ventricle

Narrow gyri

Occluded internal carotid artery

Figure 22–1. Coronal section through the head of a 78-year-old patient.

their efficacy could explain some of the characteristics of senescence: changes in sleep patterns, mood, appetite, neuroendocrine function, motor activity, and memory. Levels of choline acetyltransferase (the biosynthetic enzyme for acetylcholine) are strikingly reduced in some aged brains, particularly in Alzheimer's disease. There is, moreover, a drastic reduction in the total amount of those enzymes involved in the synthesis of dopamine and norepinephrine. There is often a reduction of the electroencephalographic variations in evoked potentials to auditory stimuli. In addition, recovery from brain damage is slower and less complete than in younger individuals.

DEMENTIA

The normal changes in form and function of the aged brain must be distinguished from those caused by diseases that abnormally intensify some of the aging processes. Such diseases are often characterized by an impairment of cognitive function or by dementia.

Dementia is defined as a loss of intellectual functions, such as memory, learning, reasoning, problem solving, and abstract thinking, while vegetative (involuntary) functions remain intact.

Classification

Dementia is associated with several types of diseases.

A. Dementia Associated with Medical Syndromes: These include hypothyroidism, Cushing's disease, nutritional deficiencies, AIDS dementia complex, and so forth.

B. Dementia Associated with Neurologic Syndromes: This group includes Huntington's chorea, Schilder's disease, and other demyelinative processes; Creutzfeldt-Jakob disease; brain tumors; brain trauma; brain and meningeal infections; and the like.

C. Diseases with Dementia as the Only or Prominent Sign: Alzheimer's disease and Pick's disease are in this category.

Epidemiology

In the USA, of the individuals over 65 years of age (30 million and increasing) almost 15% show moderate mental impairment; about 5% of this age group is seriously demented and about 50%–60% of this 5% probably have Alzheimer's disease (1.5 million individuals). Another 13% (4 million) are mildly de-

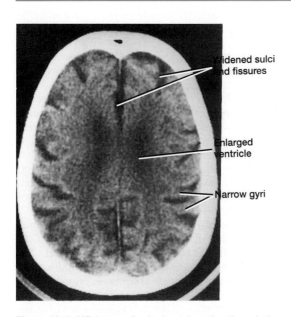

Figure 22–2. MR image of a horizontal section through the head of an 80-year-old patient.

mented. About 25% of the over-80 age group show significant dementia. The economic burden imposed on society by dementia is heavy, both because of the cost of care and because of the decreased quality of life for afflicted individuals, who often become dependent on the immediate family (which exacts a further cost). Once dementia becomes fully developed, life expectancy is less than five years; this means that at least 200,000 demented patients die each year in the USA.

Senile Dementia of the Alzheimer Type

A. Characteristics: **Alzheimer's disease** is a common type of dementia whose cause is unknown. Autopsy studies reveal that more than half of patients

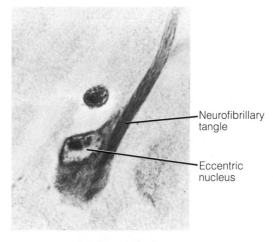

Figure 22–4. Micrograph of a nerve cell containing a neurofibrillary tangle. (Silver stain, × 800.)

who died of **senile dementia** had the Alzheimer-type disease (Fig 22–6). In most patients, gross brain weight at the time of autopsy is much lower and the ventricles and sulci are much larger than normal for that age. Demyelination and increased water content of brain tissue have been found adjacent to the lateral ventricles and in a few other areas deep in the cerebral hemispheres in elderly patients, especially those suffering from Alzheimer's disease. (This form of demyelination can be distinguished from that of multiple sclerosis on the basis of age and distribution: Patients with multiple sclerosis are much younger, and plaques, in which

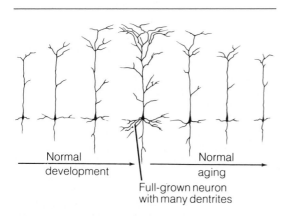

Figure 22–3. Schematic illustration of the increase in the size and number of dendrites and the decrease that occur with approaching age.

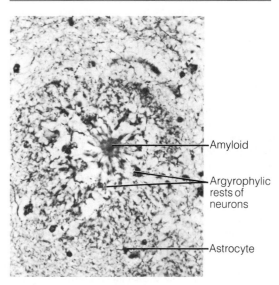

Figure 22–5. Micrograph of a senile plaque, showing an amyloid-containing center amid remnants of nerve processes and glial cells. (Silver stain, × 800.)

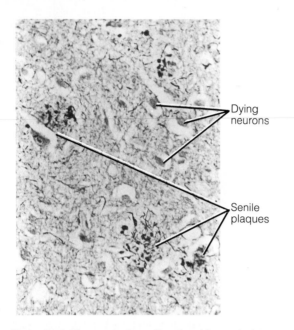

Dying neurons

Senile plaques

Figure 22–6. Micrograph of a small section of the cerebral cortex of a patient suffering from senile dementia; multiple plaques are seen amid dying neurons. (Silver stain, × 200.)

there is inflammatory demyelination, are present in many areas other than the hemispheres.)

In patients with senile dementia of the Alzheimer's type, there is a dramatic increase (in comparison with normal elderly patients) in the number of **neurofibrillary tangles** and **neuritic plaques.** Neurofibrillary tangles and neuritic plaques are present in both the normal aged brain and in Alzheimer's disease, but there are more neurofibrillary tangles and plaques in Alzheimer's disease brains. Neurofibrillary tangles and neuritic plaques are first seen, and occur in the greatest numbers, in the hippocampus, particularly the CA1 region, but are found later throughout the cerebral cortex, especially the association cortex.

Neuritic plaques consist of a central core of amyloid, surrounded by abnormal axons and dendrites together with microglial cells and reactive astrocytes. Recent research has focused on a protein fragment, approximatley 40 amino acids long, referred to as the **amyloid beta protein,** as the major component of amyloid within neuritic plaques. Amyloid beta protein is neurotoxic, and recent studies suggest (but have not yet conclusively proved) that deposition of abnormal amyloid beta protein triggers neuronal death in Alzheimer's disease. Amyloid beta protein appears to be produced by abnormal processing of a larger (695-amino acid) membrane-spanning protein, generally referred to as the **beta amyloid precursor protein** (beta-APP).

The beta-APP gene is located on chromosome 21. At least one form of **familial Alzheimer's disease (FAD)** seems to be caused by a defect on chromosome 21 (which, interestingly, is the chromosome involved in Down's syndrome, in which neuritic plaques and neurofibrillary tangles are also found). However, mutations on other genes appear to be associated with other forms of familial Alzheimer's disease and sporadic cases are common. A multi-factorial etiology, with several genetic and metabolic defects all leading to deposition of beta amyloid, is possible. The genetics, molecular biology, and metabolism of beta-APP and beta amyloid are being further studied in an effort to understand the role of these molecules in the etiology of Alzheimer's disease, with the goal of developing treatments that will prevent the development of neuritic plaques.

Alzheimer's disease is associated with a reduction in the number of cells in the **nucleus basalis** of the brain (also termed the **basal nucleus of Meynert**). The nucleus basalis has extensive cholinergic projections to large areas of the cerebral cortex; it lies in the basal forebrain below the anterior commissure (see Fig 9–7a). As expected from the involvement of the nucleus basalis in Alzheimer's disease, there is a 60–90% decrease in cortical levels of **choline acetyltransferase** (the enzyme that brings about the synthesis of acetylcholine).

Other gross or microscopic changes associated with age are often present in the brain. The presence of **proteinaceous infectious particles (prions)** in the brains of demented persons has been interpreted by some workers as suggesting that Alzheimer's disease may be an infection caused by a slow virus.

Other Diseases Associated with Dementia

Pick's disease is an often hereditary presenile dementia. Far less common than Alzheimer's disease, it is characterized grossly by circumscribed frontotemporal cerebral atrophy and associated ventricular enlargement.

Huntington's disease (Huntington's chorea) is a dominantly inherited disease of the basal ganglia and cerebral cortex that usually manifests itself in adulthood. The disease is characterized by progressive mental deterioration and **choreiform movements.** The head of the caudate nucleus may be clearly reduced in size, and greatly decreased levels of GABA and choline acetyltransferase activity are seen in patients with this disease.

Multi-infarct dementia also causes declining mental function in the elderly. It is characterized pathologically by multiple infarcts (many of them small, presumably because of ischemia in the territory of small penetrating arteries) in the cerebral hemispheres including the subcortical white matter and diencephalon. A history of step-like progression (as would be expected from repeated small strokes) can sometimes be obtained. Neurologic examination may reveal upper-motor-neuron signs (hyperreflexia, Babinski reflexes) due to involvement of both cerebral hemispheres, together with a **pseudobulbar state** characterized by dysarthria and dysphagia.

A variety of other disorders can also be associated with dementia. They include **chronic subdural hematoma,** which can be treated surgically; **normal-pressure hydrocephalus** (a form of nonobstructive hydrocephalus in which there is impaired absorption of CSF), which sometimes responds to shunting of the CSF; **brain tumors; neurosyphilis** (which can cause general paresis characterized by dementia and psychiatric abnormalitites); and **Creutzfeldt-Jakob disease** (an invariably fatal, transmissible disorder caused by a slow virus or a prion) characterized by dementia, psychiatric symptoms, abnormal motor findings, and myoclonus. **Deficiency, metabolic,** and **toxic disorders** can also cause dementia. These include, for example, B_{12} deficiency (which often causes a peripheral neuropathy together with dementia), hypothyroidism, thiamin deficiency, and various drug-induced encephalopathies. **Depression** can also produce a state that can be confused with dementia in the elderly, and can often be treated successfully with antidepressants.

NEUROTROPHIC FACTORS

Much work over the past decades has focused on **neurotrophic factors** (originally termed **growth factors**). These specialized protein molecules enhance the outgrowth of neurites from developing and regenerating neurons, and promote the survival of neurons. The number of neurotrophic factors that have been identified is growing. Each neurotrophic factor appears to have *specific* effects on particular types of neurons, with other types of neurons being unresponsive.

The first neurotrophic factor to be identified was **nerve growth factor (NGF).** The active subunit of NGF consists of paired peptides, each containing 118 amino acids. Sensory neurons derived from the neural crest (dorsal root ganglion neurons), sympathetic neurons, and CNS cholinergic cells (located in basal forebrain nucleus) are NGF-sensitive. NGF appears to be produced in target areas, where the axon terminals from these neurons terminate, and is taken up into presynaptic terminals and translocated, via axonal transport, to the neuronal cell body. Several receptors (the trk class of receptors), which bind NGF and related molecules, contain a tyrosine kinase that increases tyrosine phosphorylation after binding of the neurotrophin molecule.

Nerve growth factor is one member of a family of **neurotrophins,** which have a high degree of molecular homology. **Brain-derived neurotrophic factor (BDNF)** is produced by cells in many regions of the CNS, including the hippocampus, amygdala, cerebral cortex, and cerebellum. BDNF appears to be a neurotrophic factor for dopaminergic neurons (such as those in the substantia nigra) and cholinergic CNS neurons (such as those in basal forebrain nucleus). Two additional members of the neurotrophin family, **NT-3** and **NT-4**, have been identified and characterized. NT-3 promotes neurite outgowth from dorsal root ganglion cells and, to a smaller degree, from sympathetic neurons. The different patterns of neurotrophic action of NGF, BDNF, and NT-3 on three classes of neurons, dorsal root ganglion sensory neurons, nodose ganglion sensory neurons, and sympathetic ganglion neurons, are shown in Figure 22–7.

Still another neurotropic factor, **ciliary neurotrophic factor (CNTF),** is molecularly distinct from the neurotrophin family. CNTF is a 200-amino acid protein, related to cytokines such as interleukin-6. CNTF is neurotropic for motor neurons and, under some circumstances, may promote their survival after various pathologic injuries.

It is not known whether a deficit in the production of neurotropic factors, or the expression of receptors for these molecules, is involved in the etiology of any neurologic disease. A number of research groups are studying the survival-promoting effects of neurotrophic factors and are exploring the hypothesis that trophic factors may rescue neurons from various pathologic insults.

DEGENERATION & REGENERATION

Nerve Degeneration

A. Effects of Peripheral Nerve Lesions: The loss of a nerve's ability to conduct impulses results in impaired motor, sensory, and trophic function. Motor loss is manifested by paralysis or muscle weakness as well as atrophy of the involved muscle. Sensory involvement may be subjective or objective. Subjective sensory findings include pain and paresthesias (numbness, tingling). Objective findings include the loss of various sensibilities (analgesia, anesthesia, etc). Trophic disturbances reflect impaired nutritional and metabolic activities in tissues that are partly under neurogenic control. Most marked in the cutaneous tissues, they are manifested in numerous ways, such as dryness, cyanosis, ulcerations, hair loss, brittleness of the nails, and slow wound healing.

B. Histologic Findings: The cell body maintains the functional and anatomic integrity of the axon (Fig 22–8). If the axon is cut, the part distal to the cut degenerates **(wallerian degeneration)**, because materials for maintaining the axon (mostly proteins) are formed in the cell body and can no longer be transported down the axon **(axoplasmic transport).**

Distal to the level of axonal transection, Schwann cells dedifferentiate and divide. Together with macrophages, they phagocytize the remnants of the

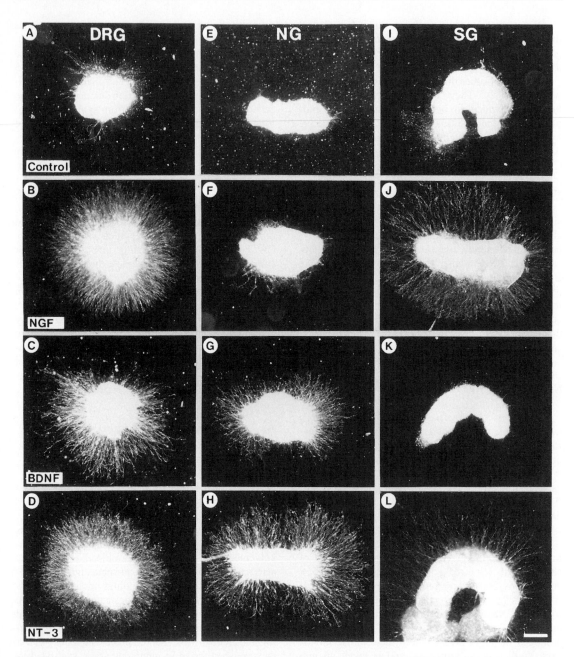

Figure 22–7. Neurotrophic factors enhance the outgrowth of axons from neurons, and accomplish this in a highly specific manner. These photomicrographs show the effects of NGF, BDNF, and NT-3 on explants of dorsal root ganglia (DRG; A-D), nodose ganglia (NG; E-H), and paravertebral sympathetic ganglia (SG; I-L) from chick embryos, maintained in culture for 24–48 hours. The neurotrophic effects are *cell-specific.* For example, NGF enhances axonal outgrowth from dorsal root ganglion cells, but not nodose ganglion neurons. In contrast, NT-3 strongly enhances neurite outgrowth from nodose ganglia. (Modified, with permission, from Maisonpierre PC et al: Neurotrophin-3: A neurotrophic factor related to NGF and BDNF. *Science* 1990;**247:**1446.)

myelin sheaths, which lose their integrity as the axon degenerates.

After injury to its axon, the neuronal cell body exhibits a distinct set of histologic changes (which have been termed the **axon reaction** or **chromatolysis**). The changes include swelling of the cell body and nucleus, which is usually displaced from the center of the cell to an eccentric location. The regular arrays of ribosome-studded endoplasmic reticulum, which characterize most neurons, are dispersed and replaced by polyribosomes (the ribosome-studded endoplasmic reticulum, which had been termed the Nissl substance by classical neuroanatomists, normally stains densely with basic dyes; the loss of staining of the Nissl sub-

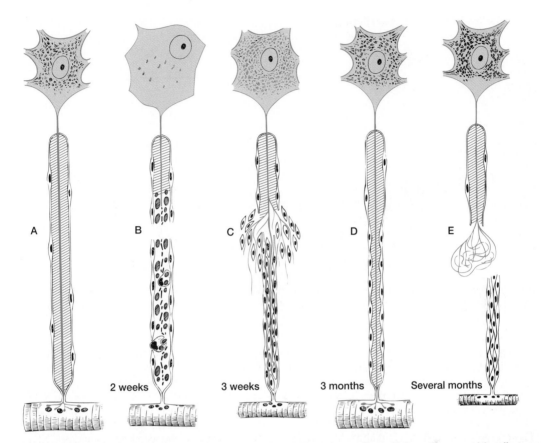

Figure 22–8. Main changes that take place in an injured nerve fiber. *A:* Normal nerve fiber, with its perikaryon and the effector cell (striated skeletal muscle). Notice the position of the neuron nucleus and the amount and distribution of Nissl bodies. *B:* When the fiber is injured, the neuronal nucleus moves to the cell periphery, and Nissl bodies become greatly reduced in number (chromatolysis), and the nerve fiber distal to the injury degenerates along with its myelin sheath. Debris is phagocytized by macrophages. *C:* The muscle fiber shows pronounced disuse atrophy. Schwann cells proliferate, forming a compact cord that is penetrated by the growing axon. The axon grows at a rate of 0.5–3 mm/d. *D:* In this example, the nerve fiber regeneration was successful, and the muscle fiber was also regenerated after receiving nerve stimuli. *E:* When the axon does not penetrate the cord of Schwann cells, its growth is not organized and successful regeneration does not occur. (Redrawn and reproduced, with permission, from Willis RA, Willis AT: *The Principles of Pathology and Bacteriology,* 3rd ed. Butterworth, 1972.)

stance, as a result of dispersion of the endoplasmic reticulum during the axon reaction, led these early scientists to use the term chromatolysis). In association with the axon reaction in some CNS neurons, there is detachment of afferent synapses, swelling of nearby astrocytes, and activation of microglia. The axon reaction may reset neuronal metabolic and biosynthetic activities in response to axonal injury in a manner that facilitates synaptic reorganization or axonal regeneration. However, successful axonal regeneration does not always occur (see following section). Many neurons appear to be dependent on connection with appropriate target cells; if the axon fails to regenerate and form a new synaptic connection with the correct postsynaptic cells, the axotomized neuron may die or atrophy.

Regeneration

A. Peripheral Nerves: Regeneration denotes a nerve's ability to repair itself, including the re-estab-

lishment of functionally useful connections (Figs 22–8 and 22–9). Shortly (1–3 days) after an axon is cut, the tips of the proximal stumps form enlargements, or growth cones, under the influence of nerve growth factor (NGF). The growth cones send out many exploratory pseudopodia that are similar to the axonal growth cones formed in normal development. Each axonal growth cone is capable of forming many branches that continue to advance away from the site of the original cut. If these branches can cross the scar tissue and enter Büngner's bands (rows of Schwann cells surrounded by basal lamina that are formed in the distal nerve stump after axonal after degeneration), in the distal nerve stump, successful regeneration with restoration of function may occur.

The importance of axonal regeneration through the Schwann cell tubes surrounded by basal lamina (Büngner's bands) in the distal stump explains the different degrees of regeneration that are seen after *nerve crush,* compared to *nerve transection.* Following a

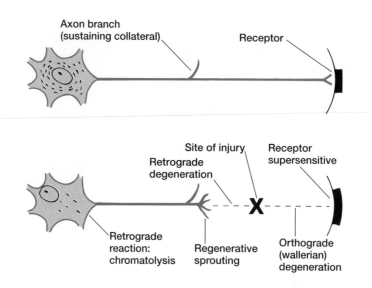

Figure 22–9. Summary of changes occurring in a neuron and the structure it innervates when its axon is crushed or cut at the point marked X. (Modified from D. Ries. Reproduced, with permission, from Ganong WF: *Review of Medical Physiology,* 16th ed. Appleton & Lange, 1993.)

crush injury to a peripheral nerve, the axons may be severed, but the Schwann cells, surrounding basal lamina, and perineurium maintain continuity through the lesion, facilitating regeneration of axons through the injured nerve. In contrast, if the nerve is cut, the continuity of these pathways is disrupted; even with meticulous surgery, it can be difficult to align the proximal and distal parts of each axon's pathway and successful regenration is, therefore, less likely.

Overproduction of branching axons occurs in the early stages of regeneration, and it is possible to see as many as 20 fine axons lying within a single Bungner's band. This number does become reduced, however. Maturation of nerve fibers and the development of a normal axon diameter is dependent upon reinnervation. The new myelin segments are thinner and shorter. Regrowth of regenerating axons occurs at the rate of about 1–4mm/d—the same rate as slow axonal transport.

In mammals, peripheral system axons will reinnervate both muscle and sensory targets; however, motor axons will not connect to sensory structures, or sensory axons to muscle. While a motor axon will reinnervate any denervated muscle, it will preferentially connect to its original muscle. Innervation of an incorrect muscle by a regenerated motor axon results in **anomalous reinnervation,** which can be accompanied by inappropriate and unwanted movements (eg, "jaw-winking," in which motor axons destined for the jaw muscles reinnervate muscles around the eye after injury).

B. Central Nervous System: Axonal regeneration is typically abortive in the central nervous system. The reasons for the failure of regeneration are not clear. Classical neuropathologists suggested that the glial scar, which is largely formed by astrocytic processes, may be partly responsible. The properties of

the oligodendroglial cells (in contrast to those of the Schwann cells of peripheral nerves) may also account for the difference in regenerative capacity: no Bungner's bands are formed. Recent work suggests that the glial scar may not present a mechanical barrier to axonal regeneration in the CNS. An inhibitory factor produced by oligodendrocytes and/or CNS myelin may interfere with regeneration of axons through the CNS. When confronted with a permissive environment (eg, when the transected axons of CNS neurons are permitted to regrow into a peripheral nerve, transplanted into the CNS as a "bridge"), CNS axons can regenerate for distances of at least a few centimeters. Moreover, some of the regenerated axons can establish synaptic connections with appropriate target cells. On the basis of this type of finding, neuroscientists are investigating the possibility of repair of the central nervous system by transplantation of appropriate cells, after injury to the CNS.

C. Remyelination: In a number of disorders of the peripheral nervous system (such as the Guillain-Barré syndrome) there is demyelination, which interferes with conduction (see Chapter 3). This is often followed by remyelination by Schwann cells, which are capable of elaborating new myelin sheaths in the PNS. In contrast, remyelination occurs much more slowly (if at all) in the CNS. There is little remyelination within demyelinated plaques within the brain and spinal cord in multiple sclerosis. A different form of plasticity, ie, the molecular reorganization of the axon membrane which acquires sodium channels in demyelinated zones, appears to underlie clinical remissions (in which there is neurologic improvement) in patients with multiple sclerosis.

D. Collateral Sprouting: This phenomenon has been demonstrated in the central nervous system as well as in the peripheral nervous system (see Fig 22–9). It occurs when an innervated structure has been partially denervated. The remaining axons then form new collaterals that reinnervate the denervated part of the end-organ. This kind of regeneration demonstrates that there is considerable plasticity in the nervous system and that one axon can take over the synaptic sites formerly occupied by another.

NEUROGENESIS

It is generally believed that neurogenesis, ie, the capability for production of neurons from undifferentiated, proliferative progenitor cells, is confined to the development period that precedes birth in mammals. Thus, following pathologic insults that result in neuronal death, the number of neurons is permanently reduced. The situation is different in some lower vertebrates such as birds and fish. In these species, **postnatal neurogenesis,** ie, the generation of neurons after birth, occurs. Moreover, in some of these species, **compensatory neurogenesis** can occur after injury to the CNS, resulting in the production of new neurons that are integrated into functional circuits.

Because neurogenesis does not occur postnatally in the mammalian CNS, it might be expected that functional recovery would not occur after pathologic insults that result in the loss of neurons. Yet in many cases some functional recovery does occur—an example is given in Clinical Illustration 22–1. While the details of the mechanisms underlying functional recovery are not understood, this recovery provides a demonstration of **neural plasticity** in humans after injury to the CNS.

CLINICAL ILLUSTRATION 22–1

This 59-year-old housewife, with a long history of hypertension, was brought to the hospital because of difficulty speaking. On admission, the patient's blood pressure was 180/100. Examination revealed that, although her speech was fluent, it was nearly devoid of content; it included nonsensical words (eg, paraphasias such as "breen" instead of "green," and neologisms such as "grenshow"). The patient had difficulty naming even simple objects, and she could not repeat even simple phrases such as "no ifs, ands, or buts." Her comprehension of spoken English was severely impaired, and she could not read. The patient also appeared to have a right homonymous hemianopsia. MRI scan of the brain showed an infarction in the left superior temporal lobe, including Wernicke's area (Fig 22–10).

During her two-week hospitalization, the patient received speech therapy. Her speech improved somewhat, but she left the hospital with significant word-finding difficulty and some difficulty with comprehension. Her deficits persisted during the next year and, although she continued to receive speech therapy, she continued to be frustrated by her impaired speech. Two years after her stroke, however, the patient began to improve markedly. On follow-up examination 2½ years after her admission, she showed significant improvement—word finding was now almost normal, she was able to read and comprehend without difficulty and to express herself completely normally.

This patient's speech disorder was because of a stroke involving Wernicke's area in the left hemi-

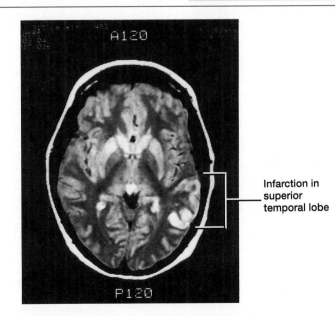

Infarction in superior temporal lobe

Figure 22–10. MR image of a horizontal section through the head showing infarction in the left superior temporal lobe (brackets).

sphere, which is responsible for important aspects of speech. Her MRI scan confirmed the presence of a lesion in this area. The clinical course in this patient provides a striking example of *functional recovery* after injury to the CNS. It is unlikely that neurogenesis accounted for this patient's recovery. Other possible mechanisms include synaptic remodeling or sprouting, strengthening of synaptic connections, and utilization of previously "silent" or unused portions of the brain. There is some evidence that pathways in the *right* hemisphere may play a role in recovery from aphasia, and these might have been recruited as this patient "relearned" to use language. Although mechanisms underlying functional recovery are not well understood, they undoubtedly play an important role in the rehabilition process.

NEURAL PLASTICITY

Neural plasticity permits the nervous system to change in response to experience, changing conditions, and repeated stimuli. Plasticity is clearly evident in developing organisms. The final definitive pattern of neural connections in the adult, for example, does not form all at once. Instead, in many parts of the central and peripheral nervous system, connections are formed more abundantly and more diffusely at first than is ultimately required. During development, these connections rearrange and refine themselves, and, eg, the amount of motor innervation matches the amount of muscle to be innervated.

The projection from the lateral geniculate nucleus to the visual cortex is refined and made more precise during development (see Chapter 15); the ocular dominance columns in layer IV of the calcarine cortex are formed by progressive segregation of the afferents from both eyes. There is a critical period in this segregation process as shown experimentally: If one eye is forced to remain closed during the period of ocular dominance formation (but not before or after), the precise pattern of the dominance columns is disrupted and remains unrecognizable for life.

Neural plasticity is evident in the ongoing fine-tuning and adjustment of our reflexes and perception. For example, a new pair of eyeglasses may make the wearer dizzy at first; after the new glasses are worn for a while, however, the dizziness disappears—and putting on the old eyeglasses will cause dizziness. This type of plasticity has been studied in a neurophysiologic experiment that showed it is possible for a person to adapt, within hours, to prismatic spectacles that displace the image on the retina. The cellular mechanisms responsible for this type of plasticity are not yet fully understood.

Neural plasticity is also evident in some examples of neural regeneration in animals. Cells in the septal complex receive afferent fibers from two distinct sources: the fibers of hippocampal origin that reach the septal nuclei via the fornix, and the axons that arise in the hypothalamus and travel to the septal nuclei in the medial forebrain bundle. The hippocampal fibers terminate almost exclusively on the dendrites of septal cells. The hypothalamic axons, on the other hand, make axosomatic as well as axodendritic synapses with septal neurons. If one of these pathways to the septum is cut and allowed to degenerate, analysis (with an electron microscope) of the remaining pathway indicates enlargement of its terminal distribution to include the postsynaptic sites previously occupied by the now degenerate pathway. Quantitative studies indicate that the rate of new synapse formation by one pathway is closely linked to the rate of degeneration in the other.

Most demonstrations of anatomic plasticity in the brain have so far been limited to rather artificial experimental situations; however, it is likely that similar organizational modifications and the tendency to form new connections participate in the clinical recovery that is seen in some patients after injury to the brain and spinal cord.

Functional imaging studies, on patients who have recovered a degree of motor control following strokes, demonstrate that new areas of the cortex may become involved in the control of movement of a particular joint or limb. Whether this involves synaptic plasticity (ie, a rewiring of the CNS) or re-routing of neural information through pre-existing, previously unused, circuits is not yet known. There will undoubtedly be rapid progress in this area.

CASE 29

A 67-year-old single woman who lived alone had been reasonably well until some three years previously, when her friends noticed changes in her behavior and mental ability: She began to be unable to carry out simple tasks (writing, telephoning, cooking), and she was depressed and sometimes confused. The patient complained of forgetfulness and of inability to find the right words. Her worried friends urged her to see a physician and brought her to the hospital.

Neurologic examination demonstrated marked confusion and disorientation with regard to person and place, memory defects (especially for recent events), aphasia, and a tendency toward perseveration. Generalized muscular weakness and atrophy were present, and there was apraxia for washing and dressing.

A provisional diagnosis was made, and the patient was referred to a nursing home. Three years later she developed severe bronchopneumonia and upon re-admission to the hospital seemed totally forgetful and apathetic.

Which neuroradiologic procedure would aid in the diagnosis? What is the differential diagnosis? What is the most likely diagnosis?

Cases are discussed further in Chapter 25. Questions and answers pertaining to Section IV (Chapters 13 through 22) can be found in Appendix D.

REFERENCES

Aguayo AJ, Rasminsky M, Bray GM et al: Degenerative and regenerative responses of injured neurons in the central nervous system of adult mammals. *Philo Trans, Roy Soc Lond B* 1991;**331:**337.

Anderson MJ, Waxman SG: Neurogenesis in adult vertebrae spinal cord *in situ* and *in vitro;* a new model system. *Ann NY Acad Sci* 1985;**457:**213.

Ip NY, Maisonpierre P, Alderson R et al: The neurotrophins and CNTF: Specificity of action toward PNS and CNS neurons. *J Physiol (Paris)* 1991;**85:**123.

Price DL, Koo EH, Unterbeck A: Cellular and molecular biology of Alzheimer's disease. *BioEssays* 1989;**10:**69.

Schwab ME: Nerve fiber regeneration after traumatic lesions of the CNS: Progress and problems. *Philos Trans, Roy Soc Lond B* 1991;**331:**303.

Seil FJ (editor): *Neuronal Regeneration and Transplantion.* AR Liss, 1989.

Selkoe DJ: The molecular pathology of Alzheimer's disease. *Neuron* 1991;**6:**487.

Terry RD: Alzheimer's disease. In: *Textbook of Neuropathology.* Davis DL, Robertson DM (editors). Williams & Wilkins, 1990.

Thoenen H: The changing scene of neurotrophic factors. *Trends Neurosci* 1991;**14:**165.

Van Horn G: Dementia. *Am J Med* 1987;**83:**101.

Waxman SG (editor): *Molecular and Cellular Approaches to the Treatment of Neurological Disease.* Raven, 1993.

Weiller C, Ramsay SC, Wise RJS, Friston KJ et al: Individual patterns of functional reorganization in the human cerebral cortex after capsular infarction. *Ann Neurol* 1993;**33:**181.

REFERENCES

Imaging of the Brain

23

Scientists have tried for many decades to obtain an image of the skull and brain. The first successful effort was in 1895, when Wilhelm C. Roentgen produced an image (a roentgenogram, or x-ray film) of the skull. In 1927, Egas Moniz injected contrast material into the cerebral arteries of a patient before making a roentgenogram; this was the first cerebral arteriogram. It is only with the modern computer-aided techniques developed by G.N. Hounsfield and A.M. Cormack in the 1960s (and first used in the United States in 1973) that success was achieved in obtaining an image of the brain itself.

Images of the skull, the brain and its vessels, and spaces in the brain containing cerebrospinal fluid can aid immeasurably in the localization of lesions, especially after a complete history taking and physical examination. In emergency cases, images of unconscious patients may be the only diagnostic information available. Traditionally, the views shown in most images have been lateral, anteroposterior (frontal), or oblique. Since the introduction of computed tomography, magnetic resonance imaging, and other methods that display sections of the head, the sagittal, coronal (frontal), and horizontal (axial) planes are commonly used. These are shown in Figure 23–1.

ROENTGENOGRAPHY

Although now limited in its general use, skull radiography with x-rays remains an excellent means of imaging calcium and its distribution in and around the brain when more precise methods are unavailable. Plain films of the skull, taken in various planes, can be used to define the extent of a skull fracture and a possible depression or determine the presence of calcified brain lesions, foreign bodies, or tumors involving the skull. They can also detect asymmetry of brain volume, found by locating the calcified pineal body in an anteroposterior view; chronically increased intracranial pressure, accompanied by thinning of the dorsum sellae; and abnormalities in the size and shape of sella turcica, which suggest large pituitary tumors. Skull films are sometimes used to screen for metal objects before beginning magnetic resonance imaging of the head.

When modern imaging methods were not available, **pneumoencephalography** was used to study patients with epilepsy, cerebral atrophies, congenital brain lesions, and posttraumatic cerebral disorders. The technique involves replacing measured quantities of cerebrospinal fluid with air or some other suitable gas introduced by means of lumbar puncture (or, more rarely, by cisternal or C1–C2 puncture). Most air is absorbed in 48 hours.

Headache, nausea, and vomiting are common complications that may occur after pneumoencephalography; they usually respond well to symptomatic therapy and resting flat in bed. Disturbances of intracranial pressure may lead to herniation of the brain. Thus, pneumoencephalography is hazardous in the presence of elevated cerebrospinal fluid pressure.

ANGIOGRAPHY

Cerebral Angiography

Angiography (arteriography) of the head and neck is a neurodiagnostic procedure used especially in cases

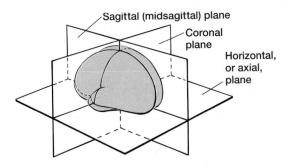

Figure 23–1. Planes used in modern imaging procedures.

Sagittal (midsagittal) plane

Coronal plane

Horizontal, or axial, plane

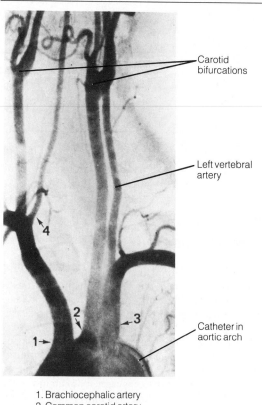

1. Brachiocephalic artery
2. Common carotid artery
3. Left subclavian artery
4. Right vertebral artery

Figure 23–2. Angiogram of the aortic arch and stem vessels. Normal image. **1:** Brachiocephalic artery; **2:** common carotid artery; **3:** left subclavian artery; **4:** right vertebral artery. (Reproduced, with permission, from Peele TL: *The Neuroanatomical Basis for Clinical Neurology.* Blakiston, 1954.)

in which a vessel abnormality such as occlusion, malformation, or aneurysm is suspected (Figs 23–2 to 23–12; see also Chapter 12). Angiography can also be used to determine whether the position of the vessels in relation to intracranial structures is normal or pathologically changed. Arteriovenous fistulas or vascular malformations can be treated by interventional angiography using balloons, a quickly coagulating solution that act as a glue, or small, inert pellets that act like emboli.

A standard set of angiograms, usually in at least two projections, or views (anteroposterior, oblique, or lateral), consists of a series of x-ray films showing contrast material introduced into a major artery (eg, via a catheter in the femoral) under fluoroscopic guidance. Arterial-phase films are followed by capillary and venous-phase films (Figs 23–6 to 23–10). Right and left internal carotid and vertebral angiograms may be complemented by other films, eg, by an external carotid series in cases of meningioma or arteriovenous malformation. The films are often presented as subtracted, ie, as reversal prints superimposed on a plain film of the skull.

Digital Subtraction Angiography

Since the introduction of computed tomography of the head, angiography has been used less frequently as a diagnostic tool. A modern form of angiography, digital subtraction angiography (extraneous tissue in the image is erased, or subtracted), makes use of selective venous or arterial injections of contrast material (Fig 23–12). The digitally enhanced x-ray images are slightly less detailed than traditional angiograms, but complications are less frequent because catherization of the carotids and vertebral arteries is not necessary. This method is frequently used to inspect large vessels in the neck or at the base of the skull.

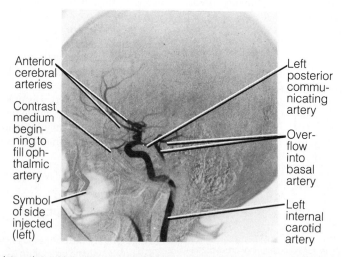

Figure 23–3. Left internal carotid angiogram, early arterial phase, lateral view. Normal image (compare with Fig 23–4).

ULTRASONOGRAPHY

In contrast to x-ray equipment, ultrasonic imaging equipment produces no tissue ionization. In addition to being harmless and fast, ultrasonography is relatively simple and requires no elaborate machinery; newer systems use computers to clean up the pictures obtained.

In ultrasonography, information about structures is obtained by analyzing the time and intensity of echoes from mechanical waves directed into the tissues. The clinical use of ultrasonography for depicting brain structures is severely limited by the dense echoes of the surrounding skull. This method may be used, however, in a young child (up to 18 months) who has open fontanelles (Figs 23–13 and 23–14), in a patient who has had a craniotomy in preparation for brain surgery, and in the rare patient whose skull flap has not healed. Ultrasonography is used extensively for evaluation of the carotid arteries and other vessels irrigating the brain, where changes caused by plaque formation or decreased blood flow may be detected.

COMPUTED TOMOGRAPHY

Computed tomography (CT), also called computed axial tomography (CAT), affords the possibility of inspecting cross sections of the skull, brain, ventricles, cisterns, large vessels, falx, and tentorium. Since its development in the 1960s, the CT scan has become a primary tool for demonstrating the presence of abnormal calcifications, brain edema, hydrocephalus, many types of tumors and cysts, hemorrhages, large aneurysms, vascular malformations, and other disorders.

CT scanning is noninvasive, fast, and safe. Although it has a high degree of sensitivity, its specificity is relatively limited. Therefore, in the presence of an abnormality, correlation with the clinical history and physical examination is an absolute requirement. Often, angiography or another neurodiagnostic procedure is required later to define and characterize a lesion better. In the case of a subarachnoid hemorrhage, for example, while a CT scan may quickly localize the areas containing blood, angiography is often required to determine whether the cause was an aneurysm or an arteriovenous malformation.

The CT scanning apparatus rotates a narrow x-ray beam around the head, and the amount of x-ray transmitted is precisely measured. Using an algorithm that consists of a series of simultaneous equations, the quantity of x-ray absorbed in small volumes (voxels [volume elements, or units]) of brain—measuring approximately 0.5 mm square by 1.5 or more millimeters in length—is computed. The exact amount of x-ray absorbed in any slice of the head can be thus determined and depicted in various ways as pixels (picture elements) in a matrix. In most cases, absorption is proportional to the density of the tissue. A digital-analog converter translates the numeric value of each pixel to a gray scale. Black-and-white pictures of head slices are then displayed, with black representing low-density structures and white representing high-density structures (Table 23–1). The thickness of the slices can be varied, from 1.5 mm to 1 cm. The range of numerical absorption values that the gray scale represents can also be varied; although a setting at which brain tissue is distinguished best is commonly used, in some cases bone, fat, or air need to be defined in great detail.

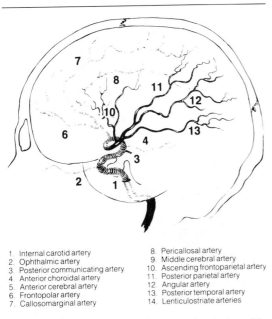

1. Internal carotid artery
2. Ophthalmic artery
3. Posterior communicating artery
4. Anterior choroidal artery
5. Anterior cerebral artery
6. Frontopolar artery
7. Callosomarginal artery
8. Pericallosal artery
9. Middle cerebral artery
10. Ascending frontoparietal artery
11. Posterior parietal artery
12. Angular artery
13. Posterior temporal artery
14. Lenticulostriate arteries

Figure 23–4. Schematic drawing of a normal angiogram of the internal carotid artery, arterial phase, lateral projection. (Redrawn and reproduced, with permission, from List, Burge, Hodges: Intracranial angiography. *Radiology* 1945;45:1.)

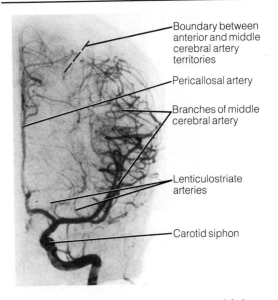

Boundary between anterior and middle cerebral artery territories

Pericallosal artery

Branches of middle cerebral artery

Lenticulostriate arteries

Carotid siphon

Figure 23–5. Left internal carotid angiogram, arterial phase, lateral view. Normal image (compare with Fig 23–6).

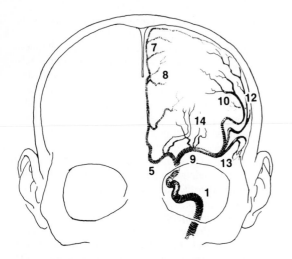

Figure 23–6. Schematic drawing of a normal angiogram of the internal carotid artery, arterial phase, frontal projection. (For significance of numbers see Fig 23–4. Redrawn and reproduced, with permission, from List, Burge, Hodges: Intracranial angiography. *Radiology* 1945;**45**:1.)

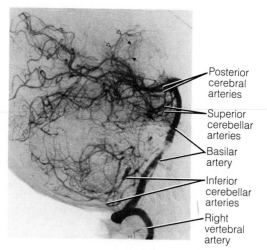

Figure 23–8. Vertebral angiogram, arterial phase, right lateral view. Normal image. Arrows indicate posterior choroidal arteries.

A series of 10–20 scans, each reconstructing a slice of brain, is usually required for a complete study. The plane of these sections is the orbitomeatal plane, which is parallel to both Reid's base plane and the intercommissural line used in stereotactic neurosurgery (Fig 23–15). Usually, a "scout view" similar to a lateral skull roentgenogram is taken with a CT scanner to align the planes of section (Fig 23–16). With the modern technology now available, each scan takes only a few seconds. Examples of normal and abnormal CT scans are shown in Figures 23–17 and 23–18 (see the figures in Chapter 6 also).

CT scanning of the posterior fossa is often unsatisfactory because of the many artifacts caused by dense bone. Injecting contrast material into the cisterns improves the image in some cases. This procedure of contrast enhancement has essentially replaced the pneumoencephalographic studies in which ventricles, cisterns, or both were filled with air prior to taking skull films. Images reformed by a computer from a series of thin sections allow visualization in any desired plane,

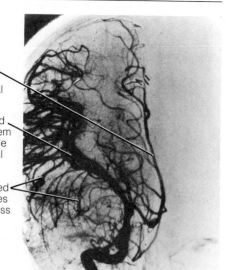

Figure 23–7. Right internal carotid angiogram, arterial phase, anteroposterior view. Abnormal image.

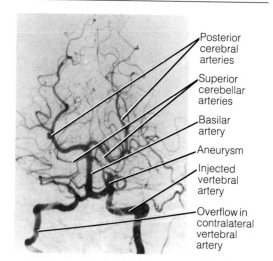

Figure 23–9. Vertebral angiogram, arterial phase, anteroposterior view, with head flexed (Towne position). An aneurysm is present, but the pattern of the vessels is normal.

eg, midsagittal (see Fig 6–17), or coronal. Coronal sections are often extremely useful for structures lying at the base of the brain, in the high convexity area, or close to the incisura. Detailed examination of orbital contents requires planes at right angles to the orbital axis.

Tissue density can change pathologically (see Figs 12–12 and 12–18). Areas of hyperemia or freshly clotted hemorrhage appear more dense; edematous tissue appears less dense. In such cases, the diagnostic sensitivity of CT scanning is increased by intravenous injection of iodinated contrast agents. When there are brain abnormalities, these agents will often pass into the abnormal tissue through defects in the blood-brain barrier. Iodine in the contrast agent absorbs a large quantity of the x-rays, making the lesion highly visible (see Fig 12–21A).

MAGNETIC RESONANCE IMAGING

Nuclear magnetic resonance (NMR) has been used in physical chemistry since the 1950s. In medicine, the magnetic resonance imaging method (MRI or MR imaging) depicts protons and neutrons in a strong ex-ternal magnetic field shielded from extraneous radio signals; no radiation is used.

The spatial distribution of elements with an odd number of protons (such as hydrogen) within slices of the body or brain can be determined by their reaction to an external radio frequency signal; gradient coils are used to localize the signal (Fig 23–19). The signal of every voxel is shown as a pixel in a matrix, similar to the CT technique. The resolution of the images is comparable to that of current CT scans, and with MR imaging an image of any plane can be obtained directly; no reformation is required. Bone is poorly imaged and does not interfere with visualization of nervous tissue; thus, MRI is especially useful for imaging the spinal cord and structures within the posterior fossa.

With MR imaging, the flow of blood within medium and larger arteries and veins can be evaluated directly, with no need for intravenous injection of a contrast agent. This makes MR imaging particularly useful in coronary, renal, and cerebral vascular studies. Fast-flowing blood produces no signal; slow-flowing or turbulent blood produces a high-intensity signal (see Figs 12–4 and 12–9). Blurred images caused by heart contractions and pulse beat can be prevented by making MR images only at certain times of the heart cycle and

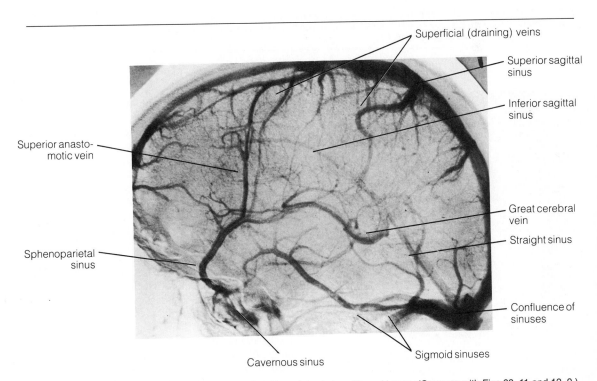

Figure 23–10. Left internal carotid angiogram, venous phase, lateral view. Normal image. (Compare with Figs 23–11 and 12–9.)

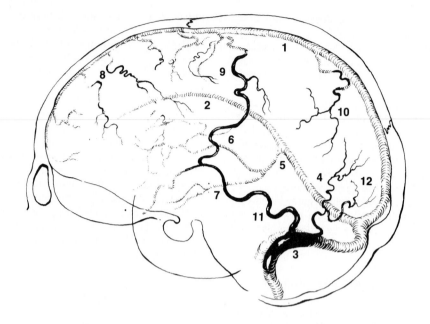

1. Superior sagittal sinus
2. Inferior sagittal sinus
3. Transverse sinus
4. Straight sinus
5. Great cerebral vein of Galen
6. Internal cerebral vein

7. Basal vein of Rosenthal
8. Frontal ascending vein
9. Rolandic vein of Trolard
10. Parietal ascending vein
11. Communicating temporal vein of Labbé
12. Descending temporo-occipital vein

Figure 23–11. Schematic drawing of normal venogram in lateral projection, obtained by carotid injection. Superficial veins are shaded more darkly than the sinuses and deep veins. (Redrawn and reproduced, with permission, from List, Burge, Hodges: Intracranial angiography. *Radiology* 1945;**45**:1.)

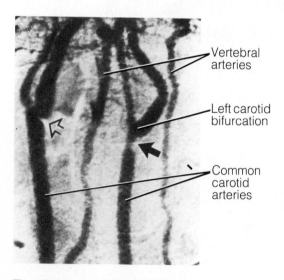

Vertebral arteries

Left carotid bifurcation

Common carotid arteries

Figure 23–12. Digital subtraction angiogram of the neck vessels, oblique anterior view. Open arrow shows small sclerotic plaque; closed arrow shows large plaque.

using a gating technique with simultaneous electrocardiographic recording.

The sequence of radio frequency excitation followed by recording of tissue disturbance (echo signals) can be varied, in both duration of excitation and sampling time. The images obtained with short time sequences differ from those obtained with longer time sequences (Fig 23–20). Normal MR images are shown in Figures 23–20 and 23–21; other MR images, both normal and abnormal, are found in Chapters 6 and 12 and elsewhere throughout this text.

The MR imaging process is relatively slow; it is safe for patients who have no ferromagnetic implants. The increasing sophistication of MR imaging technique (eg, with the use of contrast agents) is expected to broaden its clinical usefulness, and it is likely that further improvements will make the procedure faster, less costly, and more often used. Although only the distribution of water (hydrogen protons) has been thus far used for diagnostic purposes in patients, experimental work with phosphorus, nitrogen, and sodium is under

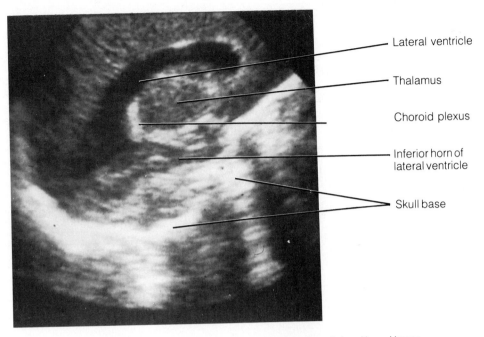

Figure 23–13. Cerebral ultrasonogram of a newborn, lateral view. Normal image.

way. MRI provides a primary method of examination, especially in cases of suspected tumors, demyelination, and infarcts. As with CT scanning, successful use of MR imaging for accurate diagnosis of an abnormality requires correlating the results with the clinical history and physical examination.

POSITRON EMISSION TOMOGRAPHY

Positron emission tomography (PET) scanning has become a major clinical research tool for the imaging of cerebral blood flow, brain metabolism, and other chemical processes (Fig 23–22). Radioisotopes are inhaled or injected, and emissions are measured with a gamma-ray-detector system. One disadvantage is the lack of detailed resolution; another is that most positron-emitting nucleides decay so rapidly that their transportation from the cyclotron (the site of production) becomes a problem. Some isotopes, such as fluorine 18 (^{18}F) and gamma-aminobutyric acid, have a sufficiently long half-life that they can be shipped by air. Some, such as ruthenium derivatives, can be made at the site of examination.

SINGLE PHOTON EMISSION COMPUTED TOMOGRAPHY

Recent advances in nuclear medicine instrumentation and radiopharmaceuticals have opened renewed interest in single photon emission computed tomogra-

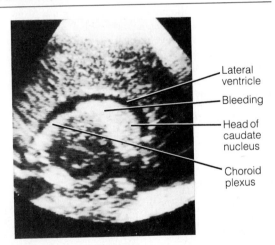

Figure 23–14. Cerebral ultrasonogram of a newborn, lateral view. Abnormal image.

Table 23–1. CT coefficients of absorption (density).

Substance	Coefficients (in Hounsfield units)
Air	–1000
Fat	–80
Water	0
Cerebrospinal fluid	0 to 16
Edematous tissue	8 to 20
White matter	24 to 36
Gray matter	30 to 50
Flowing blood	25 to 40
Clotted blood	40 to 90
Giloma (various types)	10, 60, and 400
Calcified tissue and bone	80 to 1000

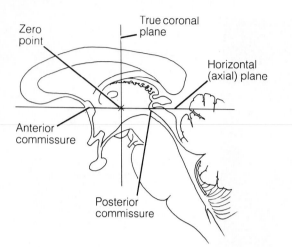

Figure 23–15. Schematic image of the zero horizontal and coronal planes. The line between anterior and posterior commissures parallels Reid's base line.

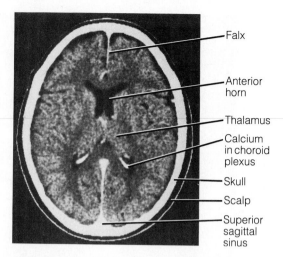

Figure 23–17. CT image, with contrast enhancement, of a horizontal section at the level of the thalamus. Normal image. Compare with Fig 13–4.

phy (SPECT) of the brain. The increasing use of investigative agents in conjunction with PET imaging has stimulated the development of diagnostic radiopharmaceuticals for SPECT; these are routinely available to clinical nuclear medicine laboratories. A Tc-99m-based compound—Tc-99m-HMPAO (Tc-99m-hexamethylpropyleneamineoxime)—is widely used. It is sufficiently lipophilic to diffuse readily across the blood-brain barrier and into nerve cells along the blood flow. It remains in brain tissue long enough to permit assessment of the relative distribution of brain blood by SPECT in 1.0–1.5 cm coronal, sagittal, and horizontal tomographic slices. SPECT studies are especially useful in patients with cerebrovascular disease (Fig 23–23).

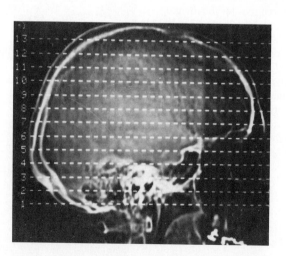

Figure 23–16. Lateral "scout view" used in CT procedure. Superimposed lines represent the levels of the images (sections). Line 1 is at the level of the foramen magnum; line 4 is at the level of the infraorbitomeatal plane.

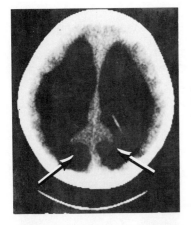

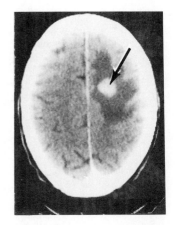

Top left: Hydrocephalus. Dilated ventricles in a 7-year-old boy who had undergone a shunting operation at age 1 year.

Top right: Brain tumor. Cerebral metastasis from carcinoma of lung in a 65-year-old man.

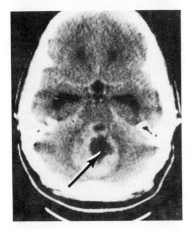

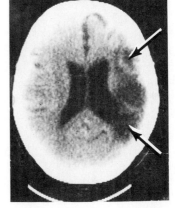

Center left: Brain tumor. Cerebellar medulloblastoma in a 16-year-old male.

Center right: Cerebral hemiatrophy History of subarachnoid hemorrhage 5 years previously in a 48-year-old woman.

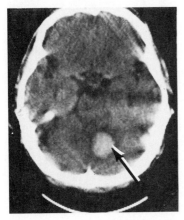

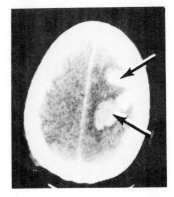

Lower left: Cerebellar hemorrhage. Eighty-one-year-old hypertensive man with acute onset of coma and quadriparesis.

Lower right: Traumatic intracerebral hemorrhage. History of a fall by an intoxicated 78-year-old man followed by confusion and hemiplegia.

Figure 23–18. Representative examples of CT images. (Courtesy of GP Ballweg.)

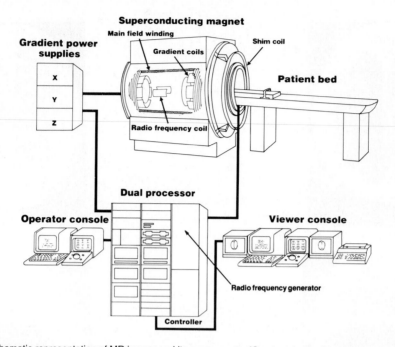

Figure 23–19. Schematic representation of MR imager and its components. (Courtesy L. Kaufmann. Reproduced, with permission, from de Groot J: *Correlative Neuroanatomy of Computed Tomography and Magnetic Resonance Imaging.* Lea & Febiger, 1984.)

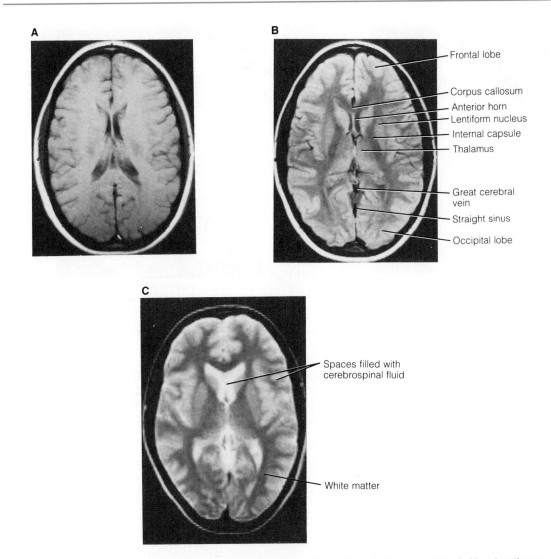

Figure 23–20. MRI of horizontal sections through the lateral ventricles. Normal images. **A:** Image obtained with a short time sequence; the gray-white boundaries are poorly defined, and the spaces filled with cerebrospinal fluid are dark. **B:** Image obtained with an intermediate time sequence. **C:** Image obtained with a long time sequence; the white matter is clearly differentiated from gray matter, and the spaces filled with cerebrospinal fluid are white.

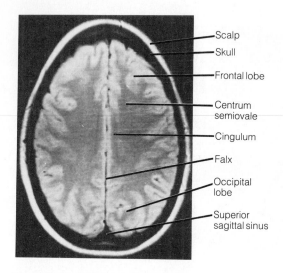

Scalp
Skull
Frontal lobe
Centrum semiovale
Cingulum
Falx
Occipital lobe
Superior sagittal sinus

Figure 23–21. MRI of a horizontal high section through the head. Normal image.

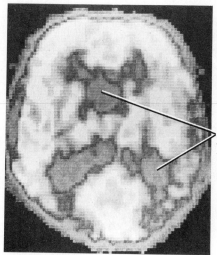
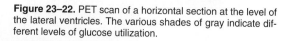

Enlarged ventricles

Figure 23–22. PET scan of a horizontal section at the level of the lateral ventricles. The various shades of gray indicate different levels of glucose utilization.

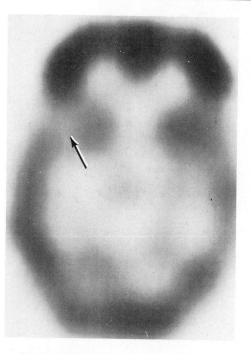

Figure 23–23. SPECT image of a horizontal section through the head at the level of the temporal lobe. An infarct (arrow) is shown as an interruption of the cortical ribbon. (Courtesy of D Price.)

REFERENCES

Brant-Zawadski M, Norman D (editors): *Magnetic Resonance Imaging of the Central Nervous System.* Raven, 1987.

deGroot J: *Correlative Neuroanatomy of Computed Tomography and Magnetic Resonance Imaging.* Lea and Febiger, 1984.

Ell PJ et al: Functional imaging of the brain. Pages 211–229 in *Seminars in Nuclear Medicine 17,* 1987.

Mazziotta JC, Gilman S: *Clinical Brain Imaging.* FA Davis, 1992.

Mills CM, deGroot J, Posin JP: *Magnetic Resonance Imaging: Atlas of the Head, Neck, and Spine.* Lea & Febiger, 1988.

Newton TH, Potts DG (editors): *Advanced Imaging Techniques.* Clavadel Press, 1983.

Oldendorf WH: *The Quest for an Image of the Brain.* Raven, 1980.

Osborn AG: *Introduction to Cerebral Angiography.* Harper & Row, 1980.

Ramsey RG: *Neuroradiology,* 2nd ed. Saunders, 1987.

24

Electrodiagnostic Tests

ELECTROENCEPHALOGRAPHY

Electroencephalography is the study of the ongoing or spontaneous electrical activity of the brain. The potentials of the brain are recorded in an electroencephalogram (EEG); they appear as periodic waves, with frequencies ranging from 0.5 to 40 cycles per second (cps or hertz [Hz]) and with an amplitude that ranges from five to several hundred μV. Because the amplitude of cerebral electrical activity is much smaller than that obtained from the heart in an electrocardiogram (ECG), sensitive (but stable) amplification is necessary to produce an undistorted record of brain activity; this requires proper grounding and electrical shielding.

Clinical Applications

Electroencephalography can provide useful information in patients with structural disease of the brain, especially when seizures occur or are suspected. EEGs can be very useful in classifying seizure disorders, and because optimal drug therapy is different for different types of seizures, the EEG findings may have important implications for treatment. Electroencephalography is also useful in evaluating cerebral abnormalities in a number of systemic disorders and in working up patients with sleep disorders.

Because CT scanning and MR imaging have higher spatial resolution and can localize lesions in three dimensions, these imaging techniques are usually used in preference to EEG for the localization of destructive lesions in the brain. When other tests are not available, an EEG can furnish considerable help in determining the area of cerebral damage. Electroencephalography has its limitations, however, and normal-appearing records can be obtained in spite of clinical evidence of severe organic brain disease. The use of **depth electrography**—the localization of a focus by recording from within the brain—may be advisable in certain cases.

Physiology

The activity recorded in the EEG originates mainly from the superficial layers of the cerebral cortex (see Chapter 10). Current is believed to flow between cortical cell dendrites and cell bodies (the dendrites are oriented in a stereotyped manner, perpendicular to the cortical surface). As a result of the synchronous activation of axodendritic synapses on many neurons, summed electrical currents flow through the extracellular space, creating the waves recorded as the EEG. The pattern of activation of cortical neurons, and thus the EEG, is modulated by inputs from the thalamus and reticular formation (which was called the *reticular activating system* by early researchers).

Technique

To detect changes in activity that may be of diagnostic importance, simultaneous recordings are obtained (when possible) from multiple analogous areas on both the left and right sides of the brain. Electrodes covered with electrolyte paste or jelly are ordinarily attached to the scalp over the frontal, parietal, occipital, and temporal areas; they are also attached to the ears (Fig 24–1).

With the subject recumbent or seated in a grounded, wire-shielded cage, a recording at least 20 minutes long is obtained; the eyes should be closed. Hyperventilation, during which the patient takes 40–50 deep breaths per minute for three minutes, is routinely employed during this time, because it frequently accentuates abnormal findings (epileptiform attacks) and may disclose latent abnormalities. Rhythmic light-flash stimulation (1–30 Hz), also termed **photic** stimulation, is carried out for two or more minutes as part of the recording routine. In some cases the EEG is continued after the patient is allowed to spontaneously fall asleep or after sedation with drugs; under these circumstances certain epileptic discharges and other focal abnormalities are more likely to be recorded.

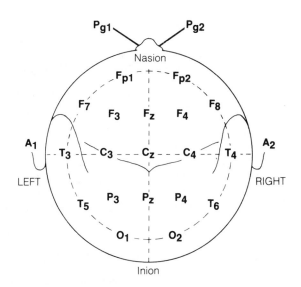

Figure 24–1. A single-plane projection of the head, showing all standard positions of electrode placement and the locations of the central sulcus (fissure of Rolando) and the lateral cerebral fissure (fissure of Sylvius). The outer circle is drawn at the level of the nasion and inion; the inner circle represents the temporal line of electrodes. This diagram provides a useful guide for electrode placement in routine recording. A, ear; C, central; Cz, central at zero, or midline; F, frontal; Fp, frontal pole; Fz, frontal at zero, or midline; O, occipital; P, parietal; Pg, nasopharyngeal; Pz, parietal at zero, or midline; T, temporal. (Courtesy of Grass Medical Instruments Co, Quincy, Mass.)

Types of Wave Forms

The **synchronized** activity of many of the dendritic units forms the wave pattern associated with **alpha rhythm** when the patient is awake, but at rest with the eyes closed. The alpha rhythm has a periodicity of 8–12Hz. **Desynchronization**—replacement of a rhythmic pattern with irregular low-voltage activity—is produced by stimulation of specific projection systems from the spinal cord and brain stem up to the level of the thalamus.

When the eyes are opened, the alpha rhythm is replaced by an **alpha block,** a fast, irregular, low-voltage activity. Other forms of sensory stimulation or mental concentration can also break up the alpha pattern. Desynchronization is sometimes termed the **arousal,** or **alerting, response,** because this breakup of the alpha pattern may be produced by sensory stimulation and is correlated with an aroused or alert state. The **beta rhythm** is characterized by low amplitude (5–20 µV) waves with a rhythm faster than 12 Hz, most prominent in the frontal regions.

Theta rhythms (4–7 Hz) are normally seen over the temporal lobes bilaterally particularly in older patients, but can also occur as a result of focal or generalized, cerebral dysfunction. **Delta activity** (1–3 Hz) is never seen in the normal EEG and indicates significant dysfunction of the underlying cortex. Brain tumors, cerebral abscesses, and subdural hematoma are often associated with focal or localized slow-wave activity. CT

scanning and MR imaging, however, can provide more information about the location and structure of the lesion and have largely replaced EEG for the diagnosis of these disorders.

Epilepsy is an expression of various groups of cortical diseases; all types are characterized by transient disturbances of brain function manifested by intermittent high-voltage waves. **Spikes** and **sharp waves** have characteristic shapes and occur either as part of seizure discharges, or interictally in patients with epilepsy; these EEG abnormalities can be diffuse or can be focal, suggesting a localized abnormality.

Absence seizures of childhood **(petit mal),** which are characterized by brief (up to 30 seconds) loss of consciousness without loss of postural tone, are associated with a characteristic three-per-second spike-and-wave abnormality on EEG. **Complex partial seizures** (which usually have a temporal lobe origin), on the other hand, can also be associated with impaired awareness, but the EEG usually shows focal temporal lobe spikes or is normal.

A number of infectious, toxic, and metabolic disorders affecting the nervous system are accompanied by characteristic EEG abnormalities. For example, in herpes simplex encephalitis, the EEG displays periodic high-voltage sharp waves over the temporal lobes at regular three-per-second intervals. In Creutzfeldt-Jakob disease (also termed subacute spongiform encephalopathy), the EEG usually shows a pattern of **burst suppression** characterized by stereotyped, high-voltage slow and sharp wave complexes superimposed on a relatively flat background. In hepatic encephalopathy, bilaterally synchronous triphasic waves are often present.

EVOKED POTENTIALS

Whereas the EEG displays ongoing or spontaneous electrical activity, evoked potential recordings permit the measurement of activity in cortical sensory areas and subcortical relay nuclei in response to stimulation of various sensory pathways. Because the electrical signals are very small, computerized averaging methods are used to extract the time-locked neural signals evoked by a large number of identical stimuli. The latency, amplitude, and waveform of the evoked potential provide information about the pathway, or group of neurons, under study.

Visual Evoked Potential

Visual evoked potential (VEP) are usually elicited by having the patient fixate on a target and flashing a reversing checkerboard pattern on a screen centered around the target. The visual evoked potential recorded in this manner are sometimes called **pattern-shift visual evoked potentials (PSVEP).** These are recorded over the left and right occipital poles (Fig 24–3). This reaction is clinically useful in detecting slight abnormalities in the visual pathways; eg, optic nerve lesions can be recognized by stimulating each eye separately because the response to stimulation of an affected optic nerve is absent or impaired. With visual pathway lesions behind the optic chiasm, a difference in response of the two cerebral hemispheres may occur. There might be a normal response in the occipital cerebral cortex of the normal cerebral hemisphere and an absent or abnormal response in the affected cerebral hemisphere (see also Chapter 15).

BRAIN STEM AUDITORY EVOKED RESPONSE

A standard brain stem auditory evoked response (BAER) consists of seven potentials that are recorded from the human scalp within 10 ms of a single appropriate acoustic stimulus. Abnormalities in the response may provide evidence suggesting clinical neurologic disorders involving the brain stem. The test has some clinical value and is useful in demonstrating structural brain stem damage caused by various disorders (see also Chapter 16).

Technique

Short-latency brain stem auditory evoked potentials can be averaged and analyzed with the aid of computer techniques (Fig 24–4). In a normal human subject with scalp electrodes placed on the vertex, a click stimulus presented to the ear may evoke typical responses with seven wave components that are believed to come from the region of the auditory nerve (wave I), dorsal cochlear nucleus (wave II), superior olive (wave III), lateral lemniscus (wave IV), and inferior colliculus (wave V). Wave VI may indicate activity of the rostral midbrain or caudal thalamus or thalamocortical projection, and wave VII originates in the auditory cortex. Peak-to-peak amplitudes and the latencies from the stimulus to each peak are all measured. At least two separate trials and averages of 2000–4000 responses are recorded for each ear.

Somatosensory Evoked Potentials

To obtain somatosensory evoked potentials (SEP), repetitive electrical stimuli are applied over the median, peroneal, and tibial nerves. This usually can be done without causing pain. Recording electrodes are placed over Erb's point above the clavicle, over the C2 spinous process, and over the contralateral somatosensory cortex for stimulation of the upper limb, and over the lumbar and cervical spine and contralateral somatosensory cortex for stimulation of the lower limb. Depending on the pattern of delay, it is possible to localize lesions within peripheral nerve (conduction delay or increased conduction time between stimulation site and Erb's point or lumbar spine), spinal roots or dorsal columns (delay between Erb's point or lumbar spine, and C2), or in the medial lemniscus and thalamic radiations (delay recorded at cortical electrode, but not at more caudal recording sites).

TRANSCRANIAL MOTOR CORTICAL STIMULATION

Methods for noninvasively stimulating the motor cortex and cervical spinal cord in humans have recently been developed and permit the evaluation of conduction in descending motor pathways. Because the largest neurons have the lowest thresholds, this technique presumably evaluates the integrity of the large upper-motor-neurons and the most rapidly conducting axons in the corticospinal system. In practice, a stimulation coil is placed over the scalp or cervical spine, and is used to excite upper-motor-neurons or motor axons. Recording electrodes are placed over various muscles, and the amplitude and latency of the response are recorded. Absent, altered, or delayed motor responses are because of damage to the upper-motor-neuron, to its axon, or to its myelin sheath.

R = right	F = frontal	P = parietal	AT = anterior temporal	T = temporal
L = left	O = occipital	Pc = precentral	Pf = posterior frontal	E = ear

Calibration: 50 μV (vertical) and 1 s (horizontal).

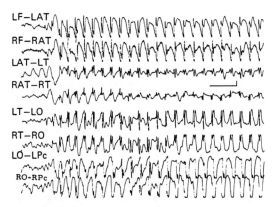

Normal Adult

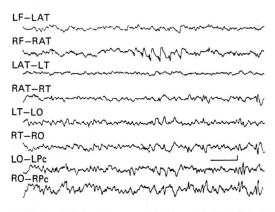

Petit Mal Epilepsy. Record of a 6-year-old boy during one of his "blank spells," in which he was transiently unaware of surroundings and blinked his eyelids during the recording.

Epilepsy. EEG of a 6-year-old child who had suffered 3 major convulsions, 2 of which appeared to start in the left extremities.

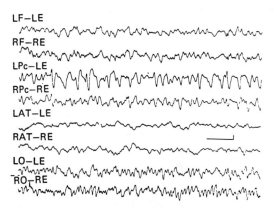

Focal Motor Epilepsy. EEG of a 47-year-old man with focal motor seizures beginning in the left hand. He stated his seizures began 20 years previously, approximately one year after a severe head injury.

Epilepsy. Record of a 6-year-old girl with frequent nocturnal major convulsions as well as daily seizures in which she became stiff, started, and shook slightly.

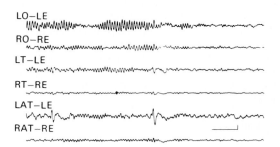

Psychomotor Epilepsy. Record of a 20-year-old man who had had monthly episodes for the previous 6 years characterized by motor automatisms and frequently followed by generalized tonic-clonic convulsions.

Figure 24–2. Representative EEGs.

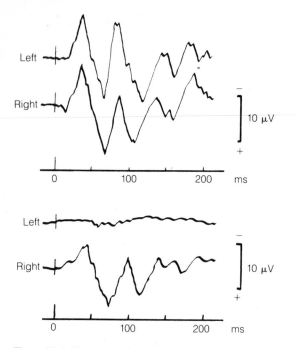

Figure 24–3. Visual evoked responses recorded from over the left and right occipital poles. **Top:** normal responses. **Bottom:** responses in a case of right homonymous hemianopia. No response is recorded over the left hemisphere. (Courtesy of M Feinsod. Reproduced, with permission, from Vaughan D, Asbury T, Tabbara KF: *General Ophthalmology*, 12th ed. Appleton & Lange, 1989.)

ELECTROMYOGRAPHY

Electromyography is concerned with the study of the electrical activity arising from muscles at rest and those that are actively contracted.

Clinical Applications

Electromyography is a particularly useful aid in diagnosing lower-motor-neuron disease or primary muscle disease and in detecting defects in transmission at the neuromuscular junction. Although it is helpful, the test does not give a specific clinical diagnosis; information from the electromyogram (EMG) must be integrated with results of other tests, muscle biopsy if necessary, clinical features, and so forth to arrive at a final diagnosis.

Physiology

Human striated muscle is composed functionally of motor units in which the axons of single motor cells in the anterior horn innervate many muscle fibers (although the size of motor units varies from muscle to muscle, in the largest motor units hundreds of muscle fibers may be innervated by a single axon). All the fibers innervated by a single motor unit respond immediately to stimulation in an all-or-none pattern, and the interaction of many motor units can produce relatively smooth motor performance. Increased motor power results from the repeated activation of a given number of motor units or the single activation of a greater number of such units.

The action potential of a muscle consists of the sum of the action potentials of many motor units; in normal muscle fibers, it originates at the motor end-plates and is triggered by an incoming nerve impulse at the myoneural junction. Clinical studies indicate that normal muscle at rest shows no action potential. In simple movements, the contracting muscle gives rise to action potentials, while its antagonist relaxes and exhibits no potentials. During contraction, different portions of the same muscle may discharge at different rates and parts may appear to be transiently inactive. In strong contractions, many motor units are simultaneously active, producing numerous action potentials.

Technique

Stimulation is usually applied over the course of the nerve or at the motor point of the muscle being tested. Muscles should always be tested at the **motor point,** which is normally the most excitable point of a muscle in that it represents the greatest concentration of nerve endings. The motor point is located on the skin over the muscle and corresponds approximately to the level at which the nerve enters the muscle belly.

A concentric (coaxial) needle, usually 24 gauge by 3–4 cm long, or a monopolar solid steel needle coated almost to the tip with insulating plastic or varnish is inserted at the motor point of a muscle and advanced by steps to several depths. Variations in electrical potential between the needle tip and a reference electrode (a metal plate) on the skin surface are amplified and displayed. The electrical activity can be displayed on a cathode-ray oscilloscope and played on a loudspeaker for simultaneous visual and auditory analysis. Observations are made in each area of the electrical activity evoked in the muscle by insertion and movement of the needle: the electrical activity of the resting muscle with the needle undisturbed, and the electrical activity of the motor units during voluntary contraction (Fig 24–5). Because various muscle fibers may respond differently, several insertions of the needle into different parts of a muscle may be necessary for adequate analysis.

Types of Activity

Insertional activity refers to the burst of action potentials that is usually observed when the EMG needle is inserted into the muscle. In normal muscle, insertional activity is short-lived, and there is usually electrical silence after the initial burst of insertional activity. Increased insertional activity is observed in

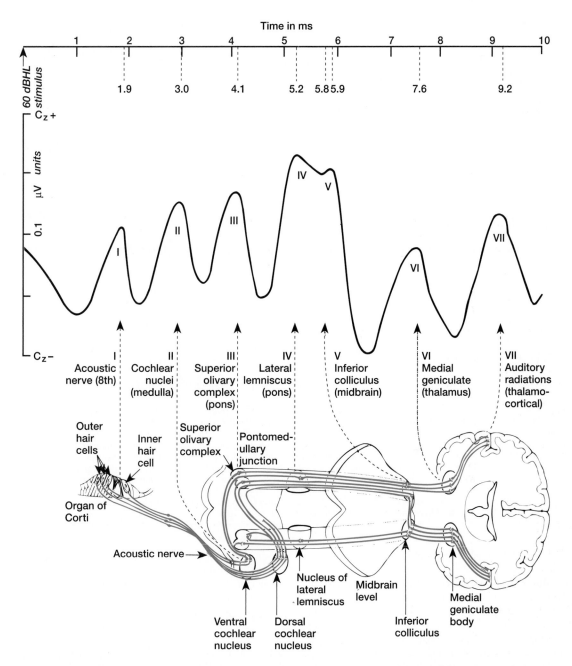

Figure 24–4. Far-field recording of brain stem auditory response latencies in humans showing proposed functional-anatomic correlations. Diagram shows normal latencies for vertex-positive brain stem auditory evoked potentials (waves I-IV) evoked by clicks of 60 dBHL (60 dB above normal hearing threshold) at a rate of 10/s. Lesions at different levels of the auditory pathway tend to produce response abnormalities beginning with the indicated components. Intermediate latency (5.8 ms) between latencies of waves IV and V is the mean peak latency of fused wave IV/V when present. C_z^+, vertex positivity, represented by an upward pen deflection, C_z-, vertex negativity, represented by a downward pen deflection. (Reproduced, with permission, from Stockard JJ, Stockard JE, Sharbrough FW: Detection and localization of occult lesions with brain stem auditory responses. *Mayo Clin Proc* 1977;**52:**761.)

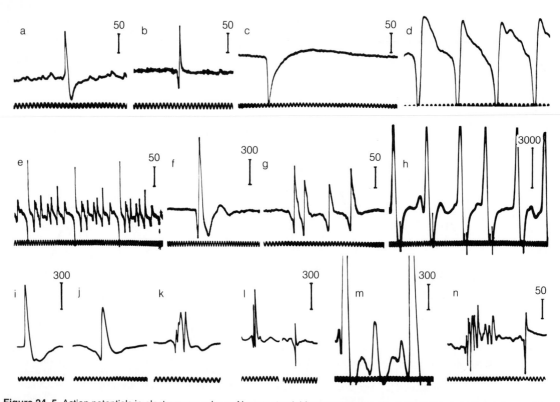

Figure 24–5. Action potentials in electromyography. **a:** Nerve potential from normal muscle; **b:** fibrillation potential and **c:** positive wave from denervated muscle; **d:** high-frequency discharge in myotonia; **e:** bizarre high-frequency discharge; **f:** fasciculation potential, single discharge; **g:** fasciculation potential, repetitive or grouped discharge; **h:** synchronized repetitive discharge in muscle cramp; **i:** diphasic, **j:** triphasic, and **k:** polyphasic motor unit action potentials from normal muscle; **l:** short-duration motor unit action potentials in progressive muscular dystrophy; **m:** large motor unit action potentials in progressive muscular dystrophy; **n:** highly polyphasic motor unit action potential and short-duration motor unit action potential during reinnervation. Calibration scale (vertical) in microvolts. The horizontal scale shows 1000 Hz waveforms. An upward deflection indicates a change of potential in the negative direction at the needle electrode. (Reproduced, with permission, from *Clinical Examinations in Neurology*, 3rd ed. Members of the Section of Neurology and Section of Physiology, Mayo Clinic and Mayo Foundation for Medical Education and Research, Graduate School, University of Minnesota, Rochester, Minnesota. Saunders, 1971.)

denervated muscles and in many forms of muscle disease.

Motor Unit Potential (MUP) are also examined by EMG, and provide important information about innervation (or denervation) of the muscle fibers within a muscle. As previously noted, the MUP in any given muscle has a characteristic size and duration. If lower-motor-neurons, roots, or nerves are injured so that motor axons are severed and muscle fibers are denervated, the number of MUPs appearing during contraction is decreased. Nevertheless, the configurations of the remaining MUPs are usually normal. The decreased number of MUPs reflects denervation of some of the muscle fibers. Later, there may be re-innervation of the previously denervated muscles, which occurs as a result of sprouting of new motor axon branches from undamaged axons, whose motor units increase in size. As a result of this, the MUPs increase in amplitude and duration, and in some cases become polyphasic. Observation of these polyphasic MUPs provides evidence of

re-innervation (and thus implies prior denervation) and can have considerable diagnostic value, providing evidence of disease involving motor neurons or their axons in the ventral roots or peripheral nerves.

Two types of spontaneous, or ongoing, activity observed by EMG have particular significance. These are termed fibrillations and fasciculations. The term **fibrillation** is reserved for spontaneous independent contractions of individual muscle fibers that are so minute that they cannot be observed through the intact skin. Denervated muscle may show electromyographic evidence of fibrillations that can persist for 1–3 weeks after losing its nerve supply. **Fasciculations,** or twitches, on the other hand, can be seen and palpated, and they can be heard with the aid of a stethoscope; they represent contractions of all (or most) of the muscle fibers of a motor unit. Spontaneous fasciculations can vary because of the length and number of muscle fibers involved; they usually result from disorders of the lower-motor-neuron. Benign fasciculations, such as those from exposure to cold or temporary ischemia (eg, caused by crossed legs), are unassociated with other clinical or electrical signs of denervation (Fig 24–5).

In a complete nerve lesion, all of the motor axons are severed, so that fibrillation potentials occur without motor unit potentials; partial nerve lesions show both fibrillation and motor unit activity from voluntary muscle contraction. Diminution or cessation of fibrillation potentials and the appearance of small, disintegrated motor unit action potentials occur with nerve regeneration. Fibrillations in a paretic muscle are increased by warmth, activity, and neostigmine; they are decreased by cold or immobilization.

After complete section of a nerve, denervation fibrillation potentials are evident (after about 18 days) in all areas of the muscles supplied by a peripheral nerve. Some motor unit discharges persist in partial nerve injuries, despite the clinical appearance of complete paralysis. Mapping the areas of denervation fibrillation potentials aids in the diagnosis of single nerve root disorders and spinal nerve root compression.

Repetitive Stimulation

In the absence of pathology, axons can conduct impulses at a high frequency and the neuromuscular junction can faithfully follow these high-frequency impulses, producing a surface muscle action potential that retains its amplitude with rates of stimulation up to 20–30 Hz for up to one minute. In contrast, in **myasthenia gravis,** the response is **decremental,** with the MUP decreasing in amplitude after several stimuli at rates as low as 3 or 4 Hz. The **Lambert-Eaton myasthenic syndrome** exhibits a different pattern; in this disorder there is a defect of neuromuscular transmission characterized by **incremental** responses, which increase in amplitude with repetitive stimulation. These distinct patterns of response to repetitive stimulation are of considerable diagnostic value.

Single-fiber Electromyography (SFEMG)

SFEMG is a relatively new technique that permits the recording of action potentials from single muscle fibers using very fine electrodes. This technique permits the measurement of muscle fiber density within a given motor unit and, thus, can be of significant value in the diagnosis of muscle disorders. Jitter (variability in the timing of action potentials for single muscle fibers comprising a given motor unit) can also be studied with this technique. Jitter appears to result from abnormalities of the preterminal part of the axons, close to the neuromuscular junction. SFEMG may be especially useful for the diagnosis of disorders involving motor neurons (eg, ALS) and the neuromuscular junction.

NERVE CONDUCTION STUDIES

By stimulating peripheral nerves through the skin and recording muscle and sensory nerve action potentials, it is possible to examine conduction velocities, distal latencies, and amplitudes of responses, which provide important information about peripheral nerve pathology. For these studies, surface electrodes are placed on the skin for stimulation of accessible peripheral nerves, and the resulting compound action potential is recorded elsewhere over the nerve, or over a muscle that is innervated by the nerve being studied. Two stimulation sites are usually used so that conduction velocity can be ascertained (by dividing the distance between the two stimulation sites by the difference in conduction times). These whole nerve conduction velocities measure the properties of the fastest-conducting (and largest) axons within the nerve and have normal values of more than 40 msec in adults. Decreased conduction velocities are seen in peripheral neuropathies characterized by demyelination (eg, Guillain-Barré syndrome, chronic inflammatory demyelinating polyneuropathy, and Charcot-Marie-Tooth disease). Slowed conduction velocities are also seen at sites of focal compression.

Measurements of amplitude, of either the muscle action potential elicited by motor axon stimulation, or of the sensory nerve action potential, can also provide useful information. Reduction of amplitude is especially pronounced in disorders characterized by loss of axons, eg, uremic and alcoholic-nutritional neuropathies. The presence, absence, or reduction of innervation can be determined by electrical stimulation of peripheral nerves, and the location of a nerve block can be shown. Anomalies of innervation can be detected by noting which muscles respond to nerve stimulation, and abnormal fatigability following repeated stimulation of the nerve can be noted.

In the presence of paralysis, a normal response of innervated muscles to stimulation of the peripheral nerve shows that the cause of paralysis is proximal to the stimulated point. On the other hand, an absent or weak response suggests further testing to detect the site and nature of the defect.

H-reflexes and F-wave

Nerve conduction studies provide information about the status of distal segments of peripheral nerves in the limbs, but do not provide information about conduction within proximal parts of the nerve or spinal roots. The H-reflex and F-wave involve conduction through spinal roots and proximal parts of peripheral nerve, and thus provide important diagnostic information about disorders that involve these areas. To elicit the H-reflex, submaximal stimuli are applied to mixed (motor-sensory) nerves at an intensity too low to produce a direct motor response; these stimuli evoke a

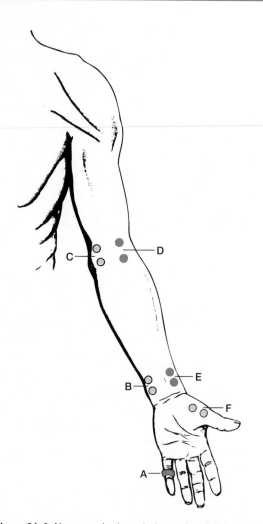

muscle contraction (H-wave) with a relatively long latency because of activation of Ia spindle afferent fibers, which travel via the dorsal roots to the spinal gray matter where they synapse with lower-motor-neurons, whose action potentials then travel through the ventral roots and then to the muscle. Absence of the H-reflex suggests pathology along this pathway, and is often a result of **radiculopathies** (disorders involving peripheral nerves) or polyneuropathies involving spinal roots or proximal parts of the peripheral nerves (eg, Guillain-Barré syndrome).

The F-wave is a long-latency response, following the direct muscle potential, that is evoked by supramaximal stimulation of motor-sensory nerves. It is produced by antidromic (retrograde) stimulation of motor axons, which results in invasion of action potentials into their cell bodies in the spinal cord and evoke a second (reflected) action potential that travels along the motor axon to muscle. As with the H-reflex, absence of the F-wave implies pathology of spinal roots or proximal parts of peripheral nerves

Figure 24–6. Nerve-conduction-velocity studies. A, B, and C are electrode placements for ulnar-nerve evoked potentials. A is a ring-shaped stimulating electrode; B and C are recording electrodes. D, E, and F are electrode placements for median-nerve motor-conduction-velocity study. D and E are points where the nerve is stimulated; F is the recording electrode. (Reproduced, with permission, from Samaha FJ: Electrodiagnostic studies in neuromuscular disease. *N Engl J Med* 1972;**285:**1244.)

REFERENCES

American EEG Society: Guidelines in EEG and evoked potentials. *J Clin Neurophysiol* 1986;**3(Supp 1):**1.

Aminoff MJ (editor): *Electrodiagnosis in Clinical Neurology,* 2nd ed. Churchill-Livingstone, 1986.

Aminoff MJ: *Electromyography in Clinical Practice,* 2nd ed. Churchill-Livingstone, 1987.

Chiappa KH: *Evoked Potentials in Clinical Medicine,* 2nd ed. Raven, 1990.

Kimura J: *Electrodiagnosis in Disease of Nerve and Muscle,* 2nd ed. FA Davis, 1989.

Moore EJ (editor): *Bases of Auditory Brain-Stem Evoked Responses.* Grune & Stratton, 1983.

Niedermeyer E, daSilva FL: *Electroencephalography,* 2nd ed. Urban & Schwarzenberg, 1987.

Porter RJ, Morselli PL (editors): *The Epilepsies.* Butterworth, 1985.

Section VII.
Discussion of Cases

Discussion of Cases

25

As outlined in Chapter 4, the important question: Where is the lesion? (What is the precise location of the deficit?), must be followed by the equally important question: What is the lesion? (What is the nature of the disease?). The answers should lead to the differential diagnosis, correct diagnosis, and prognosis, and the **patient** (the person, not the case) should benefit from appropriate treatment.

THE LOCATION OF LESIONS

In thinking about the location of the lesion, it is often helpful to systematically survey the nervous system. Lesions can be located in one or more of the following anatomic sites:

- **Muscles.** In muscle diseases, one sees weakness, sometimes together with muscle atrophy. Deep tendon reflexes are usually depressed. Diseases of muscle include the **dystrophies,** which have specific genetic patterns and stages of onset and may preferentially involve certain muscle groups; and inflammatory disorders of muscle such as **polymyositis.** Diagnosis may be aided by measuring the level of enzymes (such as creatine phosphokinase, CPK) in the serum, because damage to muscle fibers may lead to their release. Electromyography and muscle biopsy may also help with diagnosis.

- **Motor end-plates.** Disorders of the motor end-plate include **myasthenia gravis** and the **Eaton-Lambert myasthenic syndrome.** In these disorders, there is weakness, sometimes together with abnormal fatigability resulting from abnormal function (eg, decreased effect of ACh on the postjunctional muscle or decreased release of ACh) at the neuromuscular junction. Weakness may involve the limbs or trunk, or muscles involved in chewing, swallowing, or eye movements. In addition to the characteristic clinical pattern, electromyography may be helpful in diagnosis.

- **Peripheral nerves.** Peripheral nerve lesions may be differentiated from lesions of muscle or motor end-plate by clinical criteria, electrical tests or biopsy. In many disorders of peripheral nerve, both motor (lower-motor-neuron) and sensory deficits are present, although in some cases, motor or sensory function is impaired in a relatively pure way. In most peripheral neuropathies, functions subserved by the longest axons are impaired first, so that there is a "stocking-and-glove" pattern of sensory loss, together with weakness of distal musculature, ie, intrinsic muscles of the feet.

- **Roots.** A motor root lesion results in a precise segmental motor deficit, which in some cases (eg, plexus lesions) is mediated through several nerves. A single sensory deficit may be difficult to diagnose because of the adjacent overlapping dermatomes (see Fig 5–9). When a nerve root carrying axons mediating a deep tendon reflex is affected, the reflex may be depressed (see Table 5–5). Sensory root symptoms may include increased pain associated with the Valsalva maneuver, the forced expiratory effort caused by laughing, sneezing, or coughing.

- **Spinal cord.** The staggered pattern of decussation of the lateral corticospinal tract, dorsal column-medial lemniscal system, and spinothalamic tracts often permits localization of lesions within the spinal cord. Injury to the spinal cord, at a given level, may result in lower-motor-neuron signs and symptoms at that level, but will result in upper-motor-neuron abnormalities *below* the level of the lesion.

- **Brain stem.** Functional deficits in the long tracts that pass from the brain to the spinal cord or vice-versa, together with cranial nerve signs and symptoms, suggest a lesion in the brain stem. Lesions in the medulla involve the last few cranial nerves, while lesions in the pons involve nerves V, VI, and VII, and lesions of the midbrain often involve nerve III and possibly nerve IV.

- **Cerebellum.** Lesions in the cerebellum or its peduncles result in characteristic abnormalities of motor integration. There is usually impaired coordination and decreased muscle tone *ipsilateral* to a lesion in the cerebellar hemisphere.

- **Diencephalon.** Hypothalamic lesions are often complex and can cause endocrinologic disturbances as well as visual abnormality resulting from compression of neighboring optic tracts. Thalamic lesions often cause sensory dysfunction and may produce motor deficits as a result of compression of the neighboring internal capsule. Subthalamic lesions may cause abnormal movements such as hemiballismus. Epithalamic lesions are most frequently pineal region tumors, which can compress the cerebral aqueduct, thereby producing hydrocephalus.
- **Subcortical white matter.** The presence of abnormal myelin (leukodystrophy, which is more common in infants and children than in adults) or the destruction of normal myelin (which can result from inflammatory disorders such as **multiple sclerosis**) results in abnormal axonal conduction and deficits of function. Pathology may be diffuse, focal, or multifocal with a parallel pattern of clinical involvement.
- **Subcortical gray matter (basal ganglia).** A variety of movement disorders, including Parkinson's disease and Huntington's disease, occur from involvement of the basal ganglia. Tremors and other abnormal movements, abnormalities of tone (eg, cogwheel rigidity in Parkinson's disease) and slowed movements (bradykinesia) are often seen. These disorders often affect the basal ganglia bilaterally, but if there is unilateral pathology, the movement disorder will affect the contralateral limbs.
- **Cerebral cortex.** Focal lesions may produce well-circumscribed deficits such as aphasia, the hemi-inattention and neglect syndromes, or the Gerstmann syndrome (see Chapter 21). In most patients, aphasia is because of the involvement of the left hemisphere. When the primary motor cortex is involved, there is usually upper-motor-neuron weakness of the contralateral limbs. Irritative lesions of the cortex may result in seizures, which can be focal or generalized.
- **Meninges.** Hemorrhages in the subarachnoid, subdural, and epidural spaces have characteristic clinical and neuroradiologic features. Subarachnoid hemorrhage is often accompanied by severe headache ("worse headache of my life"). Subdural hemorrhages may occur acutely or chronically and can follow even trivial head injury especially in elderly patients and young children. Epidural hemorrhages are often rapidly progressive, and can produce sudden herniation of the brain. Infection of the subarachnoid space (meningitis) may present with signs of meningeal irritation (eg, stiff neck) in addition to other neurologic deficits, and the diagnosis can often be confirmed by lumbar puncture.
- **Skull, vertebral column, and associated structures.** Associated structures include the interverte-

bral disks, ligaments, and articulations. For example, metastatic tumors involving the vertebral column can produce spinal cord compression. Trauma often involves the skull and vertebral column, as well as the brain and spinal cord.

THE NATURE OF LESIONS

A variety of pathologic processes can affect the nervous system. The following is a common neuropathologic classification of disorders:

- **Vascular disorders.** Usually with a sudden onset of signs and symptoms, cerebrovascular disease often occurs in the setting of hypertension. Stenosis or occlusion of the carotid artery in the neck may be responsible. Embolism, from ulcerated plaques in the carotid or from the heart (eg, in patients with chronic atrial fibrillation) can occlude more distal vessels such as the middle cerebral. Subarachnoid hemorrhage and intraparenchymal hemorrhage (often involving the basal ganglia, thalamus, pons, or cerebellum) occur in hypertensive patients. Subdural and epidural hemorrhages occur as a result of trauma, which can be trivial (and in many cases is not remembered) in the case of subdural hematoma.
- **Trauma.** As previously noted, epidural and subdural hematomas can develop as a result of head injury. In addition, penetrating injuries can directly destroy brain tissue, produce vascular lesions, or introduce infections. Injury to the spine is a common cause of paraplegia and quadriplegia.
- **Tumors.** Primary tumors of the brain and spinal cord, as well as metastases (from, eg, breast, lung, and prostate tumors, etc) produce symptoms by direct invasion (and destruction) of neural tissue, compression of the brain and spinal cord, or compression of the ventricles and cerebral aqueduct which can lead to hydrocephalus. Classically, tumors of the CNS produce subacutely or chronically progressive deterioration, which, in contrast to vascular disorders, progresses over weeks, months, or years. Signs of increased intracranial pressure (papilledema, sixth nerve palsy, etc) may be present.
- **Infections and inflammations.** These disorders (eg, meningitis, abscess formation, encephalitis, and granulomas) may be accompanied by fever, especially if the onset is acute. Most infections and inflammations have characteristic signs, symptoms, and causes.
- **Toxic, deficiency, and metabolic disorders.** A variety of intoxications, vitamin deficiencies (eg, B_{12} deficiency) and enzyme defects leading to abnormal lipid storage in neurons are examples of this heterogeneous group of disorders. Various substances in different amounts (too much or too little) can cause selective lesions involving particular nuclei or tracts. Vitamin B_{12} deficiency, for example,

causes degeneration of axons in the dorsal and lateral columns of the spinal cord.

- **Demyelinating diseases.** Multiple sclerosis is the prototype demyelinating disease. As expected for a disorder characterized by multiple lesions in the CNS white matter, examination often provides evidence for involvement of several sites in the CNS. Evoked potentials may provide physiologic evidence for slowed axonal conduction, and the cerebrospinal fluid often shows characteristic abnormalities. MRI scans are very useful in confirming the diagnosis.

- **Degenerative diseases.** This heterogeneous group of diseases for which the cause has not yet been determined includes spinal, cerebellar, subcortical, and cortical degenerative disorders that are often characterized by specific functional deficits.

- **Congenital malformations and perinatal disorders.** Exogenous factors (eg, infection or radiation of the motor cortex) or genetic and chromosomal factors can cause abnormalities of the brain or spinal cord in newborn infants. Hydrocephalus, Chiari malformation, cortical lesions, cerebral palsy, neural tumors, vascular abnormalities, and other syndromes may persist after birth.

- **Neuromuscular disorders.** This group includes muscular dystrophies, congenital myopathies, neuromuscular junction disorders, transmitter deficiencies, and nerve lesions or neuropathies (inflammation, degeneration, and demyelination).

- **Other factors.** The nature of the lesion can also be determined by checking vital signs and body temperature and by performing blood and cerebrospinal fluid analyses, radiologic examinations, biopsies, and special tests (see Appendices A, B, and C) (Table 25–1).

CASES

Case 1, Chapter 3

Abnormal, gradual tiring of the muscles for eye movement and chewing is suggestive of fatigue at the neuromuscular junction. The neuromuscular junction can normally transmit at high frequencies so that this type of fatigue does not occur. The prominence of muscular fatigue suggested a diagnosis of **myasthenia gravis** in this patient. The absence of sensory deficits tends to confirm the diagnosis. Electromyography is a useful procedure for confirmation of the diagnosis; the muscle action potential, which provides a measure of the number of muscle cells that are contracting, decreases in size with repetitive stimulation in myasthenia gravis. In addition, antibodies to ACh receptors are often present and can provide a measure of the degree of disease activity. Injection of anticholinesterase drugs, such as neostigmine or edrophonium chloride, may reverse the fatigue and help to confirm the diagnosis. Treatment centers around the use of anticholinesterase drugs and

immunosuppressants, including corticosteroids, which decrease the rate of anti-ACh receptor antibody production. In some patients, thymectomy is effective.

Comment: Myasthenia gravis should not be confused with the **myasthenic syndrome** (Eaton-Lambert syndrome), an autoimmune disease seen in the context of systemic neoplasms (especially those affecting the lung and breast). In the myasthenic syndrome, abnormal antibodies directed against presynaptic Ca^{2+} channels, interfere with the release of ACh from the presynaptic ending at the neuromuscular junction.

Case 2, Chapter 5

The shoulder pain radiating into the left arm suggests involvement at the C5 or C6 level. The recent weakness in the left extremities, abnormal reflexes in the legs, and decreased reflexes in the left arm all suggest a lower-motor-neuron-type lesion in the left C6 ventral root and an upper-motor lesion in the corticospinal tract (probably on both sides). The sensory deficits indicate a level of C6, or perhaps C7, bilaterally. The course of the disease shows a slow progression and recent deterioration, a series of events typical of a slowly expanding mass that rather suddenly compresses the spinal cord against the hard wall of the vertebral canal. This was confirmed by imaging studies, which showed a left-sided, intradural, extramedullary mass compressing and displacing the spinal cord at the C6–C7 level.

The differential diagnosis includes a mass associated with spinal roots, meninges, and nerves; a tumor from the arachnoid **(meningioma);** and a nerve tumor (sometimes called a **neuroma**). Abscesses may form a mass, but the patient's history does not suggest an infection.

The diagnosis is a **nerve root tumor** of the left C6 nerve. During neurosurgery, the tumor was completely removed, and the C6 sensory root was sacrificed. Pathologic studies showed a schwannoma. The patient's recovery was complete and uneventful; six months later, she danced at the junior prom.

Comment: MR imaging is now usually used instead of myelography to demonstrate such root tumors (Figs 25–1 and 25–2). Especially at a time when "cost-containment" is important, it is crucial to request the **most appropriate** imaging tests. In this case, a careful examination permitted the patient's neurologist to predict the presence of a lesion compressing the spinal cord and to request radiologic examination of the spine.

Case 3, Chapter 5

The following features in the history and examination indicate extensive involvement of the motor system: weakness, atrophy, cranial motor nerve deficits (difficulty in swallowing and in speaking), and fasciculations (see Appendix A). The distribution of deficits over all the extremities suggests an extensive, generalized motor disorder. The abnormal reflexes suggest both lower- and upper-motor-neuron-type lesions. The

Table 25–1. Cerebrospinal fluid findings in various diseases.

Condition	Appearance	Pressure (in mm of water)	Cells (per μL)	Protein	Miscellaneous Findings
Tap **Normal** lumbar	Clear and color-less	70–180	0–5	15–45 mg/dL	Glucose 50–75 mg/dL
Normal ventricular	Clear and color-less	70–190	0–5 (lympho-cytes)	5–15 mg/dL	VDRL negative
Traumatic	Bloody; super-natant fluid clear	Normal	Red blood cells	4 mg/dL rise per 5000 red cells	. . .
Cerebral hemor-rhage (ventricu-lar or subarach-noid)	Bloody; super-natant fluid yellow	Slightly increased	Red blood cells	4 mg/dL rise per 5000 red cells	Blood equal in each specimen obtained
Meningitis Acute purulent	Clear, cloudy, milky, or xan-thochromic; occasional clot formation	Moderately or greatly in-creased (250–700)	Polymorphonu-clear cells, usually over 1000	Increased	Glucose de-creased early; chlorides de-creased late; or-ganisms on smear and cul-ture
Acute tubercu lous	Opalescent to turbid	Moderately in-creased (200–450)	10–500 (lym-phocytes)	Increased	Chlorides de-creased early, often before de-crease of glu-cose. Smear and culture for organisms
Brain tumor	Usually clear and colorless	Increased	Normal or in-creased	Increased	Findings depend on location and type of tumor
Brain abscess	Clear and color-less	Increased (up to 700)	Normal or in-creased	Increased	. . .
Subdural hematoma	Classically yel-low, but often clear and col-orless	Usually increased	Normal	Normal or slightly in-creased	. . .
Encephalitis	Clear and color-less	Normal	Often in-creased (mostly lym-phocytes)	Normal or slightly in-creased	Serologic tests of value in virus in-fections
Epilepsy (idio-pathic)	Normal fluid	Normal	Normal	Normal	. . .
Multiple sclerosis	Normal fluid	Normal	Normal or in-creased	Normal (in-creased gamma globulin)	Obigoclonal bands and myelin basic protein may be present
Spinal cord tumor Partial block	Clear and color-less	Normal	Normal	Slightly in-creased	. . .
Complete block	Yellow	Normal or low	Slightly in-creased	Marked rise (200–600 mg/dL)	Coagulation may occur

absence of any sensory deficit strengthens a diagnosis of a pure motor disorder, and the results of the muscle biopsy confirm this.

The diagnosis is **motor neuron disease,** also known as **amyotrophic lateral sclerosis** and popularly called **Lou Gehrig's disease.** All motor neurons in the spinal cord, brain stem, and motor cortex are gradually de-stroyed; there is no cure (Fig 25–3).

Case 4, Chapter 6

The cause—trauma—and the location—lower cer-vical spine—of the lesion are clear in this case. In the acute phase, traumatic involvement of the spinal cord usually produces spinal shock with flaccid paralysis, loss of temperature control, and hypotension. Precise neurologic localization of the extent of the lesion may

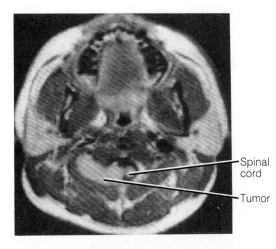

Figure 25–1. MRI of horizontal section through the neck and lower face (a different patient). The image shows a dumbbell-shaped tumor growing out of the spinal canal.

be difficult. Plain films of the spine in several projections can be used to demonstrate the location and extent of the trauma to the bony spine. Because there may be a traumatic tear in the dura, myelography is contraindicated.

The later neurologic examination showed lesions in the left corticospinal and spinothalamic tracts. There was a left lower-motor-neuron lesion around the C7 area. The lack of sensory deficit in the C7 segment can be explained by the segmental overlapping of dermatomes.

Brown-Sequard syndrome was incompletely represented in this case, because the dorsal column tract on the affected side was spared (see Figs 5–24 and 5–25).

The diagnosis is a **traumatic lesion of the spinal cord** at C7. Neurosurgical decompression of the bone fragments prevented further damage to the spinal cord, but the functional deficits caused by local cord destruction could not be corrected.

Case 5, Chapter 6

Mild trauma to the lower back, followed by pain down the sciatic region, is suggestive of **sciatica.** One of the underlying causes is herniation of the nucleus pulposus (the soft center of the intervertebral disk). The aggravation of pain by coughing, sneezing, straining, and bending backward (movements that increase abdominal pressure), and the stretching of dural root sleeves by leg raising, are highly suggestive of root involvement (right L5 nerve). The location is confirmed by the presence of paresthesia in the patient's right calf together with the absence of the Achilles tendon reflex (L5, S1). Spasm of the paravertebral muscles and tenderness along the course of the sciatic nerve are common in this disorder.

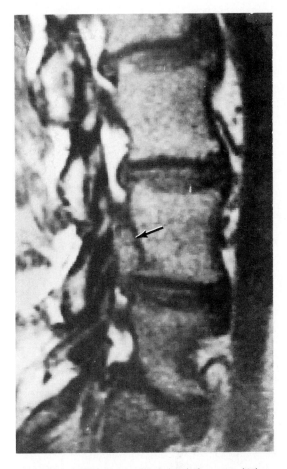

Figure 25–2. MRI (surface coil technique) of a parasagittal section through the lumbar spine in a patient with a root tumor (arrow).

Plain radiographs are useful only for showing a decrease in the height of the intervertebral disk space; myelography may show an extradural defect and root amputation. The precise location of the lesion can best be shown by CT scanning or MR imaging (Figs 25–4 and 25–5).

The diagnosis is **herniation of the nucleus pulposus** at **L5–S1.** Three weeks after the MRI study was performed, the patient underwent laminectomy with removal of the protruding disk fragment. His recovery was uneventful with minimal sequelae.

Case 6, Chapter 7

Careful analysis of the signs and symptoms shows that the following systems were involved: the vestibular system (dizziness and nystagmus); the trigeminal system, including the descending spinal tract of V (loss of pain sensation in the right half of the face); the spinothalamic system (contralateral pain deficit); the cerebellum (the inability to execute the right finger-to-nose test or to make rapid alternating movements and

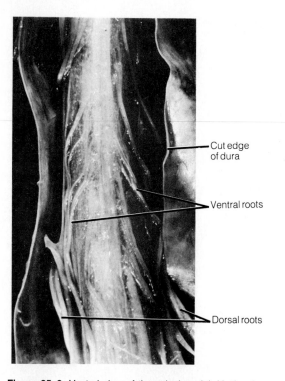

Figure 25–3. Ventral view of the spinal cord (with the dura opened) of a patient with motor neuron disease (amyotrophic lateral sclerosis). Notice the reduction in size of the ventral roots (resulting from the degeneration of the axons of motor neurons) compared with the normal dorsal roots.

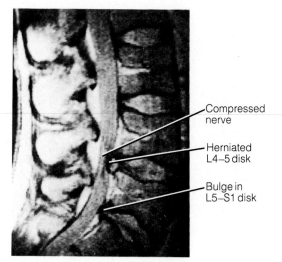

Figure 25–4. MRI (surface coil technique) of a sagittal section through the lower lumbar spine of a patient with low back pain. Note the herniation of the nucleus pulposus at L4–5 compressing the cauda equina.

the presence of intention tremor and ataxia in the right lower extremity; see Appendix A); and the vagus nerve and ambiguous nucleus (hoarseness). The combination of these findings suggests a location in the posterior cranial fossa, probably in the brain stem. The combination of miosis, ptosis, enophthalmus, and decreased sweating on one side of the face suggests Horner's syndrome, caused by interruption of the sympathetic pathway. This pathway can be interrupted in the lateral brain stem fibers that descend from higher centers in the lateral column of the upper thoracic cord, the upper sympathetic ganglia, or the postsynaptic fibers of the carotid plexus (see Fig 20–6).

Because the patient's disorder had a sudden onset and rapid course, a tumor was unlikely. The most frequent sudden neurologic deficits in the patient's age group have a vascular basis: occlusion or bleeding. Of these, occlusion (ischemic infarct) is the more common (see Chapter 12).

The only anatomic region where all these systems are contiguous is the lateral portion of the medulla; this is the site of the lesion: **lateral medullary syndrome (Wallenberg's syndrome).** Damage to the lateral medulla results from occlusion of small branches of either the posterior inferior cerebellar or the vertebral artery. In 1895, Wallenberg described six patients with

similar signs and symptoms and recognized the vascular basis of the disorder (Figs 25–6 and 25–7).

Case 7, Chapter 7

The patient's signs and symptoms during his first admission to the hospital suggest lesions in the left side of the visual system, nerve III or its nucleus, the vestibular system, the portion of the corticobulbar pathway that supplies the face, and the corticospinal tract. It would be difficult for one lesion to involve all these areas. Findings on the second admission, four months later, showed additional deficits in the cerebellum or cere-

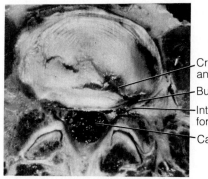

Figure 25–5. Photograph of a horizontal section through L4–5 intervertebral disk in a patient with low back pain. Note the lateral herniation of the nucleus pulposus. (Reproduced, with permission, from de Groot J: *Correlative Neuroanatomy of Computed Tomography and Magnetic Resonance Imaging.* Lea & Febiger, 1984.)

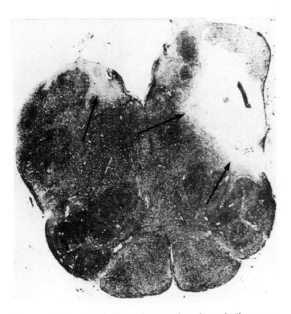

Figure 25–6. Photograph of a section through the open medulla (from Wallenberg's original publication). A large infarct is visible on the right, a smaller one on the left (arrows).

bellar peduncles as well as in the lower cranial nerves (VII, X, and XII, the nerves of articulation); once again, the lesions appeared in several systems or sites.

Signs and symptoms of multiple lesions at different times are characteristic of a disseminated infectious disease, multiple infarcts, or a multifocal demyelinating disorder. Disseminated infection was unlikely in this patient because he had no fever and was not a drug user. A CT image did not show multiple infarcts. The lumbar puncture findings were within normal limits, with a slightly increased gamma globulin level (see Table 25–1). The age of the patient (third decade), the repeated attacks, and the multifocal nature of the deficits are indicative of **multiple sclerosis,** a disease for which there is no specific cure (Figs 25–8 and 25–9). High-dose intravenous corticosteroids or other drugs may be helpful in some cases.

Comment: The risk of multiple sclerosis in populations living between latitudes 40 °N and 40 °S is low. The time course of the disease varies, with some patients remaining relatively healthy after the first episode, other patients (like the one in this case) continuing to have worsening episodes and relatively few symptom-free intervals, and yet others experiencing a course that falls between these types. The disease is usually most active in people between 10 and 45 years of age. The imaging procedure of choice is MR imaging, which readily demonstrates patches of inflammation or demyelination.

Case 8, Chapter 8

All signs and symptoms are related to a lesion in the functional components of nerve VII (see Appendix A). Because there were no long-tract signs and no other

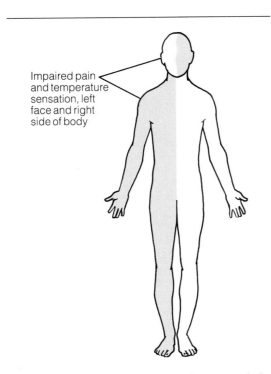

Impaired pain and temperature sensation, left face and right side of body

Figure 25–7. Left posterior inferior cerebellar artery occlusion (Wallenberg's syndrome).

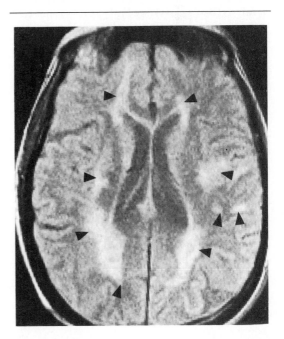

Figure 25–8. MRI of a horizontal section through the head of a 28-year-old patient, showing the lesions (arrow heads) of multiple sclerosis.

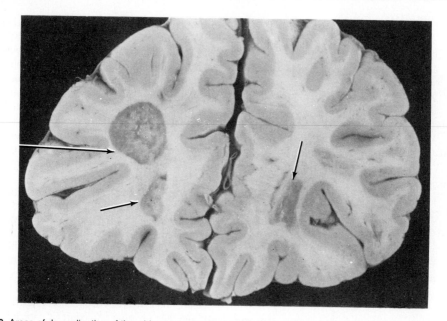

Figure 25–9. Areas of demyelination of the white matter (arrows) in the frontal lobe of a 54-year-old man with multiple sclerosis.

cranial nerve deficits, it is unlikely that the lesion was in the brain stem, where the nuclei of nerve VII occupy small, dispersed areas. Although the sudden onset of the problem may point to a vascular cause, this is unlikely because only one nerve was involved; the history suggests an isolated lesion of nerve VII.

The most probable diagnosis is **peripheral facial paralysis (Bell's palsy)** (see Fig 8–14). As in this case, the paralysis is almost always unilateral. The syndrome always includes dysfunction of the brachial efferent fibers of the facial nerve, but visceral efferent and afferent fiber functions may also be lost. In most cases, the patient recovers spontaneously.

Peripheral facial paralysis occurs commonly in diabetic patients (presumably as a result of ischemic damage to the facial nerve) and is also seen as a complication of Lyme disease. It can occur as a result of nerve damage from a tumor, or in sarcoidosis. A viral cause has been suggested in some patients.

Case 9, Chapter 8

Several causes of facial pain must be considered: pain from dental causes, sinusitis, migraine, tumors of the base of the skull and brain stem, tumors of the maxilla or nasopharynx, and other, rarer causes. Episodic facial pain can occur in multiple sclerosis. These disorders can be ruled out by careful and complete examination, including a CT scan or MR imaging of the face.

The description of brief attacks of very severe pain, triggered from a localized area in the face, in a patient who is otherwise found healthy, points to a diagnosis of **trigeminal neuralgia (tic douloureux).** Medical treatment (with carbamazepine or phenotoin) may be effective. In cases where the pain attacks persist, neurosurgical treatment is indicated.

Case 10, Chapter 9

The finding of bitemporal hemianopia is indicative of an abnormal mass located in or near the base of the brain and impinging on the optic chiasm. This may explain the complaint of worsening eyesight. The other signs and symptoms suggest pituitary dysfunction, probably of considerable duration. Additional tests could confirm this, showing lowered levels of gonadotrophic and thyrotropic hormones. The combination of headache and incipient papilledema indicated increased intracranial pressure, probably caused by a growing mass.

Differential diagnosis includes pituitary adenoma with pressure on the optic chiasm; a craniopharyngioma, a congenital tumor that can compress the pituitary gland, the optic chiasm, or both, and usually causes symptoms either before the age of 20 years or in old age; a tumor of the hypothalamus and pituitary stalk, which is unlikely because there were no other hypothalamic dysfunctions; and a gradually enlarging aneurysm of the anterior communicating artery, which is unlikely because there were endocrine dysfunctions.

Radiologic examination (CT or MR imaging) is helpful in determining the precise location, characteristics, and extent of the neoplasm (Fig 25–10). The most likely diagnosis is **pituitary adenoma.** Treatment is neurosurgical removal of the tumor and hormone-substitution therapy.

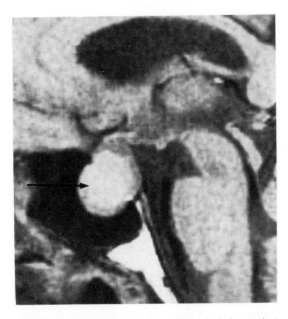

Figure 25–10. MRI through the base of the brain in a patient with a pituitary adenoma (arrow). The tumor has grown downward into the sphenoid sinus and upward to the optic chiasm.

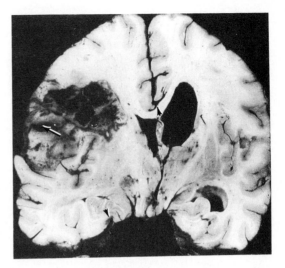

Figure 25–11. Coronal section through the brain of a patient with a hemispheric glial tumor. Histopathologic examination showed this to be a glioblastoma. Note the uncal and subfalcial herniations (arrow heads). A biopsy track is visible on the left (arrow).

Case 11, Chapter 10

The mental impairment (disorientation, confusion, distractibility, and partial loss of memory) of this patient suggests a lesion in one or both frontal lobes. The right facial signs made a left-sided lesion probable, and this was confirmed by the electroencephalogram and imaging studies. The seizure also suggested an irritative lesion in or near the motorcortex.

The differential diagnosis based on the clinical presentation must include a slow-growing tumor, an unusual type of chronic infection with no history of fever, and a degenerative disorder. The imaging studies suggested a multifocal tumor or cerebral abscesses and a brain biopsy was performed. The pathologic diagnosis was **malignant glioma.** It was unfortunate and unusual that the biopsy procedure contributed to a progressive intracranial hemorrhage, which led to brain herniation and death (Fig 25–11).

The tumor was shown to be a glioblastoma with calcifications and bleedings. The small hemorrhages found in the brain stem at autopsy were indicative of rapid herniation and were probably caused by tearing of small vessels in the midbrain and pons (Duret hemorrhages).

Comment: Gliomas are a frequent type of brain tumor in most age groups (Tables 25–2 and 25–3). Astrocytoma is considered histologically to be the most benign glioma, and glioblastoma multiforme is considered the most malignant. Modern imaging techniques are useful in determining the site, and often the type, of a mass (Figs 25–12 and 25–13).

Case 12, Chapter 10

The history of ear pain, draining ear, and fever suggests acute middle-ear infection. The subsequent worsening of the patient's condition indicates that complications had occurred: involvement of the left facial nerve (in the middle ear), headache, dysphasia, and mental deterioration. All this suggests that the infection had penetrated the cranial cavity. Electroencephalographic findings confirmed that there was abnormal electrical activity suggestive of a mass lesion in the left frontotemporal region, and CT scanning revealed a mass.

The differential diagnosis includes otitis media with meningitis, which is unlikely because there was

Table 25–2. Frequency of major types of intracranial tumors.*

Types of Tumors†		Frequency of Occurrence
Gliomas		50%
Glioblastoma multiforme	50%	
Astrocytoma	20%	
Ependymoma	10%	
Medulloblastoma	10%	
Oligodendroglioma	5%	
Mixed	5%	
Meningiomas		20%
Nerve sheath tumors		10%
Metastatic tumors		10%
Congenital tumors		5%
Miscellaneous tumors		5%

*Reproduced, with permission, from Way LW (editor): *Current Surgical Diagnosis & Treatment*, 6th ed. Lange, 1983.
†Exclusive of pituitary tumors.

Table 25–3. Brain tumor types according to age and site.*

Age	Cerebral Hemisphere	Intrasellar and Parasellar	Posterior Fossa
Childhood and adolescence	Ependymomas; less commonly, astrocytomas.	Astrocytomas, mixed gliomas, ependymomas.	Astrocytomas, medulloblastomas, ependymomas.
Age 20–40	Meningiomas, astrocytomas; less commonly, metastatic tumors.	Pituitary adenomas; less commonly, meningiomas.	Acoustic neuromas, meningiomas, hemangioblastomas; less commomly metastatic tumors.
Over age 40	Glioblastoma multiforme, meningiomas, metastatic tumors.	Pituitary adenomas; less commomly, meningiomas.	Metastatic tumors, acoustic neuromas, meningiomas.

*Reproduced, with permission, from Dunphy JE, Way LW (editors): *Current Surgical Diagnosis & Treatment,* 3rd ed. Lange, 1977.

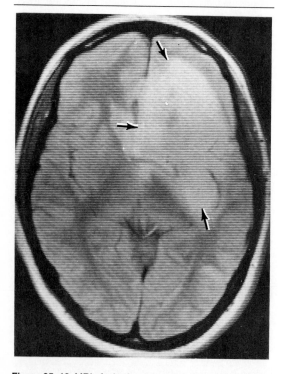

Figure 25–12. MRI of a horizontal section through the head at the level of the lentiform nucleus in a patient with a glioma surrounded by edema (arrows).

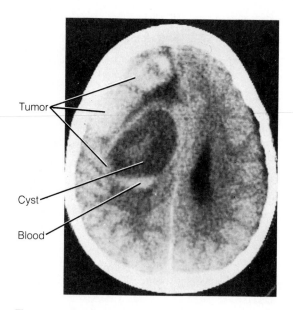

Figure 25–13. CT image of a horizontal section through the head at the level of the lateral ventricles in a patient with glioblastoma multiforma. A small amount of blood lies in the bottom of a cystic portion of the tumor.

no stiffness of the neck; encephalitis caused by an intercurrent infection, which seems too coincidental to be likely; and cerebritis (which often evolves into a cerebral abscess) as a complication of a pyogenic infection.

In this patient CT imaging confirmed the diagnosis of **cerebral abscess** (Fig 25–14; see also Table 25–1).

Comment: The high mortality rate in patients with this severe condition has been reduced by repeating the CT scan every two or three days to monitor both the effects of antibiotics and the ripening of the abscess so that surgical drainage can be performed at the right time. Patients with an impaired immune system can develop an infection in any part of the body; in the brain, the agent is often **Toxoplasma gondii** (Fig 25–15).

Case 13, Chapter 11

The history, temperature, and blood count suggest this to be an infection. Fever, poor appetite, and cough suggest a respiratory infection, and the neck stiffness points to meningeal irritation. It is likely that the initial infection had developed into septicemia and spread to the central nervous system. The lumbar puncture findings are consistent with meningitis (see Table 25–1). The low level of glucose in the cerebrospinal fluid, especially with a normal level of glucose in the blood, is characteristic of bacterial infection and a gram-stained smear showed pneumococci. The differential diagnosis is extremely limited.

The diagnosis is **pneumococcal meningitis** (Fig 25–16). Treatment consists of injecting the appropri-

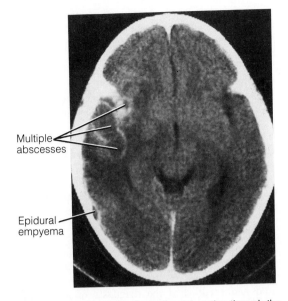

Figure 25–14. CT image of a horizontal section through the temporal lobes, showing an epidural lesion and multiple rounded confluent masses in the right lobe. Notice similarity of this lesion to that in Figure 25–13.

ate antibiotics intravenously. In addition, intrathecal injection may be considered.

Comment: Pneumococcal meningitis and other forms of purulent meningitis usually extend over the hemispheres, while tuberculous meningitis is more caseous and is often located in the basal cisterns (Fig 25–17). In both types, the circulation of cerebrospinal fluid may become impaired, leading to communicating hydrocephalus.

Case 14, Chapter 11

The history indicates trauma on the right side of the head and temporary loss of consciousness. Findings on early neurologic examination were unremarkable. At this stage, the differential diagnosis should include concussion, in which there is usually little or no loss of consciousness; contusion of the brain, which usually produces no deficits at first; and some type of intracranial hemorrhage. An immediate CT scan or MR image would have been useful to show intracranial blood. A skull film might have shown a fracture of the temporal squama but would not have shown the intracranial changes. In the absence of neuroradiologic procedures, a period of observation was indicated.

The vital signs were within normal limits at first but changed appreciably after a few hours. The combination of increasing blood pressure and decreasing pulse and respiratory rates is often indicative of increasing in-

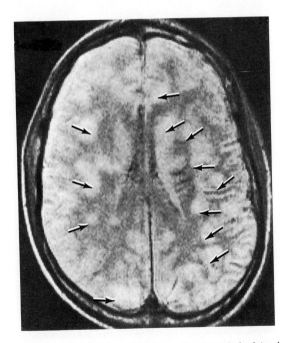

Figure 25–15. MRI of a horizontal section through the lateral ventricles in a patient with acquired immunodeficiency syndrome (AIDS). Notice the multiple high-intensity regions throughout both hemispheres, representing cerebral abscesses (arrows).

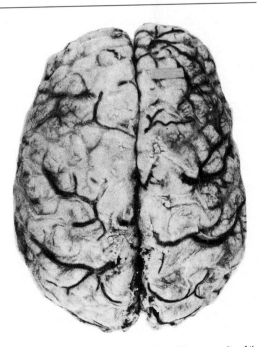

Figure 25–16. Pneumococcal meningitis. The convexity of the brain is covered by thick, yellow-green exudate in the subarachnoidal space.

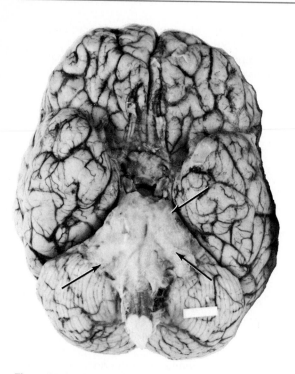

Figure 25–17. Basal view of the brain, showing tuberculous meningitis (arrows) in a 26-year-old man.

the slightly increased white blood count, and the increased erythrocyte sedimentation rate all pointed to a major abnormal vascular event, most likely a hemorrhage.

Blood in the subarachnoid space can irritate the meninges, cause neck stiffness and pain and vessel spasms, and affect the function of the cranial nerves. The motor deficits must be explained by involvement of the corticospinal tract. The most likely site is the left cerebral peduncle, where dysfunction of the cranial nerve III explains the eye findings. Severe bleeding in the subarachnoid space can also trigger displacement of the cerebrum, followed by transtentorial herniation. Compression of the cerebral peduncle and nerve III between the posterior cerebral and superior cerebellar arteries is often seen as a complication of an expanding supratentorial mass.

A lumbar puncture might have aggravated the beginning brain herniation, but if performed, it would have demonstrated frank blood in the cerebrospinal fluid and established the diagnosis of acute **subarachnoid hemorrhage** (see Table 25–1). In this case, a CT image showed a high-density area in the cisterns, particularly on the right side (see Fig 12–20). In such cases, cerebral angiography can be performed a few days later, when a clot has sealed off the bleeding site.

tracranial pressure (Cushing's phenomenon). This patient should have been re-examined at frequent intervals.

There was a loss of consciousness after a lucid interval. Together with the increased intracranial pressure, this suggested a rapidly growing mass on the right side and within the skull. The loss of right-sided functions of nerve III is indicative of beginning brain herniation.

The most likely diagnosis is **epidural hemorrhage,** perhaps with some intracerebral bleeding (contusion). Subdural hemorrhage is less likely because of the rapid deterioration of the patient's condition. Intracerebral hemorrhage can be ruled out by radiologic studies (Fig 25–18; see also Figs 12–26 and 12–27). CT or MR imaging, when available, is superior to lumbar puncture.

Neurosurgical treatment of the bleeding and removal of the epidural blood should be done quickly and may indeed be lifesaving.

Case 15, Chapter 12

The headache and painful stiff neck indicate a process irritating the basal meninges. This could be infectious, the result of bleeding in the subarachnoid space, or the result of meningeal spread from a primary tumor. The suddenness of the disease suggested vascular cause. Intracranial hypertensive bleeding was unlikely in this normotensive patient, and there was no history of trauma. The severity of the disease,

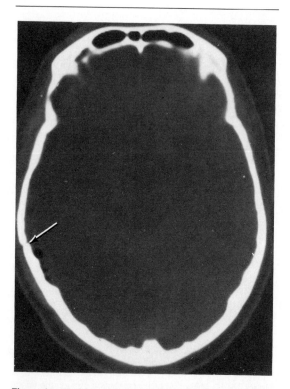

Figure 25–18. CT image through the head at the level of the external ears (bone window) in a patient with epidural hemorrhage. Note fracture site (arrow) and nearby air bubbles.

The treatment of subarachnoid hemorrhage consists of neurosurgical removal or containment of the cause of the bleeding—an aneurysm or a vascular malformation.

Case 16, Chapter 12

The history shows the patient to be an alcoholic who had possibly received trauma to the head when he fell. His level of consciousness had deteriorated, and he seemed to have had a seizure (incontinence and a bitten lip), both findings suggesting cerebral involvement. Results of the neurologic examination suggested a lesion in or near the right motor cortex, and the lumbar puncture showed xanthochromia (fresh and old blood) in the cerebrospinal fluid (see Table 25–1). All these findings indicated a hemorrhage; the time course favored subdural bleeding. Subarachnoid bleeding from a leaking aneurysm was less likely, since trauma initiated the process in this patient. An arachnoid tear could have produced the bloody cerebrospinal fluid, and subdural bleeding could occur with additional (mild) trauma. The CT image demonstrated this (see Fig 12–23). The worsening of the patient's condition was caused by imminent herniation of the brain, triggered by the blood mass, the drop in cerebrospinal fluid pressure associated with lumbar puncture, or both.

The diagnosis is subacute right-sided **subdural hemorrhage.** Treatment consists of neurosurgical removal of the blood and closure of the bleeding veins.

Comment: Most subdural hematomas cover the upper part of the hemispheres, while epidural hematomas are often more circumscribed and located lower (compare Figs 12–26 and 12–27). Bilateral hematoma is not uncommon (Fig 25–19). When bilateral hematoma is found in a youngster, child abuse may be suspected.

Case 17, Chapter 13

The history indicates a motor disorder. In the absence of cerebellar signs and of corticospinal tract deficits, an abnormality in basal ganglia system function must be suspected. This is consistent with the findings of akinesia and unilateral tremor. All observations and test results were compatible with a dysfunction of the substantia nigra or its pathways.

The most likely diagnosis was **Parkinson's disease (paralysis agitans),** and neuroradiologic examinations served only to exclude other disorders. Treatment consisted of physical therapy and appropriate administration of drugs such as levodopa. The patient had a moderately good response to therapy.

Comment: Neuropathology may confirm the diagnosis at autopsy by the finding of depigmentation of the substantia nigra (see Fig 13–8). Neuromelanin is normally absent in the midbrain and other brain stem sites up to the age of about eight years.

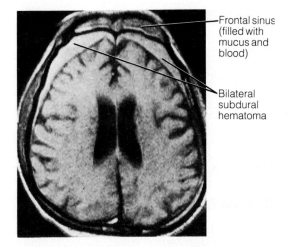

Frontal sinus (filled with mucus and blood)

Bilateral subdural hematoma

Figure 25–19. MRI of a horizontal section at the level of the lateral ventricles of a patient with bilateral subdural hematoma and congested frontal sinuses. The patient had fallen down a flight of stairs.

Case 18, Chapter 13

The suddenness of the severe neurologic deficits in a hypertensive patient most likely indicates a vascular event, probably an intracerebral hemorrhage. In cases such as this, the hematoma may be (in order of frequency) in the putamen, thalamus, pons, or cerebellum. The bleeding in this patient involved the motor system (face, tongue, and corticospinal tract dysfunction). The most likely site of bleeding was either in the putamen, with spread to the globus pallidus and internal capsule or in the pons, with involvement of the corticospinal and corticopontine systems. However, the unilaterality of the motor deficits pointed to bleeding in the basal ganglia and internal capsule, rather than in the compact pons.

A lumbar puncture could be useful in ruling out a subarachnoid hemorrhage (see case 15 and Table 25–1). Normal cerebrospinal fluid findings would not help in differentiating other types of bleeding, however, and the procedure might even contribute to herniation of the brain. The neuroradiologic procedure of choice, CT imaging, is shown in Figure 12–18. MR imaging, if available, would also be helpful.

The diagnosis is hypertensive **intracerebral hemorrhage** in the left basal ganglia and adjacent structures. Treatment includes antihypertensive therapy, intensive care, and measures to relieve symptoms.

Comment: If bleeding occurs in the putamen, the amount of blood may be small and the blood may later be reabsorbed (Fig 25–20). When the amount of blood is large, the blood may break through into the ventricles or subarachnoid space.

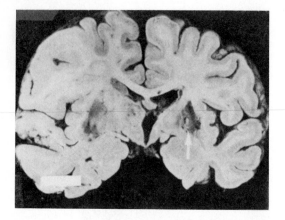

Figure 25–20. Cystic degeneration involving principally the left caudate and lenticular nuclei.

Case 19, Chapter 14

In the absence of cranial nerve signs and symptoms and cerebellar signs, the lesion must be in the spinal cord, on the right side, at the level of the lower-motor-neuron deficit, C6–C8. The numbness and tingling suggested involvement of the spinal cord on the right side. Weakness in the right hand indicated additional motor deficits of the lower-motor-neuron type. Absence of acute pain sensation was based on a lesion in the spinothalamic system. The weakness and abnormal reflexes of the extremities indicated additional involvement of the corticospinal tracts. Peripheral nerve involvement could be ruled out because the patient had upper motor neuron signs (an extensor plantar response and stronger reflexes on the right side) and a dissociated sensory deficit (the areas of loss of touch were different from those of loss of pain sensation).

The differential diagnosis includes traumatic degeneration of the spinal cord, which is unlikely because there was no history of trauma in this case; myelitis, unlikely because there was no history of fever; and bleeding or thrombosis, unlikely because of the slowly progressive course and the distribution of the deficits. A plain film of the spine is not helpful in demonstrating intrinsic cord lesions; therefore, magnetic resonance imaging, CT imaging, or myelography is preferable. An MRI study was performed and showed enlargement of the spinal cord by cavitation, or cyst formation, especially in the lower cervical segments (Fig 25–21).

The diagnosis is **syringomyelia.** The cavity extended from C4 to C7 and involved the right cuneate tract as well as portions of the ventral horns, causing atrophy of the hand muscles (Fig 5–27). Abnormal enlargement of the central canal is called **hydromyelia** and draining the cavity neurosurgically can provide relief.

Comment: MRI findings in syringomyelia must be distinguished from those in the Arnold-Chiari malformation (Fig 25–22). The latter is a congenital disorder

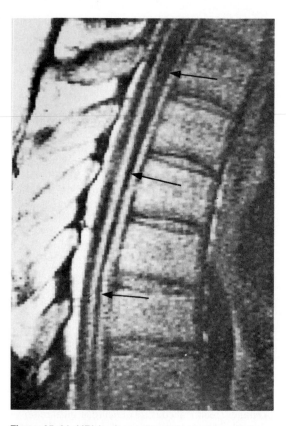

Figure 25–21. MRI (surface coil technique) of a sagittal section through the thoracic spine of a patient with syringomyelia (arrows).

characterized by downward displacement of a small cerebellum, cavitation of the spinal cord, and other abnormalities.

Case 20, Chapter 14

The patient was an alcoholic, as the history indicates. The symmetric motor deficits (lower-motor-neuron type) in all extremities and the sensory irritation or loss of sensation, especially in the distal portions, are highly suggestive of peripheral nerve involvement (Fig 25–23). The differential diagnosis could include spinal cord disease, but the distribution of the lesions is not compatible with the somatotropic organization of pathways in the cord.

The diagnosis is **polyneuropathy,** which in this case is caused by thiamine deficiency secondary to alcohol abuse. Hyperalgesia of the soles and calf muscles is characteristic of this type of nerve disease. (There are many other causes of polyneuropathy, and hyperalgesia is not always present.) The treatment in this case should include injections of vitamin B$_1$ (thiamine hydrochloride), daily ingestion of oral multivitamin pills, and institution of both a vitamin-rich diet and a therapy program for alcoholism.

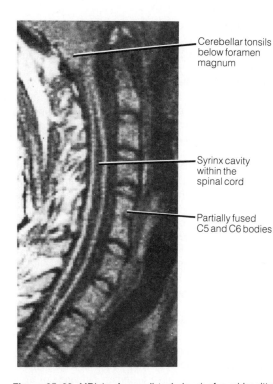

Cerebellar tonsils below foramen magnum

Syrinx cavity within the spinal cord

Partially fused C5 and C6 bodies

Figure 25–22. MRI (surface coil technique) of a midsagittal section through the upper spine of a patient with Chiari and other malformations. (Compare with Fig 7–26.)

Case 21, Chapter 15

The history of an epileptiform attack in a 50-year-old woman indicates irritation of the cerebral cortex, and the results of examination (chronic papilledema) suggest a slow-growing space-occupying lesion. The mental status is compatible with involvement of one or both frontal lobes. The loss of olfaction on the left side and the atrophy of the adjacent left optic nerve (which resulted in a pale optic disc) suggest that the lesion is located in the base of the left frontal lobe and is compressing the optic nerve. The associated cerebral edema explains the mild facial weakness and the effect on the motor pathways to the extremities.

The differential diagnosis is limited: the lesion may be an intrinsic brain tumor in the left frontal lobe or olfactory region, or it may be a meningeal tumor in that region. A CT scan or MR image would show the exact location of the tumor; however, if calcification were present in the tumor, plain skull films might also provide some useful information.

Neurosurgical removal and pathologic studies of the abnormal tissue resulted in the diagnosis of **olfactory groove meningioma** with associated **Foster Kennedy's syndrome** on the left side. This syndrome consists of contralateral papilledema and ipsilateral optic atrophy caused by a mass in the low frontal region (Fig 25–24).

Comment: Meningiomas arise from abnormal arachnoid cells; therefore, this type of tumor occurs in many intracranial locations as well as in the spinal region. Frequent sites are on the convexity of the hemisphere and along the falx (Fig 25–25).

Case 22, Chapter 16

The key to determining the site of the lesion in this case is the long-standing impairment of cranial nerve VIII, evident first in the cochlear division and more recently in the vestibular division. The ensuing signs and symptoms all related to the adjacent cranial nerves (V, VI, and VII) or their nuclei and to the brain stem (corticospinal tracts and cerebellar peduncles). The initial complaints pointed to a lesion in the pontocerebellar angle, where nerves VII and VIII lie close to the brain stem. The long period of progressive worsening and the presence of papilledema made a slow-growing tumor likely.

Differential diagnosis includes a cranial nerve tumor, a tumor of the brain stem (eg, a glioma) or the adjacent arachnoid (eg, a meningioma), or another rare neoplasm. The lesion occurring most frequently in this region is a **nerve VIII tumor.** This type of tumor usually originates just inside the proximal end of the internal auditory meatus, where it later compresses the adjacent seventh nerve and widens the meatus. The tumor (usually a schwannoma) may grow to compress

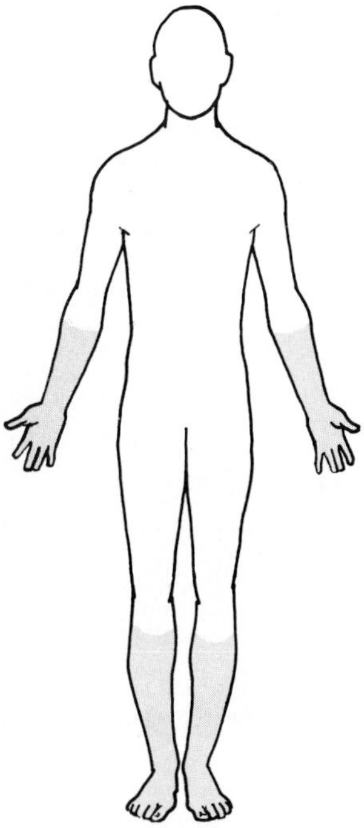

Figure 25–23. Distribution of sensory and lower-motor-neuron deficits in a patient with peripheral polyneuropathy. Notice the "stocking-and-glove" pattern of sensory loss.

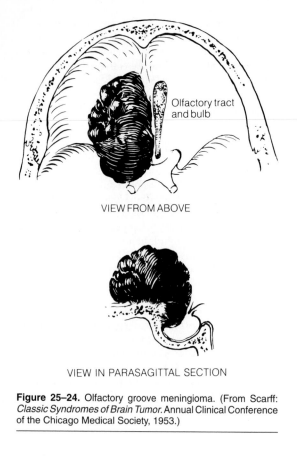

Olfactory tract
and bulb

VIEW FROM ABOVE

VIEW IN PARASAGITTAL SECTION

Figure 25–24. Olfactory groove meningioma. (From Scarff: *Classic Syndromes of Brain Tumor.* Annual Clinical Conference of the Chicago Medical Society, 1953.)

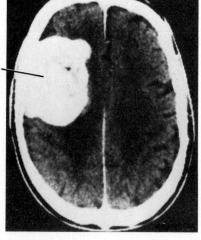

Meningioma
on the
convexity

Figure 25–25. CT image, with contrast enhancement, of a horizontal section through the cerebral hemispheres. The absence of surrounding edema suggests a slow-growing tumor, in this case a meningioma.

adjacent structures in the pontocerebellar angle (Fig 25–26). Treatment consists of surgical removal of the tumor. Function of nerve VIII may be permanently lost.

Case 23, Chapter 17

The syndrome of recurrent vertigo with tinnitus, nausea, and progressive deafness suggests an abnormality in the inner ear. Spontaneous nystagmus (horizontal or rotatory) is often present during an attack. The most likely diagnosis is **Meniere's disease** (transient ischemic attacks caused by basilar artery stenosis must first be ruled out). It is probably caused by an increase in the volume of labyrinthine fluid (endolymphatic hydrops). Bilateral involvement occurs in 50% of the patients. Caloric testing usually shows impaired vestibular function. The patient should be referred to an ENT specialist.

Medical treatment of this disease may be effective and modern surgical treatment is available.

Case 24, Chapter 18

Transient ischemic attacks are clear signals of incipient occlusive cerebrovascular disease, especially in older patients, who have a higher incidence of arteriosclerosis. The findings on neurologic examination indicated the involvement of several cranial nerves, some on the left and some on the right side: nerves III, V, VI, VII, IX, and X and the vestibular division of VIII (see Appendix A). This locates the lesion in the brain stem, which is supplied by the vertebrobasilar system of arteries. The involvement of the corticospinal system and the cerebellar deficits are all compatible with a lesion in the brain stem. The absence of visual field defects is in keeping with a lesion below the diencephalon.

The most likely diagnosis is **stenosis (narrowing) of the basilar artery,** a very serious condition that can rapidly deteriorate to complete occlusion, resulting in coma or death. If stenosis occurs rather suddenly and if the posterior communicating arteries are thin on both sides, the blood supply from anastomoses may not be adequate to prevent infarction of the brain stem, a condition that is associated with a high mortality rate. The diagnosis of stenosis may be confirmed by angiography or Doppler ultrasonography. Treatment includes anticoagulant therapy to prevent thrombosis and total occlusion.

Case 25, Chapter 19

Fever, malaise, and headache may suggest a subacute intracranial infection. The patient's "fits" indicate irritation of the cortex, possibly caused by edematous swelling of the brain. The lumbar puncture results confirmed the presence of infection and increased in-

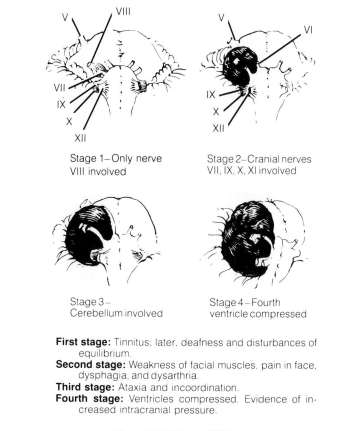

Stage 1–Only nerve VIII involved

Stage 2–Cranial nerves VII, IX, X, XI involved

Stage 3– Cerebellum involved

Stage 4–Fourth ventricle compressed

First stage: Tinnitus; later, deafness and disturbances of equilibrium.
Second stage: Weakness of facial muscles, pain in face, dysphagia, and dysarthria.
Third stage: Ataxia and incoordination.
Fourth stage: Ventricles compressed. Evidence of increased intracranial pressure.

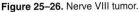

Figure 25–26. Nerve VIII tumor.

tracranial pressure; however, the basal meninges did not appear to be involved, because there was no neck stiffness.

The dysphasia and memory loss, the defects seen on the MR scan, and the electroencephalographic findings all indicated temporal lobe involvement on both sides. The CT scan findings were compatible with swelling of these sites and showed some bleeding.

The differential diagnosis includes encephalitis, cerebritis, meningitis, and subarachnoid hemorrhage. Subarachnoid hemorrhage may be associated with a moderate rise in temperature and with seizures and loss of consciousness; however, the absence of blood in the cerebrospinal fluid, the absence of neck stiffness, the presence of dysphasia, and the electroencephalographic findings make this diagnosis unlikely. Meningitis is unlikely because there was no neck stiffness and because the lumbar puncture specimen showed a white blood cell count with mostly lymphocytes rather than polymorphonuclear leukocytes (see Table 25–1). Moreover, red blood cells are not usually seen in the spinal fluid in meningitis. Although cerebritis associated with abscess formation is a possible diagnosis, it is unlikely because both temporal lobes

were simultaneously involved; there was no primary infection such as otitis media, sinusitis, or endocarditis, and the predominance of lymphocytes suggests otherwise.

The most likely diagnosis is **encephalitis** caused by a virus. Localization in both temporal lobes is typical, as are the cerebrospinal fluid results and the findings on the MR image (see Fig 19–15). The diagnosis of **herpes simplex encephalitis** was confirmed at autopsy when the herpes virus could be demonstrated in the trigeminal ganglion. In some cases patients respond well to treatment with antiviral agents such as acyclovir, although residual amnesic defects, aphasia, dementia, and seizures are common.

Case 26, Chapter 20

The history indicates a slowly progressive process involving the lower cranial nerves (VIII, X, and XII), the brain stem nuclei of these nerves, and the cerebellar pathways, all predominantly on the right side. The ataxia and the increased level of protein in the cerebrospinal fluid pointed to an intracranial location of the lesion. The hypersalivation, postural hypertension, and the cranial nerve (or nuclei) signs can be explained by involvement of the lower brain stem, where the salivatory nuclei, vasomotor center, and pertinent cranial nerve nuclei are located.

The lesion is probably a **brain stem tumor** involving the right side of the stem more than the left and characterized by a slow progression over a period of eight months. The ventricular enlargement seen on CT scan is compatible with a posterior fossa block of the cerebrospinal fluid circulation. (CT images of this region are often suboptimal because of bone artifacts; the radiologist's report in this case said, "possible enlargement of the lower brain stem.")

Treatment in this case consisted of subtotal removal of a mass that was located in the fourth ventricle and attached to the brain stem. Histopathologic studies showed that the tumor was an ependymoma (Fig 25–27).

Comment: The most common posterior fossa tumors in children are astrocytomas, medulloblastomas, and ependymomas. Different types of tumors may occur in older persons (Table 25–3; Figs 25–28 to 25–30).

Case 27, Chapter 21

The history indicates a series of transient ischemic attacks, which are highly suggestive of cerebrovascular occlusive disease. The most common cause in elderly persons is arteriosclerosis. The sudden deterioration of the patient's status may have been caused by thrombotic or embolic occlusion of a major cere-

bral vessel on the right side. The bilateral papilledema indicated an intracranial mass effect, possibly swelling of the brain associated with an ischemic infarct. The flaccid paralysis and the sensory deficits showed involvement of the blood supply to the sensory motor cortex or the underlying white matter in the right hemisphere. The left incomplete hemianopia was most likely the result of ischemia of the optic radiation.

The distribution of the deficits indicates an occlusion of an artery (not a vein or sinus). The sudden nature of the disorder and the absence of a previous history of tumors or infections tend to eliminate neoplasm and infectious mass from the differential diagnosis. The neuroradiologic examination clarified the extent of the ischemia as well as its vascular origin (Fig 25–31; see also Figs 12–12 and 12–13).

The diagnosis is **thrombosis of the right middle cerebral artery.** Treatment sometimes consists of anticoagulants and symptomatic relief. Physical therapy may be helpful in later stages.

Case 28, Chapter 21

This patient's history is consistent with a sensory seizure with predominantly visual symptoms; this suggests involvement of the occipital lobe cortex. The sudden development of a right homonymous hemianopia was probably caused by a vascular event that involved the left visual pathway behind the optic chiasm. The history of heart disease suggests embolism, in which small thrombi detach from the heart and pass into the major cerebral vessels. There was no headache, so migraine could be ruled out.

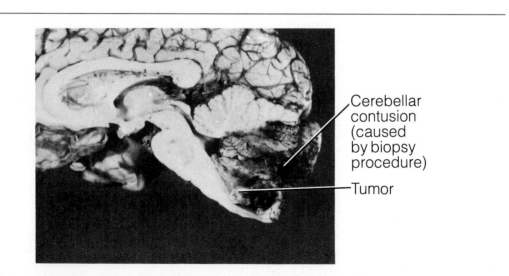

Figure 25–27. Midsagittal section through the brain of a patient with a brain stem tumor. Histologic findings showed the tumor to be an ependymoma. The biopsy track is visible (arrow).

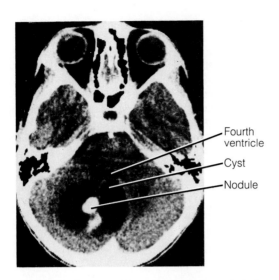

Figure 25–28. CT image, with contrast enhancement, of a horizontal section through the head. Notice the low-density cystic astrocytoma with a high-density nodule in the posterior fossa, representing a glioma of the cerebellum.

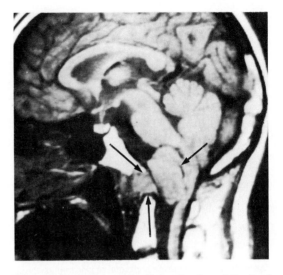

Figure 25–30. MRI of a midsagittal section through the head. The large mass that originates in the clivus and displaces the brain stem backward is a chordoma (arrows).

CT and MR imaging were helpful in confirming the diagnosis of **embolic infarction** of part of the left occipital lobe. Emboli passing to the brain often lodge in the largest vessels, the middle cerebral arteries. In this case, the infarct occurred in the territory of the posterior cerebral artery, which it may have reached by passage through a large (embryonic type) posterior communicating artery or by way of the vertebrobasilar system. Although angiography would help to determine this, there is debate about whether it should be done shortly after an infarct has occurred.

Treatment of embolic infarction consists of controlled anticoagulation to prevent further emboli.

Comment: Emboli, such as blood-borne metastases to the brain, most frequently lodge in the territory of the middle cerebral artery (Fig 25–32).

Case 29, Chapter 22

The progressively worsening mental status, the absence of clear localizing signs, and the age of the patient suggest **senile dementia of the Alzheimer type.** Other diseases with dementia (Huntington's, Creutzfeld-Jacob, and Pick's diseases) have characteristic courses and epidemiologic findings but are also difficult to diagnose without further tests. Treatable causes of dementia (eg, B_{12} deficiency, hypothy-

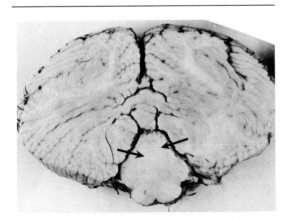

Figure 25–29. Astrocytoma of the medulla oblongata.

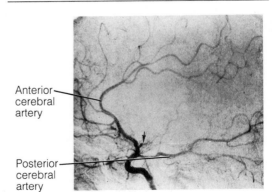

Figure 25–31. Left internal carotid angiogram, arterial phase, lateral view, showing occlusion of the middle cerebral artery (arrow). The posterior artery is well filled (compare with Fig 23–4).

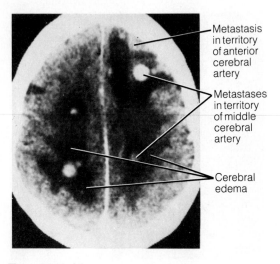

Metastasis
in territory
of anterior
cerebral
artery

Metastases
in territory
of middle
cerebral
artery

Cerebral
edema

Figure 25–32. CT image of a horizontal section through the upper hemispheres of a patient with a known bronchial carcinoma.

roidism) were considered in this woman, but were ruled out by the laboratory tests.

A CT image showed widening of the sulci and dilatation of the spaces containing cerebrospinal fluid (see Fig 22–2). This finding reinforced senile dementia of the Alzheimer's type, the most likely diagnosis. A definitive diagnosis, however, can be made only by pathologic examination of the brain.

There is no specific treatment for senile dementia of the Alzheimer type.

REFERENCES

Adams JH, Corsellis JAN, Duchen LW: *Greenfield's Neuropathology,* 4th ed. Wiley, 1984.

Adams RD, Victor M: *Principles of Neurology,* 5th ed. McGraw-Hill, 1993.

Bradley WG, Daroff RB, Fenichel, Marsden CD: *Neurology in Clinical Practice.* Butterworth-Heinemann, 1991.

Davis RL, Robertson DM (editors): *Textbook of Neuropathology,* 2nd ed. Williams & Wilkins, 1990.

Escourolle R, Poirier J: *Manual of Basic Neuropathology,* 2nd ed. Saunders, 1978.

Greenberg DA, Aminoff MJ, Simon RP: *Clinical Neurology,* 2nd ed. Appleton & Lange, 1993.

Rosenblum ML, Levy, RM, Bredesen, DE: *AIDS and the Nervous System.* Raven, 1988.

Rowland LP (editor): *Merritt's Textbook of Neurology,* 8th ed. Lea Febiger, 1989.

Appendix A:
The Neurologic Examination

EXAMINING CHILDREN & ADULTS

HISTORY

A complete history of the nature, onset, extent, and duration of the chief complaint and associated complaints must be taken. This should include previous diseases, personal and family history, occupational data, and social history. It may be desirable—or necessary—to interview relatives and friends.

Detailed information is particularly important in regard to the following:

A. Headache: Notice the duration, time of onset, location, frequency, severity, progression, precipitating circumstances, associated symptoms, and response to analgesics.

B. Seizures and Episodic Loss of Consciousness: Record the character of the individual episode, age at onset, frequency, duration, mental status during and after episodes, associated signs and symptoms, aura, and the type and effectiveness of previous treatment.

C. Visual Disturbances: The frequency, progression or remissions, scotomas, acuity changes, diplopia, field changes, and associated phenomena should be noted.

D. Pain: The onset, progression, frequency, characteristics, effect of physical measures, associated complaints, and type and effectiveness of previous treatment should be included.

THE PHYSICAL EXAMINATION

Even before beginning the formal physical examination, important information may be gleaned by carefully observing the patient while the history is given.

Is the patient well-groomed, or unkempt? Is the patient aware of and appropriately concerned about the illness? Does the patient attend equally well to stimuli on the left and right sides, ie, does the patient relate equally well to the physician when asked questions from the left, then the right? The examiner can learn much simply by interacting with the patient and observing closely.

A general physical examination should always be made. In particular, the circulatory, respiratory, genitourinary, gastrointestinal, and skeletal systems should be studied and a record of the temperature, pulse rate, respiratory rate, and blood pressure routinely made. Note especially any deformity or limitation of the head, neck, vertebral column, or joints. If there is any question of disease involving the spinal cord, determine if there is tenderness or pain on percussion over the spinal column. Inspect and carefully palpate the scalp and skull for localized thickening of the skull, clusters of abnormal scalp vessels, depressed areas, abnormal contours or asymmetry of the skull, and craniotomy and other operative scars. Percussion may disclose local scalp or skull tenderness over diseased areas and, in hydrocephalic children, a tympanic cracked-pot sound. Auscultate the skull and neck for bruits.

THE NEUROLOGIC EXAMINATION

Level of Consciousness and Alertness

The patient's level of consciousness and degree of alertness should be explicitly noted. Is the patient conscious and fully alert, lethargic, stuporous, or comatose? A depressed level of consciousness can be an important clue, eg, in patients harboring subdural hematomas.

The patient's ability to focus attention should also be noted. Is the patient fully alert or are they confused, ie, unable to maintain a coherent stream of thought? Confusional states occur with a variety of focal lesions in the brain, but are more commonly seen as a result of metabolic and toxic disorders.

Mental Status

Changes in mental status are frequently encountered in clinical neurology. Some changes in mental status have important localizing value, ie, they suggest the presence of focal brain lesions in particular areas. Wernicke's and Broca's aphasia, for example, are seen with lesions involving Wernicke's and Broca's area in the dominant cerebral hemisphere (Chapter 21). Spatial disorientation suggests disease involving the dominant parietal lobe. Hemispatial neglect, in which the patient neglects stimuli, usually in the left hand side of the world, suggests a disorder involving the right hemisphere. With some neurologic disorders (eg, brain tumor, multiple sclerosis, paralysis agitans), the insidious onset and the course of remissions and exacerbations can result in the misdiagnosis of psychogenic illness. Early neurologic disease may occur without significant physical, laboratory, radiologic, or other special diagnostic findings, and drugs used in treatment may further complicate the clinical picture.

A. General Behavior: Evaluate the patient's speech, appearance, concentration, cooperation, posture, general attitude, characteristic mannerisms, and movement.

B. Mood: Look for anxiety, depression, apathy, fear, suspicion, irritability, elation, and aggression.

C. Language: Listen to the patient's spontaneous language, and to the response to your verbal questions. Is the patient's speech fluent, nonfluent, or effortful? Is word choice appropriate? Can the patient name simple objects (pen, pencil, eraser, button, buttonhole), color (point to various objects), and body parts? Is the patient able to repeat simple words ("dog") or phrases of varying complexity ("President Kennedy"; "no ifs, ands, or buts"; "if he were here, then I would go home with him")? Check comprehension of spoken language. This can be accomplished even in the patient who cannot speak by asking the patient to "make a fist"; "show me two fingers"; "point to the ceiling"; "point to the place where I entered the room"; or by asking the patient to nod yes or no in response to questions such as "is school meant for children?" "Do helicopters eat their young?"

Check the patient's ability to read (make sure the patient is wearing reading glasses, if necessary, or use a large print newspaper) and write.

D. Orientation: Check for orientation with respect to person, place, time, or situation.

E. Level of Intelligence: Measures of intelligence include vocabulary, judgment, cultural outlook, and general information.

F. Memory: Details and dates of recent and remote events should be elicited, including such items as birth date, marriage date, names and ages of children and relatives, specific details of the past few days and from more remote times. It is best to ask about objective facts ("What happened in sports last week?" "Who won the World Series?" "Who is the president?" "Who was president before that?")

G. Ability to acquire and manipulate knowledge:

1. General information–These questions should be adapted to the patient's background. Examples are the names of prominent political and world figures, the capitals of countries and states, and current events in politics, sports, and performing arts.

2. Similarities and differences–Have the patient compare wood and coal; iron and silver; book, teacher, and newspaper; president and king; dwarf and child; man and plant; lie and mistake.

3. Calculations–The patient should count backward from 100 by 7s; ie, subtract 7s from 100 (100 − 7 = 93; 93 − 7 = 86; 86 − 7 = 79; etc). Add, multiply, or divide single numbers (eg, 3×5, 4×3, 16×3) and double digit numbers ($11 \times 17 = 187$). Calculate interest at 6% for 18 months. The examiner should make the calculations easier or more difficult depending upon the patient's background.

4. Retention–Ask the patient to repeat digits in natural or reverse order. (Normally, an adult can retain seven forward and five backward.) After instruction, ask the patient to repeat a list of three cities and three two-digit numbers after a pause of three minutes.

5. Right-left orientation; finger recognition– The patient's ability to distinguish right from left and to recognize fingers can be tested with the question "touch your left ear with your right thumb." Defective right-left orientation and inability to recognize fingers are seen (together with impaired ability to calculate and difficulty writing) in the **Gerstmann syndrome** as a result of lesions in the left angular gyrus.

6. Judgment–Ask the patient for the symbolic or specific meaning of simple proverbs such as the following: "A stitch in time saves nine." "A rolling stone gathers no moss." "People who live in glass houses should not throw stones." The content of a simple story or paragraph from a newspaper or magazine can be read and the patient's retention, comprehension, and formulation observed.

7. Memory and comprehension–The examiner tells a story, which is then retold in the patient's own words. The patient is also asked to explain the meaning of the story. The following stories are commonly used.

a. Cowboy story–A cowboy went to San Francisco with his dog, which he left at a friend's house while he went to buy a new suit of clothes. Dressed in his brand-new clothing, he came back to the dog, whistled to it, called it by name, and patted it. But the dog would have nothing to do with him in his new coat and hat. Coaxing was to no avail, so the cowboy went away and put on his old suit, and the dog immediately showed its wild joy in seeing its master as it thought he ought to be.

b. Gilded-boy story–At the coronation of one of the popes, about 300 years ago, a little boy was chosen to play the part of an angel. In order that his appearance might be as magnificent as possible, he was covered from head to foot with a coating of gold foil. The little boy fell ill, and although everything possible was done for his recovery except the removal of the fatal golden covering, he died within a few hours.

H. Content of Thought: Thought content may include obsessions, phobias, delusions, compulsions, recurrent dreams or nightmares, depersonalization, or hallucinations. Check special preoccupations and disorders of content, with attention to special topics of concern to the patient and the form they take.

Cranial Nerves

A. Olfactory Nerve (I): Use familiar odors such as peppermint, coffee, menthol, or vanilla, and avoid use of irritants such as ammonia and vinegar. A test substance is rapidly passed toward the subject from a distance of about 1 meter, and the patient must then identify the substance with eyes shut and one nostril held closed. Complete or unilateral anosmia may be significant in the absence of intranasal disorders.

B. Optic Nerve (II):

1. Visual acuity test–A Snellen chart can be used to measure visual acuity and determine whether improvement is obtained with correction. For individuals with severe defects, cruder tests may be employed, eg, the ability to count fingers, detect hand movements, and changes from dark to light.

2. Ophthalmoscopic examination–Each optic fundus must be examined as part of the neurologic examination. If necessary, dilate the pupils with drugs after the pupillary reflexes have been noted. Details of the ophthalmoscopic examination should include the color, size, and shape of the optic disk; the presence or absence of a physiologic cup; the distinctness of the optic disc edges; the size, shape, and configuration of the vessels; and the presence of hemorrhage, exudate, or pigment.

3. Visual field test–The visual fields can be roughly tested by confrontation, with the patient seated about 1 meter from the examiner. With the left eye covered, the patient looks at the examiner's left eye. The examiner slowly raises both hands upward from a position where they can barely be seen in the lower two quadrants, and the patient signifies when the examiner's moving hands first become visible. The upper quadrants are similarly tested, with the examiner's hands moving downward. The left eye of the patient is then tested against the right eye of the examiner.

More accurate visual field determination requires the use of a perimeter or tangent screen.

C. Oculomotor (III), Trochlear (IV), and Abducens (VI) Nerves: Strabismus, nystagmus, ptosis, exophthalmos, and pupillary abnormalities can be detected on initial examination. Test ocular movements by having the patient follow the movement of an object (eg, a finger or a light) to the extremes of the lateral and vertical planes.

The size and shape of each pupil are noted. The reactions of both pupils to a bright light flashed into one eye in a darkened room while the patient gazes into the distance are noted. The direct light reaction is the response of the pupil of the illuminated eye; the consensual light reaction is the reaction of the opposite pupil, which is carefully shielded from the stimulating light.

In testing the accommodation-convergence response, the examiner asks the patient to focus alternately on two objects, one distant and the other 15 cm (6 inches) from the patient's face.

The examiner should carefully note whether **nystagmus** (rhythmic, jerking movements of the eyes) is present, and if so, the direction of its fast and slow phases at rest or elicited by gaze in a particular direction. Nystagmus can indicate disease of the vestibular system, cerebellum, or brain stem.

D. Trigeminal Nerve (V): The ability to perceive a pinprick or the touch of a bit of cotton is tested over the face and anterior half of the scalp. The corneal sensation is tested by approaching the cornea from the side and touching it with a strand of cotton as the patient looks upward. Care must be taken not to touch the eyelashes or conjunctiva. Test the motor function of the trigeminal nerve by palpating the contraction of the masseter and temporalis muscles induced by a biting movement of the jaws.

E. Facial Nerve (VII): Notice facial expression, mobility, and symmetry. Assess the voluntary movements of the lower facial musculature by having the patient smile, whistle, bare the teeth, and pucker his or her lips. Maneuvers such as closing the eyes or wrinkling the forehead are ways of testing the upper facial musculature.

Test taste sensation of the anterior two-thirds of the tongue by applying small quantities of test solutions to the protruded tongue with cotton applicators. The test solutions used are sweet (sugar), bitter (quinine), salt (saline), and sour (vinegar). As each taste is perceived, the patient responds by pointing to a labeled card. Between tests, the tongue should be irrigated with water.

F. Vestibulocochlear Nerve (VIII):

1. Cochlear nerve–The patient's ability to hear the examiner's voice in ordinary conversation is noted. The ability to hear the sound produced by rubbing the thumb and forefinger together is then tested for each ear at distances up to a few centimeters. The farthest distance from either ear at which the ticking of a loud watch or the spoken voice is heard can be measured.

Use a tuning fork vibrating at 256 Hz to test air and bone conduction for each ear (see Table 16–1): In Rinne's test, the vibrating tuning fork is placed on the mastoid process and then in front of the ear. Normally, the fork is heard for several seconds longer when it is placed in front of the ear than when it is placed on the mastoid. In injury to the cochlear nerve, there may be complete or partial inability to hear the vibrating tuning fork (nerve deafness). When partial hearing remains, air conduction exceeds bone conduction. In disease of the middle ear with impaired hearing, bone conduction of the sound of the tuning fork is better than air conduction (conduction deafness).

In Weber's test, a vibrating tuning fork (256 Hz) is placed on the bridge of the nose or over the vertex of the scalp. Normally, the sound is heard equally well in both ears. In patients with unilateral deafness as a result of middle ear disease, the sound is heard best in the affected ear.

2. Vestibular nerve–The caloric test is frequently used to evaluate vestibular function. The eardrum is first examined to make certain no perforations exist. The patient is asked to sit with the head tilted slightly forward to test the vertical canals or to lie supine with the head tilted back at an angle of 60 degrees to test the horizontal canals. The examiner slowly and steadily irrigates one external auditory canal with cool (30°C) or warm (40°C) water. Normally, cool water in one ear produces nystagmus on the opposite side; warm water produces it on the same side. (A mnemonic for this is COWS: *c*ool, *o*pposite; *w*arm, *s*ame.) Irrigation is continued until the patient complains of nausea or dizziness or until nystagmus is detected. This normally takes 20–30 seconds. If no reaction occurs after three minutes, the test is discontinued.

G. Glossopharyngeal Nerve (IX): Taste over the posterior third of the tongue is tested in a manner similar to that described above for the anterior two-thirds of the tongue. Sensation (usually touch) is tested on the soft palate and pharynx. The pharyngeal response (gag reflex) is tested bilaterally.

H. Vagus Nerve (X): Test the swallowing function by noting the patient's ability to drink water and eat solid food. The pharyngeal wall contraction is observed as part of the gag reflex. Movement of the median raphe of the palate and uvula when the patient says "ah" is recorded. In unilateral paralysis of the vagus nerve, the raphe and uvula move toward the intact side, and the posterior pharyngeal wall of the paralyzed side moves like a curtain toward the intact side. The character, volume, and sound of the patient's voice are recorded. Using a dental mirror, the position of the vocal cords can be observed by indirect laryngoscopy. The resting heart rate and the bradycardia produced by pressure on the eyeball (oculocardiac reflex) or pressure on the carotid sinus may be influenced by lesions involving the vagus nerve.

I. Accessory Nerve (XI): Instruct the patient to rotate his or her head against resistance applied to the side of the chin. This tests the function of the opposite sternocleidomastoid muscle. To test both sternocleidomastoid muscles together, the patient flexes the head forward against resistance placed under the chin. Shrugging a shoulder against resistance is a way of testing trapezius muscle function.

J. Hypoglossal Nerve (XII): Examine the tongue for atrophy and for fasciculations or tremors when it is protruded and when it is lying at rest in the mouth. Note any deviation of the tongue on protrusion; a lesion of the hypoglossal nerve or nucleus causes deviation to the same side.

Motor System

The power of muscle groups of the extremities, neck, and trunk is tested. Where there is an indication of diminished strength, test smaller muscle groups and individual muscles (see Appendix B). Atrophy or hypertrophy of muscles is judged by inspection and palpation and, in the case of the musculature of the extremities, by measuring the circumferences of the limbs. The differences between the circumferences on the two sides may be related to the handedness or occupation of the patient but are often because of atrophy. Notice abnormal movements, and record the influence upon them of postural and emotional change, intention, and voluntary movements.

Muscle tone is judged by palpation of the muscles of the extremities and by passive movements of the joints by the examiner. Carefully describe increased or decreased resistance to passive movement. Note tone alterations, including clasp-knife spasticity, plastic or cogwheel rigidity, spasms, contractures, and hypotonia.

Pendulousness is the motion of a passively displaced extremity when it is permitted to swing freely. It is increased in hypotonia, markedly reduced in rigidity of extrapyramidal origin, and irregular in pattern (though normal or slightly diminished in duration) in spasticity. Notice and describe involuntary movements, including tremors, athetosis, chorea, tics, and myoclonus.

Coordination, Gait, & Equilibrium

A. Simple Walking Test: Observe posture, gait, coordinated automatic movements (swinging arms), and ability to walk a straight line and to make rapid turning movements as the patient walks. Record a detailed and full description of the gait.

B. Romberg Test: Have the patient stand with heels and toes together and eyes closed. Increased swaying commonly occurs in patients with dysfunction of cerebellar or vestibular mechanisms. Patients with disease of the posterior columns of the spinal cord may fall when their eyes are closed, although they are able to maintain their position well with the eyes open.

C. Finger-to-Nose and Finger-to-Finger Tests: In the finger-to-nose test, the patient places the tip of a finger on his or her nose. In the finger-to-finger test, the patient attempts to approximate the tips of the index fingers after the arms have been extended forward. Dysmetria, with overshooting of the mark, is often observed in cerebellar disorders.

D. Heel-to-Shin Test: The patient places one heel on the opposite knee and then moves the heel along the shin. Dysmetria, with overshooting the mark, is often observed in cerebellar disorders.

E. Rapidly Alternating Movements: In this test, the patient rapidly flexes and extends the fingers or taps the table rapidly with extended fingers. Test supination and pronation of the forearm in continuous rapid alternation. The inability to perform these movements quickly and smoothly is a feature of dysdiadochokinesia, an indication of cerebellar disease.

Reflexes

The following reflexes are routinely tested, and the response elicited is graded from 0 to 4+ (2+ is normal).

A. Deep Reflexes:

1. Biceps reflex–When the patient's elbow is flexed at a right angle, the examiner places a thumb on the patient's biceps tendon and then strikes the thumb. Normally, a slight contraction of the biceps muscle occurs.

2. Triceps reflex–With the patient's elbow supported in the examiner's hand, the triceps tendon is sharply percussed just above the olecranon. Contraction of the triceps muscle, with extension of the forearm, usually results.

3. Knee reflex–The patellar tendon is located by palpation and tapped lightly with a percussion hammer or fingers. Increase the force of the tapping until contraction of the quadriceps muscle can be elicited. The patient is usually seated on the edge of a table or bed, with the legs hanging loosely. For patients who are bedridden, the knees can be flexed over the supporting arm of the examiner, with the heels resting lightly on the bed.

4. Ankle reflex–This is best elicited by having the patient kneel on a chair, with ankles and feet projecting over the edge of the chair. The Achilles tendon is then struck with a percussion hammer.

B. Superficial Reflexes:

1. Abdominal reflex–With the patient lying supine with relaxed abdominal muscles, stroke the skin of each quadrant of the abdomen briskly with a pin from the periphery toward the umbilicus. Normally, the local abdominal muscles contract, causing the umbilicus to move toward the quadrant stimulated.

2. Cremasteric reflex–In men, stroking the skin of the inner side of the proximal third of the thigh causes retraction of the ipsilateral testicle.

3. Plantar response–With the thigh in slight external rotation, stroke the outer surface of the sole of the foot lightly with a large pin or wooden applicator from the heel toward the base of the little toe and then inward across the ball of the foot. The normal plantar response consists of plantar flexion of all toes, with slight inversion and flexion of the distal portion of the foot. In abnormal responses, there may be extension of the great toe, with fanning and flexion of the other toes (Babinski's reflex).

C. Clonus: Clonus (repeated reflex muscular movements) may be elicited in patients with exaggerated reflexes. Wrist clonus is sometimes elicited by forcible flexion of the wrist. Patellar clonus can be elicited by sudden downward movement of the patella, with consequent clonic contraction of the quadriceps muscle. Ankle clonus is tested by quickly flexing the foot dorsally, producing clonic contractions of the calf muscles.

Sensory System

Sensory examination can be a difficult and tiring procedure for both the patient and the examiner. The patient should be well rested and must be reassured and in a cooperative frame of mind before a sensory examination is attempted. Abnormalities, especially of minor degree, should be checked by reexamination. The following modalities are tested and charted.

A. Pain: Test the patient's ability to perceive pinprick or deep pressure.

B. Temperature: To check for the ability to detect and distinguish between warm and cold, use a test tube of warm water and one of cold water.

C. Touch: Test the ability to perceive light stroking of the skin with cotton.

D. Vibration: The patient should be able to feel the buzz of a tuning fork (at a frequency of 128 Hz) applied to the bony prominences. After the tuning fork has been set into maximum vibration, the duration of the patient's perception of the vibration is timed with the base of the fork applied to the malleoli, patellas, iliac crests, vertebral spinous processes, and ulnar prominences.

E. Sense of Position: This is tested by having the patient determine the position of toes and fingers when these are grasped by the examiner. A digit is grasped on the sides, and the patient, with eyes closed, attempts to determine whether it is moved upward or downward. Test the larger parts of the extremities if impairment is demonstrated in the digits.

F. Perception of Passive Motion: Check the patient's ability to perceive passive movements of the extremities, especially the distal portions.

G. Stereognosis: To test the patient's capacity to recognize the forms, sizes, and weights of objects, place a familiar object (eg, a coin, key, or knife) in the patient's hand and ask him or her to identify the object without looking at it.

H. Two-Point Discrimination: The shortest distance between two separate points of a compass or calipers at which the patient perceives two stimuli is compared for homologous areas of the body. (Normal: finger tips, 0.3–0.6 cm; palms of hands and soles of feet, 1.5–2 cm; dorsum of hands, 3 cm; shin, 4 cm.)

I. Topognosis: After making sure that the patient's eyes are closed, the examiner touches the patient's body. The patient then points to the spot touched, thereby enabling the examiner to assess the patient's ability to localize tactile sensation. Similar areas of both sides of the body are compared. *Extinction on double simultaneous stimulation* (eg, the ability to perceive tactile sensation on the right hand when presented alone, but not when presented simultaneously with a stimulus to the left hand) suggests a disorder involving the contralateral parietal lobe.

EXAMINING NEONATES

The neonatal neurologic examination is usually performed 36–60 hours after birth. Repeat examinations at weekly intervals may be desirable. The examination should be planned with little stimulation of the infant occurring initially so that spontaneous behavior can be observed.

GENERAL STATUS

Observe the motor pattern and supine and prone body posture and evaluate the reflexes throughout the examination.

In normal infants, the limbs are flexed, the head may be turned to the side, and there may be kicking movements of the lower limbs. Extension of the limbs can occur with intracranial hemorrhage, opisthotonos with kernicterus, and asymmetry of the upper limbs with brachial plexus palsy. Paucity of movements may occur with brachial plexus palsy and meningomyelocele.

Infants normally become more active and cry during the examination. In cases of anoxia or intracerebral hemorrhage, the infant reacts very little.

THE NEUROLOGIC EXAMINATION

Cranial Nerves

A. Optic Nerve (II): Test the infant's blink response to light. Ophthalmoscopic examination should be made at the end of the examination.

B. Oculomotor (III), Trochlear (IV), and Abducens (VI) Nerves: Check the size, shape, and equality of the pupils and pupillary responses to light. Lateral rotation of the head causes rotation of the eyes in the opposite direction (doll's eye reflex).

C. Trigeminal (V) and Facial (VII) Nerves: The sucking reflex is elicited by placing a finger or nipple between the infant's lips. In the rooting reflex, the infant's mouth will open and turn toward the stimulus if a fingertip touches the infant's cheek.

D. Vestibulocochlear Nerve (VIII): The blink response occurs in reaction to loud noise. To test the labyrinthine reflex, the infant is carried and held up by the examiner, who makes several turns to the right and then to the left. A normal infant will look ahead in the direction of rotation; when rotation stops, the infant will look back in the opposite direction.

E. Glossopharyngeal (IX) and Vagus (X) Nerves: Notice the infant's ability to swallow.

Motor System & Reflexes

Spontaneous and induced motor activity are noted. If the infant is inactive and quiet, the Moro reflex (see below) may be used or the infant may be placed in the prone position to induce movement.

A. Incurvation Reflex (Galant's Reflex): With the infant prone, tactile stimulation of the normal thoracolumbar paravertebral zone with a finger produces contraction of the ipsilateral long muscles of the back, so that the head and legs curve towards the stimulated area and the trunk moves away from the stimulus.

B. Muscle Tone: Assess muscle tone by palpating muscles during activity and relaxation. Resistance to passive extension of the elbows and knees is noted.

C. Limb Motion: Determine the infant's ability to move a limb from a given position. Notice any asymmetries in movements of the right versus left limbs.

D. Joint Motion: Flex the infant's hip and knee joints to check the pull of gravity when the infant is briefly held head down in vertical suspension.

E. Grasp Reflex: Stimulation of the ulnar palmar surfaces causes the infant to grasp the examiner's hands forcefully.

F. Traction Response: Contraction of shoulder and neck muscles occurs when a normal infant is pulled from the supine to a sitting position.

G. Stepping Response: The normal infant makes stepping movements when held upright with the feet just touching the table.

H. Placing and Supporting Reactions: Drawing the dorsum of the infant's foot across the lower edge of a moderately sharp surface (eg, the edge of the examining table) normally produces flexion at the knee and hip, followed by extension at the hip (placing reaction). If the plantar surface comes in contact with a flat surface, extension of the knee and hip may occur (positive supporting reaction).

I. Moro Reflex (Startle Response): The Moro reflex is present in normal infants. A sudden stimulus (eg, a loud noise) causes abduction and extension of all extremities, with extension and fanning of digits except for flexion of the index finger and thumb. This is followed by flexion and adduction of the extremities.

J. Other Reflexes and Responses: Knee-jerk, plantar response (normal response is extensor), abdominal reflex, and ankle clonus are tested with the infant quiet and relaxed.

Sensory System

Withdrawal of the stimulated limb and sometimes also the unstimulated limb may be caused by pinprick of the sole of the foot.

Appendix B:
Testing Muscle Function

Muscle testing depends upon a thorough understanding of which muscles are used in performing certain movements. Testing is best performed when the patient is warm, rested, comfortable, attentive, and relaxed. Because several muscles may function similarly, it is not always easy for the patient to contract a single muscle upon request. Positioning or fixation of parts can emphasize the contraction of a particular muscle while other muscles of similar function are inhibited. The effect of gravity must be considered, since it can enhance or reduce certain movements. Testing of individual muscles is useful for evaluating peripheral nerve and muscle function and dysfunction.

Two techniques of testing can be used: active motion against the examiner's resistance and resistance against a movement performed by the examiner. The degree of impairment of muscle function may be difficult to estimate by inspection. It is helpful to palpate the body or tendon of a muscle for evidence of contraction or movement. The normal or least affected muscles should be tested first to gain the cooperation and confidence of the patient. The strength of the muscle tested should always be compared with that of its contralateral muscle.

The strength of various muscles should also be graded and charted. Scales of various types are used, most commonly grading strength from 0 (no muscle contraction) to 5 (normal).

See Tables B–1 and B–2 and Figs B–1 to B–54.

Notice that in all the figures, white arrows indicate the direction of movement in testing the given muscle. Black arrows indicate the direction of resistance, and the blocks show the site of application of resistance.

Table B–1. Grading muscle **strength.**

0:	No muscular contraction
1:	A flicker of contraction, either seen or palpated, but insufficient to move joint
2:	Muscular contraction sufficient to move joint horizontally but not against the force of gravity
3:	Muscular contraction sufficient to maintain a position against the force of gravity
4:	Muscular contraction sufficient to resist the force of gravity plus additional force
5:	Normal motor power

Modified from: *Aids to the Investigation of Peripheral Nerve Inquiries.* Her Majesty's Royal Stationary Office. London, 1953.

Table B–2. Motor function.*

Action to Be Tested	Muscle	Cord Segment	Nerves	Plexus
Shoulder Girdle and Upper Extremity				
Flexion of neck	Deep neck muscles (stern-ocleidomastoid and trapezius also participate)	C1–4	Cervical	Cervical
Extension of neck				
Rotation of neck				
Lateral bending of neck				
Elevation of upper thorax	Scaleni	C3–5	Phrenic	
Inspiration	Diaphragm			
Adduction of arm from behind to front	Pectoralis major and minor	C5–8, T1	Pectoral (thoracic; from medial and lateral cords of plexus)	Brachial
Forward thrust of shoulder	Serratus anterior	C5–7	Long thoracic	
Elevation of scapula	Levator scapulae	C3–5	Dorsal scapular	
Medial adduction and elevation of scapula	Rhomboids	C4, 5		
Abduction of arm	Supraspinatus	C4–6	Suprascapular	
Lateral rotation of arm	Infraspinatus	C4–6		
Medial rotation of arm	Latissimus dorsi, teres major, and subscapularis	C5–8	Subscapular (from posterior cord of plexus)	
Adduction of arm from front to back				
Abduction of arm	Deltoid	C5, 6	Axillary (from posterior cord of plexus)	
Lateral rotation of arm	Teres minor	C4, 5		
Flexion of forearm	Biceps brachii	C5, 6	Musculocutaneous (from lateral cord of plexus)	
Supination of forearm				
Adduction of arm	Coracobrachialis	C5–7		
Flexion of forearm				
Flexion of forearm	Brachialis	C5, 6		
Ulnar flexion of hand	Flexor carpi ulnaris	C7, 8; T1	Ulnar (from medial cord of plexus)	
Flexion of all fingers but thumb	Flexor digitorum profundus (ulnar portion)	C7, 8; T1		
Adduction of metacarpal of thumb	Adductor pollicis	C8, T1		
Abduction of little finger	Abductor digiti quinti	C8, T1		
Opposition of little finger	Opponens digiti quinti	C7, 8; T1		
Flexion of little finger	Flexor digiti quinti	C7, 8; T1		
Flexion of proximal phalanx, extension of 2 distal phalanges, adduction and abduction of fingers	Interossei	C8, T1		
Pronation of forearm	Pronator teres	C6, 7	Median (C6, 7 from lateral cord of plexus; C8, T1 from medial cord of plexus)	
Radial flexion of hand	Flexor carpi radialis	C6, 7		
Flexion of hand	Palmaris longus	C7, 8; T1		
Flexion of middle phalanx of index, middle, ring, or little finger	Flexor digitorum superficalis	C7, 8; T1		
Flexion of hand				
Flexion of terminal phalanx of thumb	Flexor pollicis longus	C7, 8; T1		
Flexion of terminal phalanx of index or middle finger	Flexor digitorum profundus (radial portion)	C7, 8; T1		
Flexion of hand				

(continued)

Table B–2 (cont'd). Motor function.*

Action to Be Tested	Muscle	Cord Segment	Nerves	Plexus
Shoulder Girdle and Upper Extremity (cont.)				
Abduction of metacarpal of thumb	Abductor pollicis brevis	C7, 8; T1	Median (C7, 8 from lateral cord of plexus; C8, T1 from medial cord of plexus	Brachial
Flexion of proximal phalanx of thumb	Flexor pollicis brevis	C7, 8; T1		
Opposition of metacarpal of thumb	Opponens pollicis	C8; T1		
Flexion of proximal phalanx and extension of the 2 distal phalanges of index, middle, ring, or little finger	Lumbricales (the 2 lateral)	C8; T1		
	Lubricales (the 2 medial)	C8; T1	Ulnar	
Extension of forearm	Triceps brachii and anconeus	C6–8	Radial (from posterior cord of plexus)	
Flexion of forearm	Brachioradialis	C5, 6		
Radial extension of hand	Extensor carpi radialis	C6–8		
Extension of phalanges of index, middle, ring, or little finger	Extensor digitorum	C7–8		
Extension of hand				
Extension of phalanges of little finger	Extensor digiti quanti proprius	C6–8		
Extension of hand				
Ulnar extension of hand	Extensor carpi ulnaris	C6–8		
Supination of forearm	Supinator	C5–7	Radial (from posterior cord of plexus)	
Abduction of metacarpal of thumb	Abductor pollicis longus	C7, 8; T1		
Radial extension of hand				
Extension of thumb	Extensor pollicis brevis	C7, 8		
Radial extension of hand	Extensor pollicis longus	C6-8		
Extension of index finger	Extensor indicis proprius	C6–8		
Extension of hand				
Trunk and Thorax				
Elevation of ribs	Thoracic, abdominal, and back	T1–L3	Thoracic and posterior lumbosacral branches	Brachial
Depression of ribs				
Contraction of abdomen				
Anteroflexion of trunk				
Lateral flexion of trunk				
Hip Girdle and Lower Extremity				
Flexion of hip	Iliopsoas	L1–3	Femoral	Lumbar
Flexion of hip (and eversion of thigh)	Sartorius	L2, 3		
Extension of leg	Quadriceps femoris	L2–4		
Adduction of thigh	Pectineus	L2, 3	Obturator	
	Adductor longus	L2, 3		
	Adductor brevis	L2–4		
	Adductor magnus	L3, 4		
	Gracilis	L2–4		
Adduction of thigh	Obturator externus	L3, 4		
Lateral rotation of thigh				

(*continued*)

Table B–2 (cont'd). Motor function.*

Action to Be Tested	Muscle	Cord Segment	Nerves	Plexus
Abduction of thigh	Gluteus medius and minimus	L4, 5; S1	Superior gluteal	Sacral
Medial rotation of thigh				
Flexion of thigh	Tensor fasciae latae	L4, 5		
Lateral rotation of thigh	Pirlformis	S1, 2	. . .	
Abduction of thigh	Gluteus maximus	L4, 5; S1, 2	Inferior gluteal	
Lateral rotation of thigh	Obturator internus	L5, S1,	Muscular branches from sacral plexus	
	Gemelli	L4, 5; S1		
	Quadratus femoris	L4, 5; S1		
Flexion of leg (assist in extension of thigh)	Biceps femoris	L4, 5; S1, 2	Sciatic (trunk)	Sacral
	Semitendinosus	L4, 5; S1		
	Semimembranosus	L4, 5; S1		
Dorsal flexion of foot	Tibialis anterior	L4, 5	Deep peroneal	
Supination of foot				
Extension of toes 2–5	Extensor digitorum longus	L4, 5; S1		
Dorsal flexion of foot				
Extension of great toe	Extensor hallucis longus	L4, 5; S1		
Dorsal flexion of foot				
Extension of great toe and the 3 medial toes	Extensor digitorum brevis	L4, 5; S1		
Plantar flexion of foot in pronation	Peroneus longus and brevis	L5; S1	Superficial peroneal	
	Gastrocnemius	L5; S1, 2	Tibial	
Plantar flexion of foot in supination	Tibialis posterior and triceps surae	L5, S1		
Plantar flexion of foot in supination	Flexor digitorum longus	S1; 2		
Flexion of terminal phalanx of toes II–V				
Plantar flexion of foot in supination	Flexor hallucis longus	L5; S1, 2		
Flexion of terminal phalanx of great toe				
Flexion of middle phalanx of toes II–V	Flexor digitorum brevis	L5; S1		
Flexion of proximal phalanx of great toe	Flexor hallucis brevis	L5; S1, 2		
Spreading and closing of toes	Small muscles of foot	S1, 2		
Flexion of proximal phalanx of toes				
Voluntary control of pelvic floor	Perineal and sphincters	S2–4	Pudendal	

*Modified and reproduced, with permission, from JC McKinley

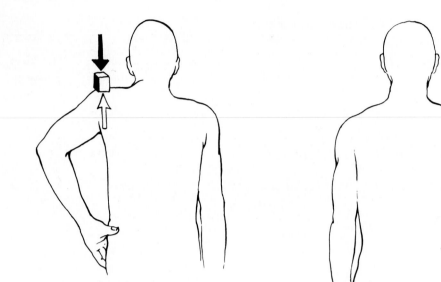

Figure B–1. Trapezius, upper portion (C3, 4; spinal accessory nerve). The shoulder is elevated against resistance.

Figure B–3. Rhomboids (C4, 5; dorsal scapular nerve). The shoulder is thrust backward against resistance.

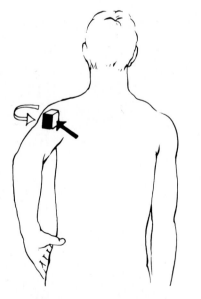

Figure B–2. Trapezius, lower portion (C3, 4; spinal accessory nerve). The shoulder is thrust backward against resistance.

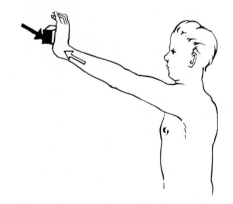

Figure B–4. Serratus anterior (C5–7; long thoracic nerve). The patient pushes hard with outstretched arms; the inner edge of the scapula remains against the thoracic wall. (If the trapezius is weak, the inner edge may move from the chest wall.)

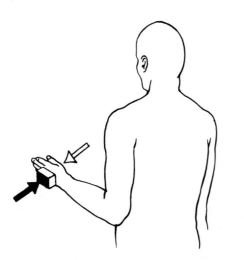

Figure B–5. Infraspinatus (C4–6; suprascapular nerve). With the elbow flexed at the side, the arm is externally rotated against resistance on the forearm.

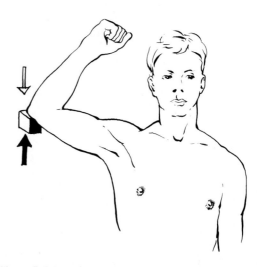

Figure B-7. Latissimus dorsi (C5–8; subscapular nerve). The arm is adducted from a horizontal and lateral position against resistance.

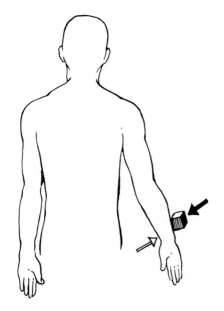

Figure B–6. Supraspinatus (C4–6; suprascapular nerve). The arm is abducted from the side of the body against resistance.

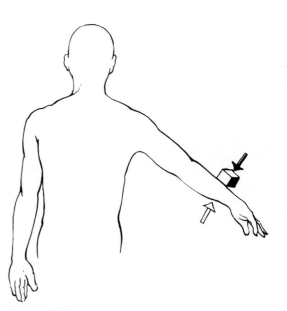

Figure B–8. Deltoid (C5, 6; axillary nerve). Abduction of laterally raised arm (30–75 degrees from body) against resistance.

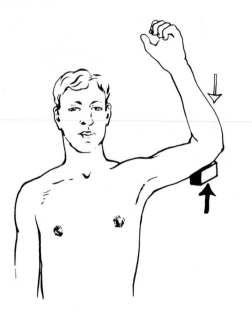

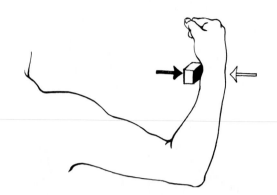

Figure B–11. Biceps (C5, 6; musculocutaneous nerve). The supinated forearm is flexed against resistance.

Figure B–9. Pectoralis major, upper portion (C5–8; T1; lateral and medial pectoral nerves). The arm is adducted from an elevated or horizontal and forward position against resistance.

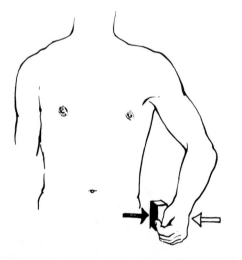

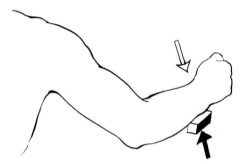

Figure B–12. Triceps (C6–8; radial nerve). The forearm, flexed at the elbow, is extended against resistance.

Figure B–10. Pectoralis major, lower portion (C5–8, T1; lateral and medial pectoral nerves). The arm is adducted from a forward position below the horizontal level against resistance.

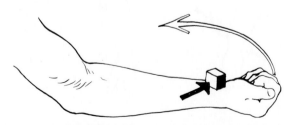

Figure B–13. Brachioradialis (C5, 6; radial nerve). The forearm is flexed against resistance while it is in neutral position (neither pronated nor supinated).

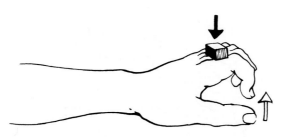

Figure B–14. Extensor digitorum (C7, 8; radial nerve). The fingers are extended at the metacarpophalangeal joints against resistance.

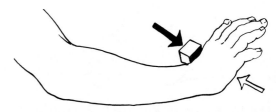

Figure B–16. Extensor carpi radialis (C6–8; radial nerve). The wrist is extended to the radial side against resistance; fingers remain extended.

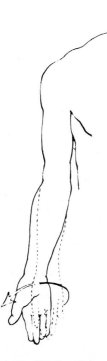

Figure B–15. Supinator (C5–7; radial nerve). The hand is supinated against resistance, with arms extended at the side. Resistance is applied by the grip of the examiner's hand on the patient's forearm near the wrist.

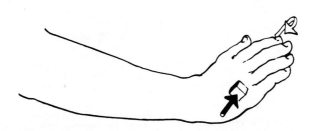

Figure B–17. Extensor carpi ulnaris (C6–8; radial nerve). The wrist joint is extended to the ulnar side against resistance.

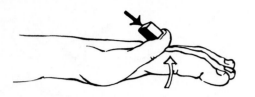

Figure B–18. Extensor pollicis longus (C7, 8; radial nerve). The thumb is extended against resistance.

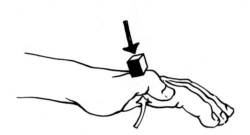

Figure B–19. Extensor pollicis brevis (C7, 8; radial nerve). The thumb is extended at the metacarpophalangeal joint against resistance.

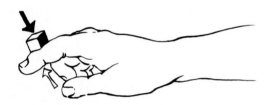

Figure B–20. Extensor indicis proprius (C6–8; radial nerve). The index finger is extended against resistance placed on the dorsal aspect of the finger.

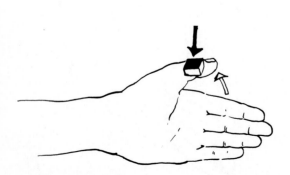

Figure B–21. Abductor pollicis longus (C7, 8; T1; radial nerve). The thumb is abducted against resistance in a plane at a right angle to the palmar surface.

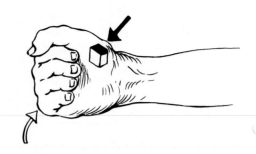

Figure B–22. Flexor carpi radialis (C6, 7; median nerve). The wrist is flexed to the radial side against resistance.

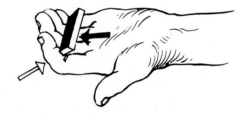

Figure B–23. Flexor digitorum superficialis (C7, 8, T1; median nerve). The fingers are flexed at the first interphalangeal joint against resistance; proximal phalanges remain fixed.

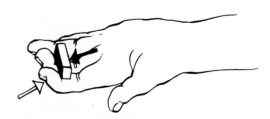

Figure B–24. Flexor digitorum profundus (C7, 8; T1; median nerve). The terminal phalanges of the index and middle fingers are flexed against resistance while the second phalanges are held in extension.

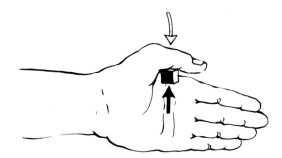

Figure B–28. Flexor pollicis brevis (C7, 8; T1; median nerve). The proximal phalanx of the thumb is flexed against resistance placed on its palmar surface.

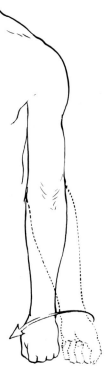

Figure B–25. Pronator teres (C6, 7; median nerve). The extended arm is pronated against resistance. Resistance is applied by the grip of the examiner's hand on the patient's forearm near the wrist.

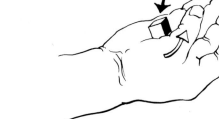

Figure B–29. Opponens pollicis (C8, T1; median nerve). The thumb is crossed over the palm against resistance to touch the top of the little finger, with the thumbnail held parallel to the palm.

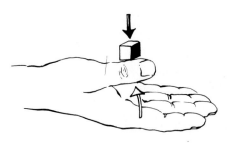

Figure B–26. Abductor pollicis brevis (C7, 8; T1; median nerve). The thumb is abducted against resistance in a plane at a right angle to the palmar surface.

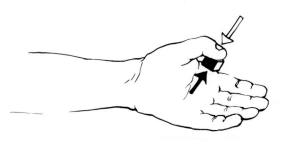

Figure B–27. Flexor pollicis longus (C7, 8; T1; median nerve). The terminal phalanx of the thumb is flexed against resistance as the proximal phalanx is held in extension.

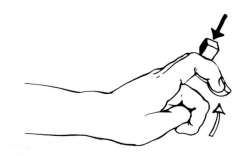

Figure B–30. Lumbricales-interossei, radial half (C8, T1; median and ulnar nerves). The second and third phalanges are extended against resistance; the first phalanx is in full extension. The ulnar has the same innervation and can be tested in the same manner.

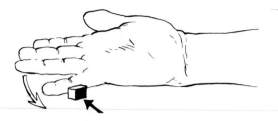
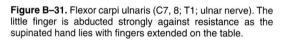

Figure B–31. Flexor carpi ulnaris (C7, 8; T1; ulnar nerve). The little finger is abducted strongly against resistance as the supinated hand lies with fingers extended on the table.

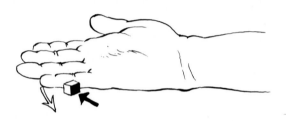
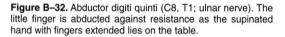

Figure B–32. Abductor digiti quinti (C8, T1; ulnar nerve). The little finger is abducted against resistance as the supinated hand with fingers extended lies on the table.

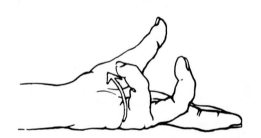

Figure B–33. Opponens digiti quinti (C7, 8; T1; ulnar nerve). With fingers extended, the little finger is moved across the palm to the base of the thumb.

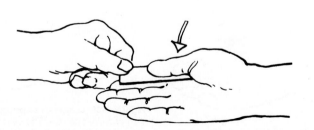

Figure B–34. Adductor pollicis (C8, T1; ulnar nerve). A piece of paper grasped between the palm and the thumb is held against resistance with the thumbnail kept at a right angle to the palm.

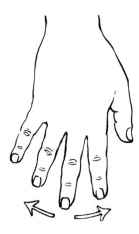

Figure B–35. Dorsal interossei (C8, T1; ulnar nerve). The index and ring fingers are abducted from the midline against resistance as the palm of the hand lies flat on the table.

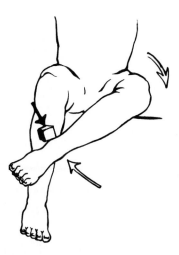

Figure B–37. Sartorius (L2, 3; femoral nerve). With the patient sitting and the knee flexed, the thigh is rotated outward against resistance on the leg.

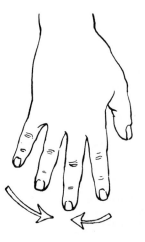

Figure B–36. Palmar interossei (C8, T1; ulnar nerve). The abducted index, ring, and little fingers are adducted to the midline against resistance as the palm of the hand lies flat on the table.

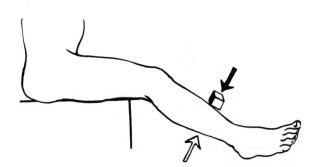

Figure B–38. Quadriceps femoris (L2–4; femoral nerve). The knee is extended against resistance on the leg.

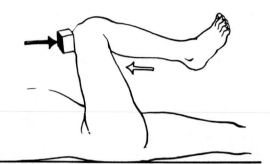

Figure B–39. Iliopsoas (L1–3; femoral nerve). The patient lies supine with the knee flexed. The flexed thigh (at about 90 degrees) is further flexed against resistance.

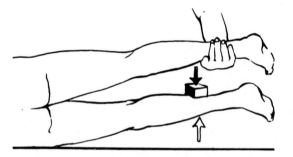

Figure B–40. Adductors (L2–4; obturator nerve). With the patient on one side with knees extended, the lower extremity is adducted against resistance; the upper leg is supported by the examiner.

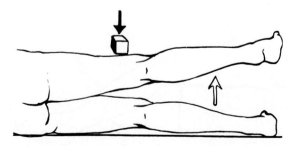

Figure B–41. Gluteus medius and minimus; tensor fasciae latae (L4, 5; S1; superior gluteal nerve). Testing abduction: With the patient lying on one side and the thigh and leg extended, the uppermost lower extremity is abducted against resistance.

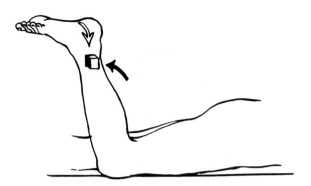

Figure B–42. Gluteus medius and minimus; tensor fasciae latae (L4, 5; S1; superior gluteal nerve). Testing rotation: With the patient prone and the knee flexed, the foot is moved laterally against resistance.

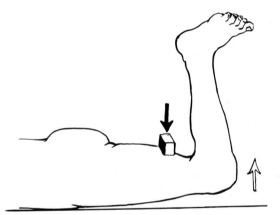

Figure B–43. Gluteus maximus (L4, 5; S1, 2; inferior gluteal nerve). With the patient prone, the knee is lifted off the table against resistance.

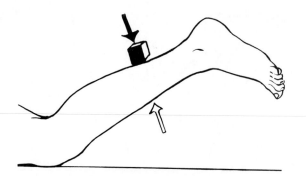

Figure B–44. Hamstring group (L4, 5; S1, 2; sciatic nerve). With the patient prone, the knee is flexed against resistance.

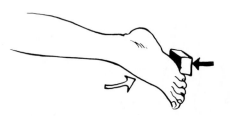

Figure B–45. Gastrocnemius (L5; S1, 2; tibial nerve). With the patient prone, the foot is plantar-flexed against resistance.

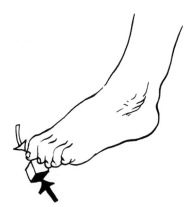

Figure B–47. Flexor hallucis longus (L5; S1, 2; tibial nerve). The great toe is plantar-flexed against resistance. The second and third toes are also flexed.

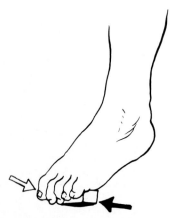

Figure B–46. Flexor digitorum longus (S1, 2; tibial nerve). The toe joints are plantar-flexed against resistance.

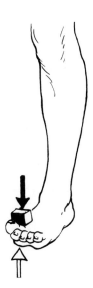

Figure B–48. Extensor hallucis longus (L4, 5; S1; deep per-oneal nerve). The large toe is dorsiflexed against resistance.

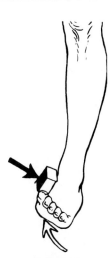

Figure B–50. Tibialis anterior (L4, 5; deep peroneal nerve). The foot is dorsiflexed and inverted against resistance applied by gripping the foot with the examiner's hand.

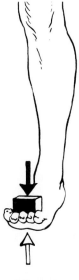

Figure B–49. Extensor digitorum longus (L4, 5; S1; deep per-oneal nerve). The toes are dorsiflexed against resistance.

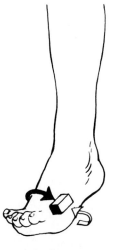

Figure B–51. Peroneus longus and brevis (L5, S1; superficial peroneal nerve). The foot is everted against resistance applied by gripping the foot with the examiner's hand.

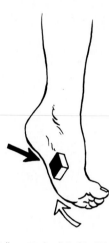

Figure B–52. Tibialis posterior (L5, S1; tibial nerve). The plantar-flexed foot is inverted against resistance applied by gripping the foot with the examiner's hand.

Appendix C:
Spinal Nerves & Plexuses

SENSORY LEVELS

MOTOR LEVELS

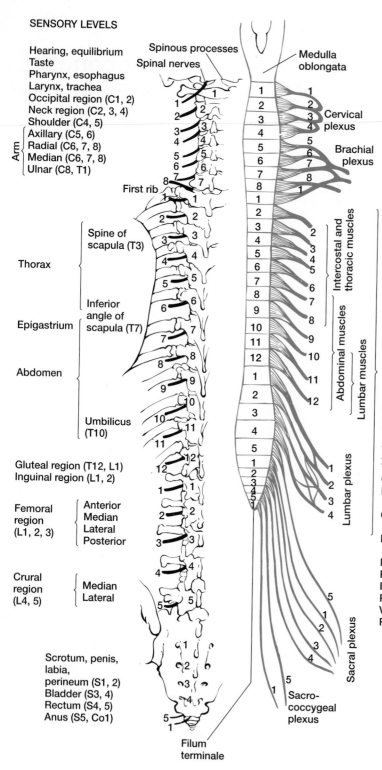

Hearing, equilibrium
Taste
Pharynx, esophagus
Larynx, trachea
Occipital region (C1, 2)
Neck region (C2, 3, 4)
Shoulder (C4, 5)

Arm {
Axillary (C5, 6)
Radial (C6, 7, 8)
Median (C6, 7, 8)
Ulnar (C8, T1)
}

First rib

Spine of scapula (T3)

Thorax

Inferior angle of scapula (T7)

Epigastrium

Abdomen

Umbilicus (T10)

Gluteal region (T12, L1)
Inguinal region (L1, 2)

Femoral region (L1, 2, 3) {
Anterior
Median
Lateral
Posterior
}

Crural region (L4, 5) {
Median
Lateral
}

Scrotum, penis, labia, perineum (S1, 2)
Bladder (S3, 4)
Rectum (S4, 5)
Anus (S5, Co1)

Spinous processes
Spinal nerves

Medulla oblongata

Cervical plexus

Brachial plexus

Intercostal and thoracic muscles

Abdominal muscles

Lumbar muscles

Lumbar plexus

Sacral plexus

Sacro-coccygeal plexus

Filum terminale

Facial muscles VII
Pharyngeal, palatine muscles X
Laryngeal muscles XI
Tongue muscles XII
Esophagus X
Sternocleidomastoid XI (C1, 2, 3)
Neck muscles (C1, 2, 3)
Trapezius (C3, 4)
Rhomboids (C4, 5)
Diaphragm (C3, 4, 5)
Supra-, infraspinatus (C4, 5, 6)

Deltoid, brachioradialis, and biceps (C5, 6)
Serratus anterior (C5, 6, 7)
Pectoralis major (C5, 6, 7, 8) } Arm
Teres minor (C4, 5)
Pronators (C6, 7, 8, T1)
Triceps (C6, 7, 8)
Long extensors of carpi and digits (C6, 7, 8) } Forearm
Latissimus dorsi, teres major (C5, 6, 7, 8)
Long flexors (C7, 8, T1)
Thumb extensors (C7, 8) } Hand
Interossei, lumbricales, thenar, hypothenar (C8, T1)

Iliopsoas (L1, 2, 3)
Sartorius (L2, 3)
Quadriceps femoris (L2, 3, 4)
Gluteal muscles (L4, 5, S1)
Tensor fasciae latae (L4, 5)
Adductors of femur (L2, 3, 4)
Abductors of femur (L4, 5, S1)
Tibialis anterior (L5)
Gastrocnemius, soleus (L5, S1, 2)
Biceps, semitendinosus, semimembranosus (L4, 5, S1)
Obturator, piriformis, quadratus femoris (L4, 5, S1)
Flexors of the foot, extensors of toes (L5, S1)
Peronei (L5, S1)
Flexors of toes (L5, S1, 2)
Interossei (S1, 2)
Perineal muscles (S3, 4)
Vesicular muscles (S4, 5)
Rectal muscles (S4, 5, Co1)

Figure C–1. Motor and sensory levels of the spinal cord.

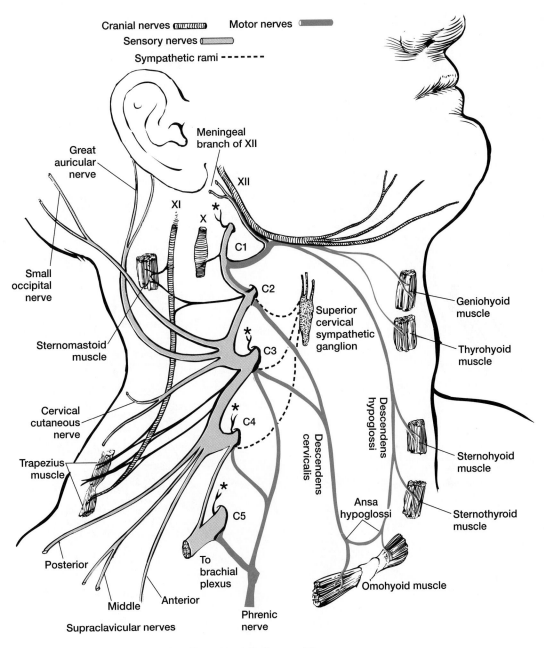

Cranial nerves
Motor nerves
Sensory nerves
Sympathetic rami - - - - - -

Meningeal branch of XII

Great auricular nerve

XII

XI

X

C1

Small occipital nerve

C2

Superior cervical sympathetic ganglion

Geniohyoid muscle

Sternomastoid muscle

C3

Thyrohyoid muscle

Cervical cutaneous nerve

C4

Descendens cervicalis

Descendens hypoglossi

Sternohyoid muscle

Trapezius muscle

C5

Ansa hypoglossi

Sternothyroid muscle

Posterior

To brachial plexus

Omohyoid muscle

Middle   Anterior

Supraclavicular nerves

Phrenic nerve

★ To adjacent vertebral musculature

Figure C–2. The cervical plexus.

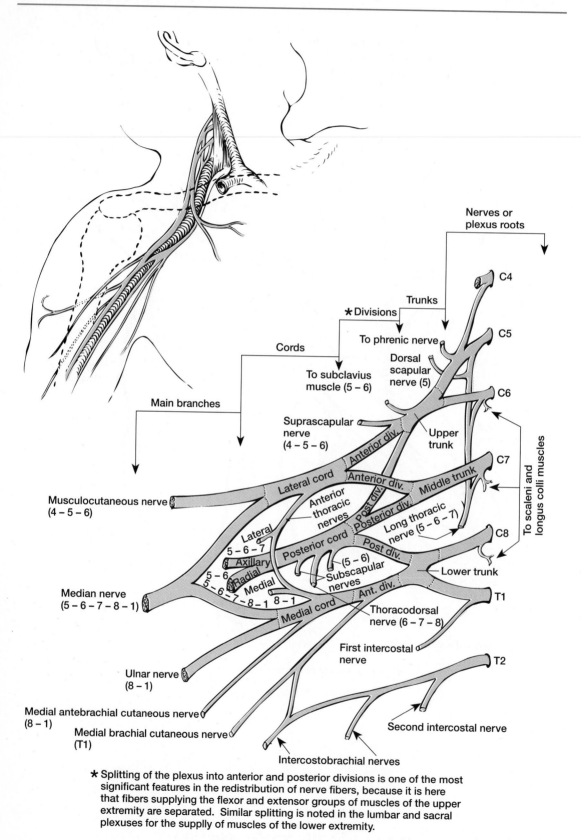

* Splitting of the plexus into anterior and posterior divisions is one of the most significant features in the redistribution of nerve fibers, because it is here that fibers supplying the flexor and extensor groups of muscles of the upper extremity are separated. Similar splitting is noted in the lumbar and sacral plexuses for the supplly of muscles of the lower extremity.

Figure C–3. The brachial plexus.

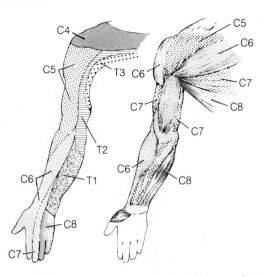

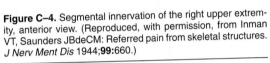

Figure C–4. Segmental innervation of the right upper extremity, anterior view. (Reproduced, with permission, from Inman VT, Saunders JBdeCM: Referred pain from skeletal structures. *J Nerv Ment Dis* 1944;**99**:660.)

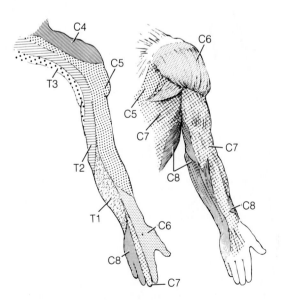

Figure C–5. Segmental innervation of the right upper extremity, posterior view. (Reproduced, with permission, from Inman VT, Saunders JBdeCM: Referred pain from skeletal structures. *J Nerv Ment Dis* 1944;**99**:660.)

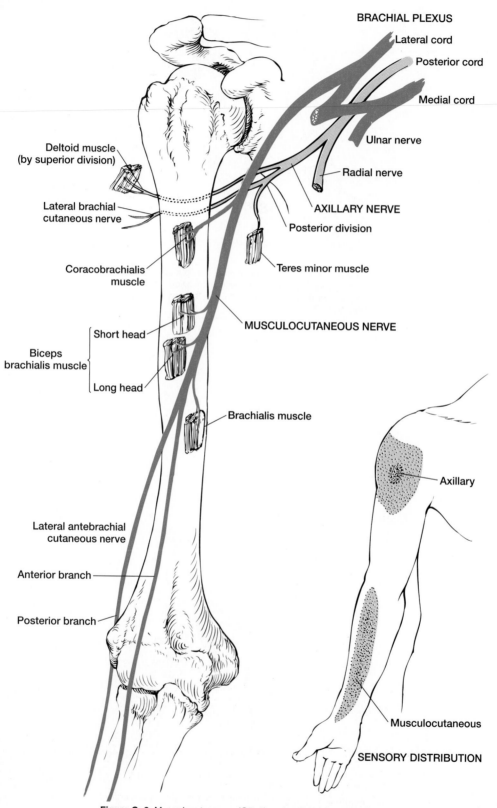

Deltoid muscle
(by superior division)

Lateral brachial
cutaneous nerve

Coracobrachialis
muscle

Short head

Biceps
brachialis muscle

Long head

Lateral antebrachial
cutaneous nerve

Anterior branch

Posterior branch

BRACHIAL PLEXUS

Lateral cord

Posterior cord

Medial cord

Ulnar nerve

Radial nerve

AXILLARY NERVE

Posterior division

Teres minor muscle

MUSCULOCUTANEOUS NERVE

Brachialis muscle

Axillary

Musculocutaneous

SENSORY DISTRIBUTION

Figure C–6. Musculocutaneous (C5, 6) and axillary (C5, 6) nerves.

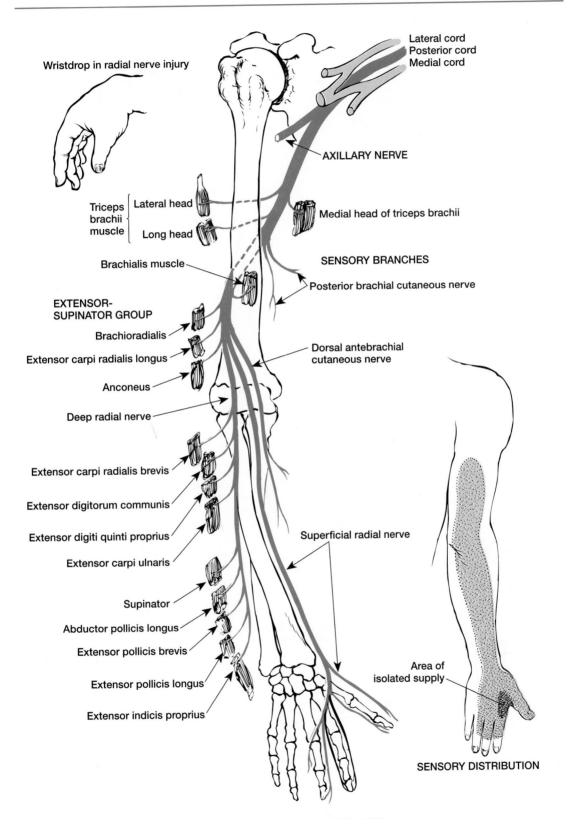

Wristdrop in radial nerve injury

Lateral cord
Posterior cord
Medial cord

AXILLARY NERVE

Triceps brachii muscle { Lateral head / Long head

Medial head of triceps brachii

Brachialis muscle

SENSORY BRANCHES

Posterior brachial cutaneous nerve

EXTENSOR-SUPINATOR GROUP

Brachioradialis

Extensor carpi radialis longus

Anconeus

Dorsal antebrachial cutaneous nerve

Deep radial nerve

Extensor carpi radialis brevis

Extensor digitorum communis

Extensor digiti quinti proprius

Extensor carpi ulnaris

Superficial radial nerve

Supinator

Abductor pollicis longus

Extensor pollicis brevis

Extensor pollicis longus

Area of isolated supply

Extensor indicis proprius

SENSORY DISTRIBUTION

Figure C–7. The radial nerve (C6–8, T1).

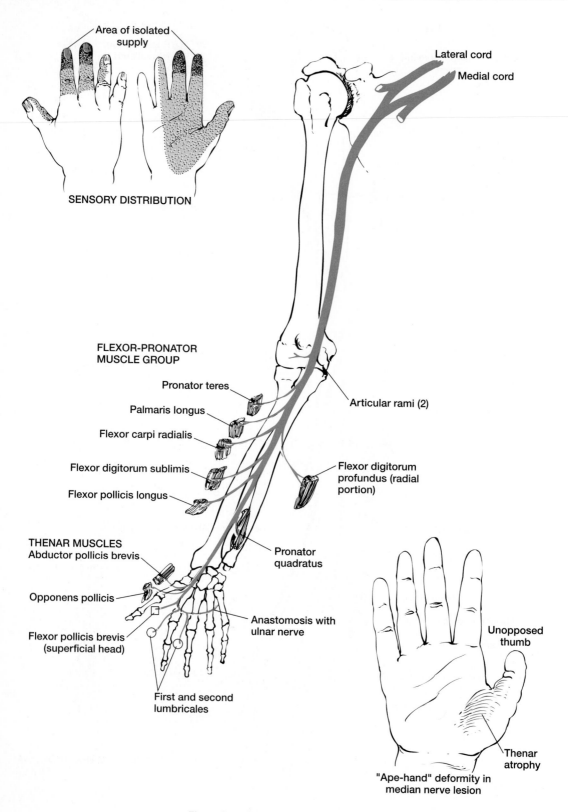

Figure C–8. The median nerve (C6–8, T1).

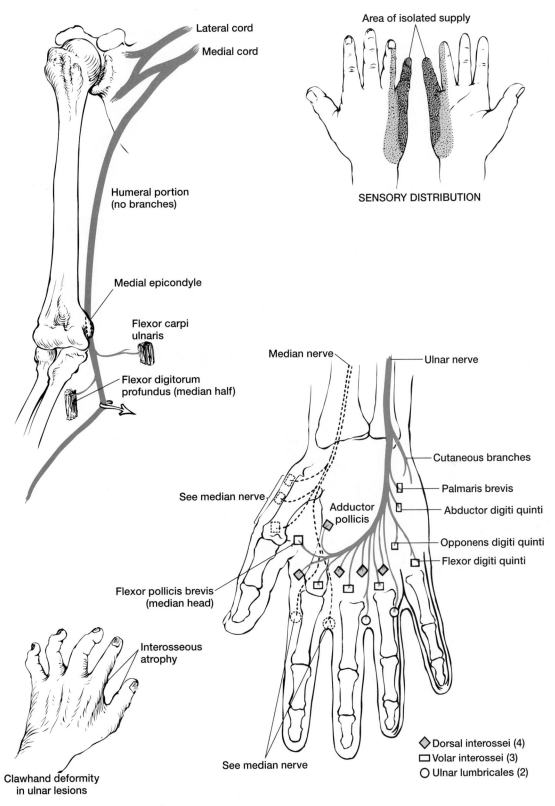

Lateral cord

Medial cord

Humeral portion
(no branches)

Medial epicondyle

Flexor carpi
ulnaris

Flexor digitorum
profundus (median half)

Area of isolated supply

SENSORY DISTRIBUTION

Median nerve

Ulnar nerve

See median nerve

Adductor
pollicis

Cutaneous branches

Palmaris brevis

Abductor digiti quinti

Opponens digiti quinti

Flexor digiti quinti

Flexor pollicis brevis
(median head)

Interosseous
atrophy

See median nerve

Clawhand deformity
in ulnar lesions

◆ Dorsal interossei (4)
▢ Volar interossei (3)
◯ Ulnar lumbricales (2)

Figure C–9. The ulnar nerve (C8, T1).

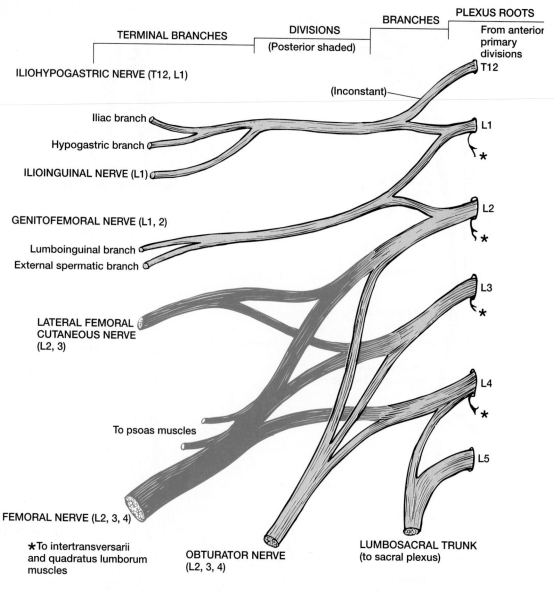

Figure C–10. The lumbar plexus.

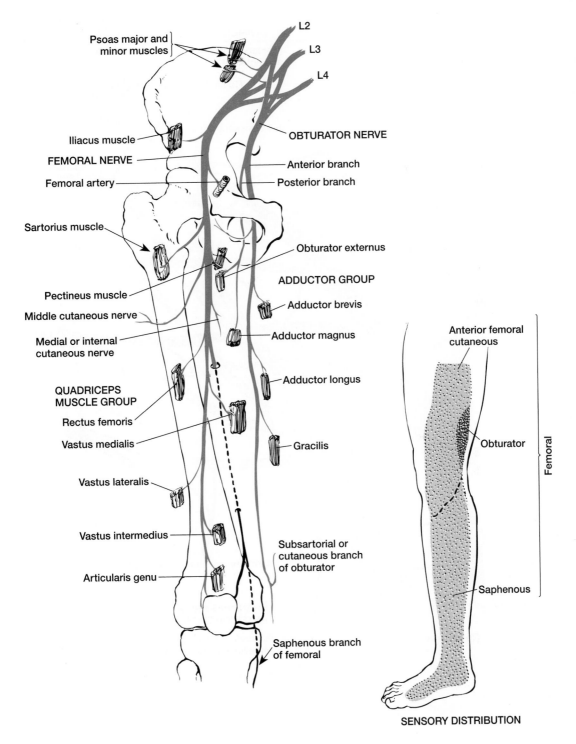

Figure C–11. The femoral (L2–4) and obturator (L2–4) nerves.

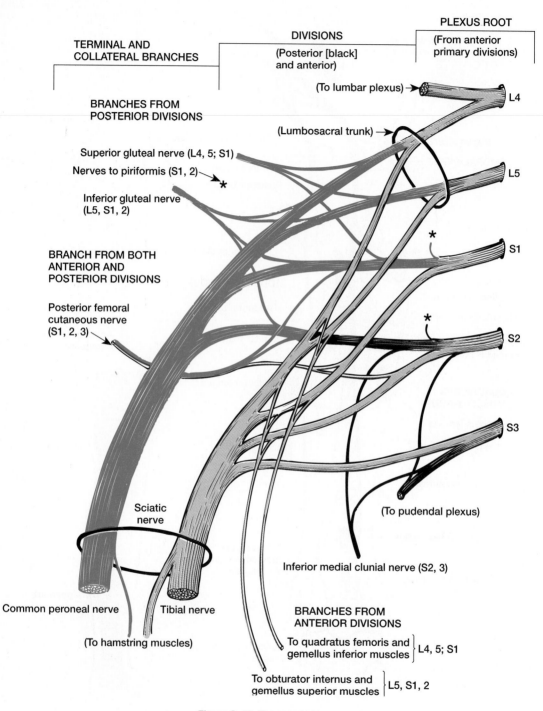

BRANCHES FROM
POSTERIOR DIVISIONS

Superior gluteal nerve (L4, 5; S1)
Nerves to piriformis (S1, 2)

Inferior gluteal nerve
(L5, S1, 2)

BRANCH FROM BOTH
ANTERIOR AND
POSTERIOR DIVISIONS

Posterior femoral
cutaneous nerve
(S1, 2, 3)

TERMINAL AND
COLLATERAL BRANCHES

DIVISIONS

(Posterior [black]
and anterior)

PLEXUS ROOT

(From anterior
primary divisions)

(To lumbar plexus) → L4

(Lumbosacral trunk) →

L5

S1

S2

S3

(To pudendal plexus)

Inferior medial clunial nerve (S2, 3)

Sciatic
nerve

Common peroneal nerve   Tibial nerve

(To hamstring muscles)

BRANCHES FROM
ANTERIOR DIVISIONS

To quadratus femoris and   } L4, 5; S1
gemellus inferior muscles

To obturator internus and   } L5, S1, 2
gemellus superior muscles

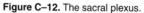

Figure C–12. The sacral plexus.

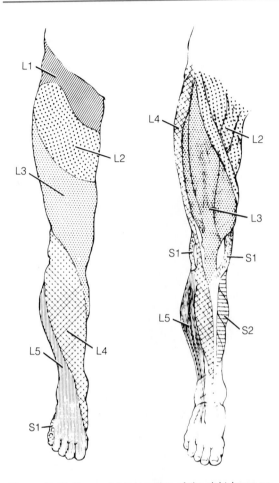

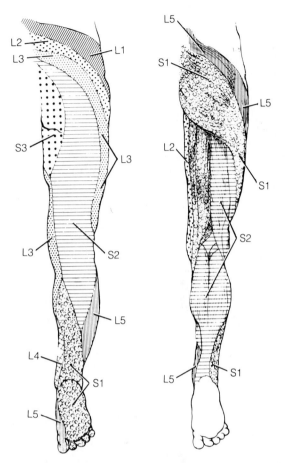

Figure C–13. Segmental innervation of the right lower extremity, anterior view. (Reproduced, with permission, from Inman VT, Saunders JBdeCM: Referred pain from skeletal structures. *J Nerv Ment Dis* 1944;**99:**660.)

Figure C–14. Segmental innervation of the right lower extremity, posterior view. (Reproduced, with permission, from Inman VT, Saunders JBdeCM: Referred pain from skeletal structures. *J Nerv Ment Dis* 1944;**99:**660.)

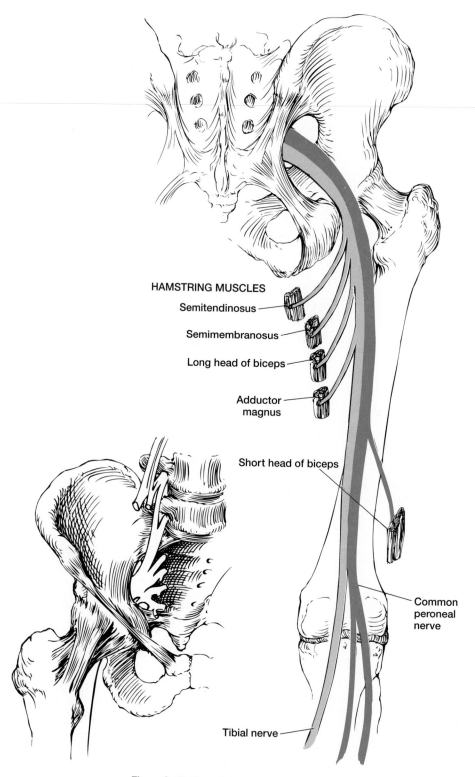

HAMSTRING MUSCLES

Semitendinosus

Semimembranosus

Long head of biceps

Adductor magnus

Short head of biceps

Common peroneal nerve

Tibial nerve

Figure C–15. The sciatic nerve (L4, 5; S1–3).

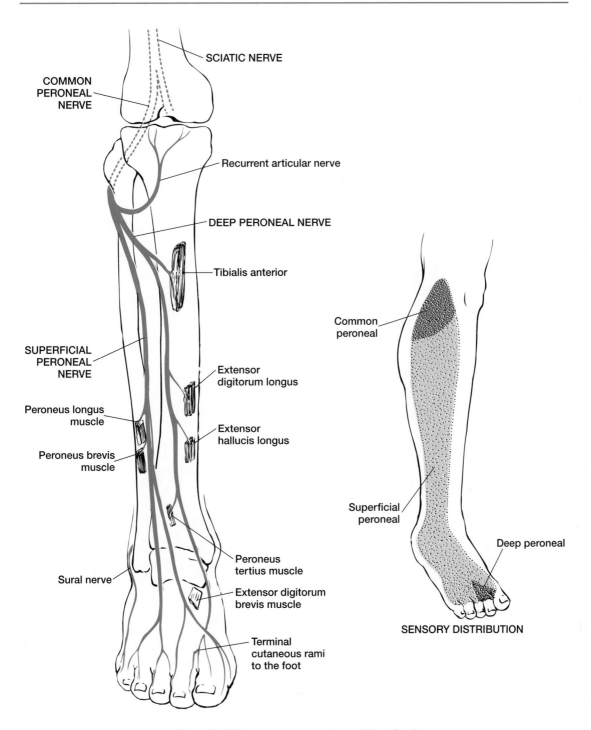

Figure C–16. The common peroneal nerve (L4, 5; S1, 2).

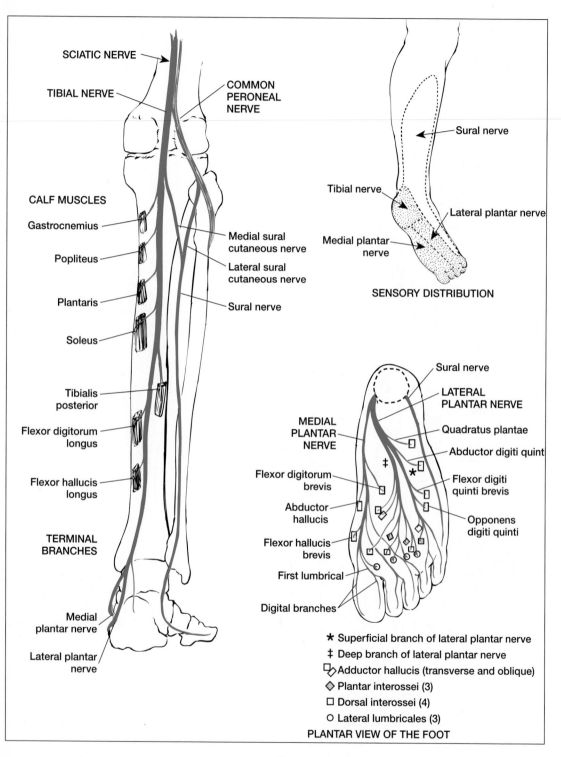

SCIATIC NERVE

TIBIAL NERVE

COMMON PERONEAL NERVE

Sural nerve

Tibial nerve

Lateral plantar nerve

Medial plantar nerve

SENSORY DISTRIBUTION

CALF MUSCLES

Gastrocnemius

Medial sural cutaneous nerve

Popliteus

Lateral sural cutaneous nerve

Plantaris

Sural nerve

Soleus

Sural nerve

LATERAL PLANTAR NERVE

MEDIAL PLANTAR NERVE

Quadratus plantae

Abductor digiti quint

Tibialis posterior

Flexor digitorum brevis

Flexor digiti quinti brevis

Flexor digitorum longus

Abductor hallucis

Opponens digiti quinti

Flexor hallucis longus

Flexor hallucis brevis

TERMINAL BRANCHES

First lumbrical

Digital branches

Medial plantar nerve

Lateral plantar nerve

∗ Superficial branch of lateral plantar nerve
‡ Deep branch of lateral plantar nerve
⬒◇ Adductor hallucis (transverse and oblique)
◆ Plantar interossei (3)
□ Dorsal interossei (4)
○ Lateral lumbricales (3)

PLANTAR VIEW OF THE FOOT

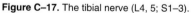

Figure C–17. The tibial nerve (L4, 5; S1–3).

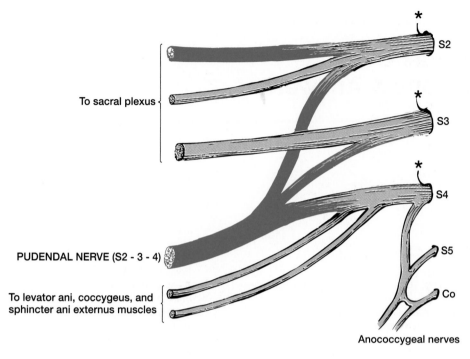

To sacral plexus

*

S2

*

S3

*

S4

S5

Co

PUDENDAL NERVE (S2 - 3 - 4)

To levator ani, coccygeus, and
sphincter ani externus muscles

Anococcygeal nerves

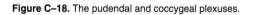

★ Visceral branches

Figure C–18. The pudendal and coccygeal plexuses.

Appendix D:
Questions & Answers

Section I: Chapters 1, 2, and 3

In the following questions, select the single best answer.

1. The basic neuronal signaling unit is–
    A. the equilibrium potential
    B. the action potential
    C. the resting potential
    D. the supernormal period

2. In a motor neuron at rest, an excitatory synapse produces an EPSP of 15 mV, and an inhibitory synapse produces an IPSP of 5 mV. If both the EPSP and IPSP occur simultaneously, then the motor neuron would–
    A. depolarize by about 10 mV.
    B. depolarize by 20 mV.
    C. depolarize by more than 20 mV
    D. change its potential by less than 1 mV.

3. The equilibrium potential for K^+ in neurons is ordinarily nearest–
    A. the equilibrium potential for Na^+
    B. resting potential
    C. reversal potential for the EPSP
    D. the peak of the action potential

4. Generation of the action potential–
    A. depends on depolarization caused by the opening of K^+ channels
    B. depends on hyperpolarization caused by the opening of K^+ channels
    C. depends on depolarization caused by the opening of Na^+ channels
    D. depends on hyperpolarization caused by the opening of Na^+ channels
    E. depends on second-messengers

5. The cerebrum consists of the–
    A. thalamus and basal ganglia
    B. telencephalon and midbrain
    C. telencephalon and diencephalon
    D. brain stem and prosencephalon
    E. cerebellum and prosencephalon

6. The somatic nervous system innervates the–
    A. blood vessels of the skin
    B. blood vessels of the brain
    C. muscles of the heart
    D. muscles of the body wall
    E. muscles of the viscera

7. The peripheral nervous system–
    A. includes the spinal cord
    B. is sheathed in fluid-filled spaces enclosed by membranes
    C. includes cranial nerves
    D. does not include spinal nerves
    E. is surrounded by bone

8. ATP provides an essential energy source in the CNS for–
    A. division of neurons
    B. maintenance of ionic gradients via ATPase
    C. generation of action potentials
    D. EPSPs and IPSPs

9. Myelin is produced by–
    A. oligodendrocytes in the CNS and Schwann cells in the PNS
    B. Schwann cells in the CNS and oligodendrocytes in the PNS
    C. oligodendrocytes in both CNS and PNS
    D. Schwann cells in both CNS and PNS

In the following questions, one or more answers may be correct. Select–
    A if **1, 2,** and **3** are correct
    B if **1** and **3** are correct
    C if **2** and **4** are correct
    D if only **4** is correct
    E is **all** are correct

10. A spinal motor neuron in an adult–
    1. maintains its membrane potential via the active transport of sodium and potassium ions
    2. synthesizes protein only in the cell body and not in the axon
    3. does not synthesize DNA for mitosis
    4. does not regenerate its axon following section of its peripheral portion

11. The myelin sheath is–
    1. produced within the central nervous system by oligodendrocytes

2. produced within the peripheral nervous system by Schwann cells
3. interrupted periodically by the nodes of Ranvier
4. composed of spirally wrapped plasma membrane

12. Astrocytes–
   1. may function to buffer extracellular K^+
   2. are interconnected by gap junctions
   3. can proliferate to form a scar following an injury
   4. migrate to the central nervous system from bone marrow

13. The cell body of most neurons–
   1. cannot divide in the adult
   2. is the main site of protein synthesis in the neuron
   3. is the site of the cell nucleus
   4. contains synaptic vesicles

14. Most synaptic terminals of axons that form chemical synapses in the central nervous system contain–
   1. synaptic vesicles
   2. presynaptic densities
   3. neurotransmitter(s)
   4. rough endoplasmic reticulum

15. Na, K-ATPase–
   1. utilizes ATP
   2. acts as an ion pump
   3. maintains the gradients of Na^+ and K^+ ions across neuronal membranes
   4. consumes more than 25% of cerebral energy production

16. In axoplasmic transport–
   1. some macromolecules move away from the cell body at rates of several centimeters per day
   2. mitochondria move along the axon
   3. microtubules seem to be involved
   4. some types of molecules move toward the cell body at rates of up to 300 mm per day

17. The brain stem includes–
   1. the midbrain (mesencephalon)
   2. pons
   3. medulla oblongata
   4. telencephalon

18. A ganglion is defined as a–
   1. part of the basal ganglia
   2. group of nerve cell bodies within the hypothalamus
   3. layer of similar cells in the cerebral cortex
   4. group of nerve cell bodies outside the neuraxis

19. Neurotransmitters found in the brain stem include–
   1. acetylcholine
   2. norepinephrine
   3. dopamine
   4. serotonin

20. The cell layer around the central canal of the spinal cord–
   1. is called the ventricular zone
   2. is the same as the pia

3. encloses cerebrospinal fluid
4. is called the marginal zone

21. Norepinephrine is found in the–
   1. sympathetic nervous trunk
   2. locus ceruleus
   3. lateral tegmentum of the midbrain
   4. neuromuscular junction

22. Glutamate–
   1. is the transmitter at the neuromuscular junction
   2. may be involved in excitotoxicity
   3. is a major inhibitory transmitter in the CNS
   4. is a major excitatory transmitter in the CNS

23. Decussations are–
   1. aggregates of tracts
   2. fiber bundles in a spinal nerve
   3. horizontal connections crossing within the central nervous system from the dominant to non-dominant side
   4. vertical connections crossing within the central nervous system from left to right or vice-versa.

24. Inhibitory transmitters in the CNS include–
   1. glutamate (presynaptic inhibition)
   2. GABA (presynaptic inhibition)
   3. glutamate (postsynaptic inhibition)
   4. GABA (postsynaptic inhibition)

25. The neurotransmitter dopamine–
   1. is produced by neurons that project from the substantia nigra to the caudate and putamen
   2. mediates transmission at the neuromuscular junction
   3. is depleted in Parkinson's disease
   4. is the major excitatory transmitter in the CNS

Section III: Chapters 5 and 6

In the following questions, select the single best answer.

1. The lateral column of the spinal cord contains the–
   A. lateral corticospinal tract
   B. direct corticospinal tract
   C. Lissauer's tract
   D. Gracile tract

2. A sign of an upper-motor-neuron lesion in the spinal cord is–
   A. severe muscle atrophy
   B. hyperactive deep tendon reflexes
   C. flaccid paralysis
   D. absence of pathologic reflexes
   E. absence of withdrawal responses

3. The following fiber systems in the spinal cord are ascending tracts except for the–
   A. cuneate tract
   B. ventral spinocerebellar tract
   C. spinothalamic tract
   D. spinoreticular tract
   E. reticulospinal tract

4. Axons in the spinothalamic tracts decussate–
   A. in the medullary decussation

B. in the medullary lemniscus

C. within the spinal cord, 5–6 segments above the level where they enter

D. within the spinal cord, within 1–2 segments of the level where they enter

E. in the medial lemniscus

5. The spinal subarachnoid space normally–
   A. lies between the pachymeninx and the arachnoid
   B. lies between the pia and the arachnoid
   C. ends at the cauda equina
   D. communicates with the peritoneal space
   E. is adjacent to the vertebrae

6. The subclavian artery gives rise directly to the–
   A. lumbar radicular artery
   B. great ventral radicular artery
   C. anterior spinal artery
   D. vertebral artery

7. The dorsal nucleus (of Clarke) in the spinal cord–
   A. receives contralateral input from dorsal root ganglia
   B. terminates at the L-2 segment
   C. terminates in the midbrain
   D. terminates in the ipsilateral cerebellum
   E. receives fibers from the external cuneate nucleus

8. A patient complains of unsteadiness. Examination shows a marked diminution of position sense, vibration sense, and stereognosis of all extremities. He is unable to stand without wavering for more than a few seconds when his eyes are closed. There are no other abnormal findings. The lesion most likely involves the–
   A. lateral columns of the spinal cord, bilaterally
   B. inferior cerebellar peduncles, bilaterally
   C. dorsal columns of the spinal cord, bilaterally
   D. spinothalamic tracts, bilaterally
   E. corticospinal tracts

In the following questions, one or more answers may be correct. Select–

A if **1, 2**, and **3** are correct
B if **1** and **3** are correct
C if **2** and **4** are correct
D if only **4** is correct
E if **all** are correct

9. Fine diameter dorsal root axons of L-5 on one side terminate in the–
   1. marginal layer of the ipsilateral dorsal horn
   2. ipsilateral substantia gelatinosa
   3. ipsilateral lamina V of the dorsal horn
   4. ipsilateral dorsal nucleus (of Clarke)

10. Axons in the spinothalamic tract–
    1. carry information about pain and temperature (lateral spinothalamic tract) and light touch (anterior spinothalamic tract)

2. carry information about pain (lateral spinothalamic tract) and temperature (anterior spinothalamic tract)

3. decussate within the spinal cord, within 1–2 segments of their origin

4. synapse in the gracile and cuneate nuclei

11. The dorsal spinocerebellar tract–
    1. arises in the dorsal nucleus of Clarke and, above C-8, in the accessory cuneate nucleus
    2. carries information arising in the muscle spindles, Golgi tendon organs, touch and pressure receptors
    3. ascends to terminate in the cerebellar cortex
    4. projects without synapses to the basal ganglia and cerebellum

12. Second-order neurons in the dorsal column system–
    1. convey information about pain and temperature
    2. cross within the lemniscal decussation
    3. cross within the pyramidal decussation
    4. convey well-localized sensations of fine touch, vibration, 2-point discrimination, and proprioception

13. The following rules about dermatomes are correct–
    1. the C-4 and T-2 dermatomes are contiguous over the anterior trunk
    2. the nipple is at the level of C-8
    3. the thumb, middle finger, and 5th digit are within the C-6, C-7 and C-8 dermatomes, respectively
    4. the umbilicus is at the level of L-2

14. Signs of upper-motor-neuron lesions include–
    1. Babinski's sign
    2. hypoactive deep tendon reflexes and hyporeflexia
    3. spastic paralysis
    4. severe muscle atrophy

15. A-delta and C peripheral afferent fibers–
    1. terminate in laminas I and II of the dorsal horn
    2. convey the sensation of pain
    3. terminate in lamina V of the dorsal horn
    4. convey the sensation of light touch

16. The following are correct–
    1. the diaphragm is innervated via the C-3 and C-4 roots
    2. the deltoid and triceps are innervated via the C-5 root
    3. the biceps is innervated via the C-5 root
    4. the gastrocnemius is innervated via the L-4 root

17. The long-term consequences of a left hemisection of the spinal cord at midthoracic level would include–
    1. loss of voluntary movement of the left leg

2. loss of pain and temperature sensation in the right leg
3. diminished position and vibration sense in the left leg
4. diminished deep tendon reflexes in the left leg

18. The spinal nerve roots—
    1. exit below the corresponding vertebral bodies in the cervical spine
    2. exit above the corresponding vertebral bodies in the cervical spine
    3. exit above the corresponding vertebral bodies in the lower spine
    4. exit below the corresponding vertebral bodies in the lower spine

19. Gamma-efferent motor neurons—
    1. are located in the intermedial lateral cell column of the spinal cord
    2. cause contraction of intrafusal muscle fibers
    3. provide vasomotor control to blood vessels in muscles
    4. are modulated by axons in the vestibulospinal tract

20. The dorsal column system of one side of the spinal cord—
    1. is essential for normal 2-point discrimination on that side
    2. arises from both dorsal root ganglion cells and dorsal horn neurons
    3. synapses upon neurons of the ipsilateral gracile and cuneate nuclei
    4. consists primarily of large, myelinated, rapidly conducting axons

21. Large-diameter dorsal root axons of one side of L-5 terminate in the—
    1. marginal layer of the ipsilateral dorsal horn
    2. ipsilateral gracile nucleus
    3. ipsilateral cuneate nucleus
    4. ipsilateral dorsal nucleus (of Clarke)

22. The fibers carrying information from the spinal cord to the cerebellum—
    1. can arise from Clarke's column cells (dorsal nucleus)
    2. represent the contralateral body half in the dorsal spinocerebellar tract
    3. can arise from cells of the external cuneate nucleus
    4. are important elements in the conscious sensation of joint position

23. The intermediolateral gray column—
    1. contains preganglionic neurons for the autonomic nervous system
    2. is prominent in the thoracic region
    3. is prominent in upper lumbar regions
    4. is prominent in cervical regions

24. In adults—
    1. there is very little myelin in the spinal cord

2. the dorsal columns and lateral columns are heavily myelinated
3. the spinal cord terminates at the level of the S-5 vertebrae
4. the spinal cord terminates at the level of the L-1 or L-2 vertebra

25. In humans, the spinothalamic tract—
    1. carries information from the ipsilateral side of the body
    2. exhibits topographic organization
    3. arises principally from neurons of the same side of the cord
    4. mediates information about pain and temperature

Section IV: Chapters 7 through 12

In the following questions, select the single best answer.

1. Examination of a patient revealed a drooping left eyelid, together with weakness of adduction and elevation of the left eye, loss of the pupillary light reflex in the left eye, and weakness of the limbs and lower facial muscles on the right side. A single lesion most likely to produce all these signs would be located in the—
   A. medial region of the left pontomedullary junction
   B. basomedial region of the left cerebral peduncle
   C. superior region of the left mesencephalon
   D. dorsolateral region of the medulla on the left side
   E. periaqueductal gray matter on the left side

2. A neurologic syndrome is characterized by loss of pain and thermosensitivity on the left side of the face and on the right side of the body from the neck down; partial paralysis of the soft palate, larynx, and pharynx on the left side; ataxia on the left side; and hiccuping. This syndrome could be expected from infarction in the territory of the—
   A. basilar artery
   B. right posterior inferior cerebellar artery
   C. left posterior inferior cerebellar artery
   D. right superior cerebellar artery
   E. left superior cerebellar artery

3. Hemiplegia and sensory deficit on the right side of the body may be caused by infarction in the territory of the—
   A. left middle cerebral artery
   B. right anterior cerebral artery
   C. left posterior cerebral artery
   D. left superior cerebellar artery
   E. anterior communicating artery

4. If the oculomotor nerve (III) is sectioned, each of the following may result except for—
   A. partial ptosis
   B. abduction of the eyeball
   C. dilation of the pupil

D. impairment of lacrimal secretion

E. paralysis of the ciliary muscle

5. Structures in the ventromedial regions of the medulla receive their blood supply from the–

A. posterior spinal and superior cerebellar arteries

B. vertebral and anterior spinal arteries

C. posterior spinal and posterior cerebral arteries

D. posterior spinal and posterior inferior cerebellar arteries

E. posterior and anterior inferior cerebellar arteries

6. The efferent axons of the cerebellar cortex arise from–

A. Golgi cells

B. vestigial nucleus cells

C. granule cells

D. Purkinje cells

E. pyramidal cells

7. A lesion in the nucleus of cranial nerve IV would produce a deficit in the–

A. upward gaze of the ipsilateral eye

B. upward gaze of the contralateral eye

C. downward gaze of the contralateral eye

D. downward gaze of the ipsilateral eye

8. Sensory input for taste is carried by–

A. the vestibulocochlear (VIII) nerve

B. the facial (VII) nerve for the entire tongue

C. the facial (VII) and glossopharyngeal (IX) nerves for the anterior 2/3 and posterior 1/3 of the tongue, respectively

D. the glossopharyngeal (IX) and vagus (X) nerves for the anterior 2/3 and posterior 1/3 of the tongue, respectively

9. In central facial paralysis resulting from damage of the facial (VII) nucleus there is–

A. paralysis of all ipsilateral facial muscles

B. paralysis of all contralateral facial muscles

C. paralysis of ipsilateral facial muscles except the buccinator

D. paralysis of all contralateral muscles except the buccinator

E. paralysis of contralateral facial muscles except the frontalis and orbicularis oculi

10. Within the internal capsule, descending motor fibers for the face–

A. are located in front of fibers for the arm, in the anterior part of the anterior limb

B. are located posterior to the fibers for the leg, in the posterior 1/2 of the posterior limb

C. are located in front of the fibers for the arm, in the anterior part of the posterior limb

D. travel within the corticovestibular tract

E. synapse in the capsular nucleus

11. Brodmann's area 4 corresponds to the–

A. primary motor cortex

B. premotor cortex

C. Broca's area

D. primary sensory cortex

E. striate cortex

12. In a stroke affecting the territory of the middle cerebral artery–

A. weakness and sensory loss are most severe in the contralateral leg

B. weakness and sensory loss are most severe in the contralateral face and arm

C. weakness and sensory loss are most severe in the ipsilateral leg

D. weakness and sensory loss are most severe in the ipsilateral face and arm

E. akinetic mutism is often seen

In the following questions, one or more answers may be correct. Select–

A if **1, 2,** and **3** are correct

B if **1** and **3** are correct

C if **2** and **4** are correct

D if only **4** is correct

E if **all** are correct

13. Cortical area 17–

1. is also termed the striate cortex

2. is involved in the processing of auditory stimuli

3. receives input from the lateral geniculate body

4. receives input from the medial geniculate body

14. Within the cerebellum–

1. climbing fibers and mossy fibers carry afferent information

2. Purkinje cells provide the primary output from the cerebellar cortex

3. Purkinje cells project to the ipsilateral deep cerebellar nuclei

4. efferents from the deep cerebellar nuclei project to the contralateral red nucleus and thalamic nuclei

15. In a patient with a missile wound involving the left cerebral hemisphere, the following might be expected–

1. dense neglect of stimuli on the left side

2. hemiplegia involving the right arm and leg

3. hemiplegia involving the left arm and leg

4. aphasia

16. The striatum includes–

1. the caudate nucleus

2. the globus pallidus

3. the putamen

4. the substantia nigra

17. The ventroposterior medial nucleus of the thalamus–

1. receives axons from neurons located in the contralateral cuneate nucleus in the medulla
2. receives axons from neurons located in area 4 on the medial surface of the ipsilateral cerebral hemisphere
3. contains neurons that respond to olfactory stimuli applied ipsilaterally
4. contains neurons whose axons project to the somatosensory cortex of the ipsilateral cerebral hemisphere

18. A healthy 25-year-old man had an episode of blurred vision in the left eye that lasted two weeks and then resolved. Six months later he developed difficulty walking. Examination showed decreased visual acuity in the left eye, nystagmus, loss of vibratory sensation and position sense at the toes and knees bilaterally, and hyperactive deep tendon reflexes with a Babinski reflex on the right. Three years later, the man was admitted to the hospital with dysarthria, intention tremor of the left arm, and urinary incontinence. The clinical features are consistent with–
  1. myasthenia gravis
  2. a series of strokes
  3. a cerebellar tumor
  4. multiple sclerosis

19. The vagus (X) nerve contains–
  1. visceral afferent fibers
  2. visceral efferent fibers
  3. branchial efferent fibers
  4. somatic efferent fibers

20. Lesions of the cerebral cortex on one side can result in a deficit in muscles innervated by the–
  1. contralateral spinal motor neurons
  2. ipsilateral spinal motor neurons
  3. contralateral facial (VII) nerve
  4. ipsilateral facial (VII) nerve

21. The trigeminal nuclear complex–
  1. has somatic afferent components
  2. participates in certain reflex responses of cranial muscles
  3. has a branchial efferent component
  4. receives projections of axons coursing with nerve X

22. The solitary nucleus–
  1. serves visceral functions, none of which are consciously perceived
  2. gives rise to preganglionic parasympathetic axons
  3. mediates pain arising from the heart during myocardial ischemia
  4. receives axons running with nerve VII

23. Sensory nuclei of the thalamus include–
  1. lateral geniculate
  2. superior geniculate
  3. ventral posterior, lateral
  4. ventral anterior

24. Axon pathways that decussate before they terminate include the–
  1. optic nerve (II) fibers from the temporal halves of the two retinas
  2. gracile fasciculus
  3. cuneate fasciculus
  4. olivocerebellar fibers

25. A 55-year-old patient presented with an eight month history of gradually progressive incoordination in the right arm and leg. Examination revealed hypotonia and ataxia in the limbs on the right side. The most likely diagnosis is–
  1. a stroke
  2. a tumor
  3. in the left cerebellar hemisphere
  4. in the right cerebellar hemisphere

Section V: Chapters 13 through 22

In the following questions, select the single best answer.

1. A lesion of the right frontal cortex (area 8) produces–
  A. double vision (diplopia)
  B. impaired gaze to the right
  C. impaired gaze to the left
  D. dilated pupils
  E. no disturbances of the ocular motor system

2. Axons in the optic nerve originate from–
  A. rods and cones
  B. retinal ganglion cells
  C. amacrine cells
  D. all of the above

3. Meyer's loop carries optic radiation fibers representing–
  A. the upper part of the contralateral visual field
  B. the lower part of the contralateral visual field
  C. the upper part of the ipsilateral visual field
  D. the lower part of the ipsilateral visual field

4. Which of the following statements about the auditory system is not true?
  A. the lateral lemniscus carries information from both ears
  B. it has a major synaptic delay in the midbrain
  C. it has a major synaptic delay in the thalamus
  D. it has a major synaptic delay in the inferior olivary nucleus
  E. crossing fibers pass through the trapezoid body

5. The hippocampal formation consists of the–
  A. dentate gyrus
  B. hippocampus

C. subiculum

D. all of the above

6. Which of the following is not part of the Papez circuit?

    A. hippocampus

    B. mammillary bodies

    C. posterior thalamic nuclei

    D. cingulate gyrus

    E. parahippocampal gyrus

7. Wernicke's aphasia is usually caused by–

    A. a lesion in the superior temporal gyrus

    B. a lesion in the inferior temporal gyrus

    C. a lesion in the inferior frontal gyrus of the dominant hemisphere

    D. lesions in the midbrain

    E. alcohol abuse

8. Which of the following statements about the globus pallidus is not true?

    A. it is located adjacent to the internal capsule

    B. it receives excitatory axons from the caudate and putamen

    C. it is the major outflow nucleus of the corpus striatum

    D. it sends inhibitory axons to the thalamus

9. In a patient with hemi-Parkinsonism (unilateral Parkinson's disease) affecting the right arm, a lesion is most likely in the–

    A. right subthalamic nucleus

    B. left subthalamic nucleus

    C. right substantia nigra

    D. left substantia nigra

    E. right globus pallidus

    F. left globus pallidus

10. Complex cells in the visual cortex have receptive fields that–

    A. are smaller than the receptive fields of simple cells

    B. respond to lines or edges with a specific orientation, only when presented at one location in the visual field

    C. respond to lines or edges with a specific orientation, presented anywhere within the visual field

    D. contain "on" or "off" centers

In the following questions one or more answers may be correct. Select–

    A if **1, 2,** and **3** are correct

    B if **1** and **3** are correct

    C if **2** and **4** are correct

    D if only **4** is correct

    E if **all** are correct

11. Auditory stimuli normally cause impulses to pass through the–

    1. trapezoid body

    2. inferior olivary nucleus

    3. medial geniculate nucleus

    4. medial lemniscus

12. The principal neurotransmitter(s) released by synaptic terminals of sympathetic axons is/are–

    1. epinephrine

    2. norepinephrine

    3. acetylcholine

    4. gamma-aminobutyric acid

13. Alzheimer's disease is characterized by–

    1. neurofibrillary tangles

    2. loss of neurons in the basal forebrain (Meynert) nucleus

    3. senile plaques

    4. severe pathology in CA1

14. Destruction of the lower cervical and upper thoracic ventral roots on the left side leads to–

    1. dilated right pupil

    2. constricted right pupil

    3. dilated left pupil

    4. constricted left pupil

15. Following transection of the peripheral nerve, the–

    1. axons and Schwann cells distal to the cut undergo degeneration and disappear

    2. sensory axons distal to the cut survive, but motor axons degenerate

    3. motor neurons whose axons were cut degenerate and disappear

    4. surviving axons of the proximal stump will send out new growth cones to attempt regeneration

16. The Klüver-Bucy syndrome–

    1. is characterized by hyperorality and hypersexuality

    2. is characterized by psychic blindness and personality changes

    3. is seen in patients with bilateral temporal lobe lesions

    4. is seen in patients with lesions of the anterior thalamus

17. Pain sensation–

    1. is carried in large myelinated (A-alpha) axons

    2. is carried by small myelinated and unmyelinated (A-delta and C) axons

    3. is carried upward in the dorsal columns of the spinal cord

    4. is carried upward in the spinothalamic tract and spinoreticulothalamic system

18. Parasympathetic fibers are carried in–

    1. cranial nerve III and VII

    2. cranial nerve IX and X

    3. sacral roots S2–S4

    4. thoracic roots T8–T12

19. A 68-year-old hypertensive teacher complained of a severe headache and was taken to the hospital. Examination revealed that he could write normally, but could not read. His speech was normal. The lesion(s) mostly likely involved the–

1. corpus callosum
2. Broca's area
3. left visual cortex
4. left angular gyrus

20. In the patient described in question No. 19–
    1. the left anterior cerebral artery was probably involved
    2. there was probably a right homonymous hemianopia
    3. the left middle cerebral artery was probably involved
    4. the left posterior cerebral artery was probably involved

21. The extrastriate cortex–
    1. is Brodmann's areas 18 and 19
    2. receives input from area 17
    3. is the visual association cortex
    4. is the primary auditory cortex

22. The corticospinal tract passes through–
    1. the internal capsule
    2. the crus cerebri
    3. the pyramids of the medulla
    4. the lateral and anterior columns of the spinal cord

23. The homunculus in the motor cortex–
    1. contains magnified representations of the face and hand
    2. represents the face highest on the convexity of the hemisphere
    3. is located largely within the territory of the middle cerebral artery
    4. gives rise to all of the axons that descend as the corticospinal tract

24. The optic chiasm–
    1. is located close to the pineal and is often compressed by pineal tumors
    2. is located close to the pituitary and is often compressed by pituitary tumors
    3. contains decussating axons that arise in the temporal halves of the retinas
    4. contains decussating axons that arise in the nasal halves of the retinas

In the following question, select the single best answer.

25. A 54-year-old accountant, who worked until the day of his illness, was found on the floor, with a right hemiparesis (arm and face more severely affected than the leg) and severe aphasia. The diagnosis is most likely–

A. a tumor involving the thalamus on the left
B. a large tumor of the left cerebral hemisphere
C. a stroke involving the right middle cerebral territory
D. a stroke involving the right anterior cerebral territory
E. a stroke involving the left middle cerebral territory
F. a stroke involving the left anterior cerebral territory

ANSWERS

Section I

1. B	6. D	11. E	16. E	21. A
2. A	7. C	12. A	17. A	22. C
3. B	8. B	13. A	18. D	23. D
4. C	9. A	14. A	19. E	24. C
5. C	10. A	15. E	20. B	25. B

Section III

1. A	6. D	11. A	16. B	21. C
2. B	7. D	12. D	17. A	22. B
3. E	8. C	13. B	18. C	23. A
4. D	9. A	14. B	19. C	24. C
5. B	10. B	15. A	20. E	25. C

Section IV

1. B	6. D	11. A	16. B	21. A
2. C	7. D	12. B	17. D	22. D
3. A	8. C	13. B	18. D	23. B
4. D	9. E	14. E	19. A	24. D
5. B	10. C	15. C	20. B	25. C

Section V

1. C	6. C	11. B	16. A	21. A
2. B	7. A	12. A	17. C	22. E
3. A	8. B	13. E	18. A	23. B
4. D	9. D	14. D	19. B	24. C
5. D	10. C	15. D	20. C	25. E

Index